*This book is dedicated to those who taught me
about knee arthroplasty,
Chitranjan Ranawat, John Insall, Michael Freeman,
and to my family.*

T.P.S.

*I dedicate this book to my family, and to my teachers,
Leonardo Gui and Michael Freeman*

E.A.M.

The roots of culture
are bitter,
but its fruit is sweet

ARISTOTLE

Thomas P. Sculco   Ermanno A. Martucci (eds.)

KNEE
ARTHROPLASTY

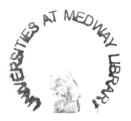

SpringerWienNewYork

Thomas P. Sculco, M.D.
Hospital for Special Surgery
New York, NY, USA

Ermanno A. Martucci, M.D.
Rizzoli Orthopedic Institute
Bologna, Italy

Italian Edition by:
TIMEO Editore s.r.l., Rastignano - Bologna (Italy)
ISBN 88-86891-96-7

© 2001 Springer-Verlag/Wien
Printed in Italy

Typesetting: ASLAY Fotocomposizione s.r.l., Rastignano, Bologna (Italy)
Printing and binding: LITOSEI s.r.l., Rastignano, Bologna (Italy)

Printed on acid-free and chlorine-free bleached paper

SPIN: 10773095

With numerous Figures

ISBN 3-211-83531-8 Springer-Verlag Wien New York

Foreword

After a first phase of doubt, knee prostheses like hip prostheses revealed their effectiveness with a more than 90% survival rate after 15 to 20 years.

Currently, more than 200,000 knee prostheses are implanted annually in the United States, and about 20,000 knees are revised.

The success of surgical treatment is essentially due to three factors: the correctness of surgical indications, the correct choice of the type of implant, and the correct surgical technique.

The development of studies on biomechanics, on prosthetic design, and on material used, have led to the progressive evolution of implants, making them more and more suited to increasing the survival rate.

If the criteria that guide surgical indications and surgical method are mostly standardized, the choice of the type of prosthesis and thus of prosthetic design, of the type of fixation and thus of whether or not to use cement, of whether or not to resurface the patella, regarding the retention or removal of the posterior cruciate ligament, are all related to the surgeon's experience.

For this reason, the text takes into consideration the biomechanical features, indications, and surgical methods used in prostheses where there is preservation or sacrifice of the posterior cruciate ligament, and also of constraint models in case of severe instability of the periarticular soft tissues. Particular attention is paid to the use of prostheses with a mobile surface. Recently, indications for the use of these prostheses have increased to attempt to obtain a more physiological joint kinematics, to reduce polyethylene wear, and stress at the prosthesis/bone or prosthesis/cement/bone interface.

The type of prosthetic design and above all the presence of a mobile surface requires of the surgeon to obtain, during surgery, correct balancing of the soft tissues, thus allowing for joint kinematics that are compatible with joint function, suited to carrying out common daily activities, and above all compatible with prosthetic materials, in order to minimize polyethylene wear and to guarantee good fixation of the implant.

A rise in indications for the treatment of degenerative pathology of the knee through the prosthesis has inevitably led to a rise in surgical and mechanical complications, and thus to a rise in the number of revisions.

Thus, a wide view of the most common complications and surgical techniques that may be adopted in these cases is presented.

The subjects dealt with are purposely separated into sections to ease in-depth conceptual, technical and scientific knowledge.

Thus, I am honored to present this very thorough study on the subject. My warmest congratulations go to the two Editors, Thomas Sculco and Ermanno Martucci, who have written numerous chapters and who have gathered the experience of authors of international renown.

This text was brought about with the contribution of all, and it is the State of the Art on knee arthroplasty.

SANDRO GIANNINI
Rizzoli Orthopaedic Institute - Bologna

Introduction

Knee arthroplasty as it is currently defined became a part of clinical practice about twenty-five years ago. The intuitions and the experiences developed separately by Michael Freeman and John Insall have brought about an essential change in this delicate area of orthopaedic surgery; moreover, thanks to the contribution of other authors, it has formidably and gradually expanded. The number of patients submitted each year to knee replacement surgery has constantly risen, until it has even exceeded, in the USA, that of patients submitted to hip replacement. It is, in fact, true that arthritis of the knee involves a high, and ever-increasing, number of elderly persons: arthroplasty allows for the regression of pain and the recovery of joint function, thus, in the final analysis, for a better and more independent life. Over the years, significant progress has been made in the quality of materials used, in the accuracy and reliability of surgical instruments, and also in prosthetic design. To this regard, however, it is important to emphasize that modern prostheses are not characterized by revolutionary differences, as compared to the Total Condylar prosthesis developed at the Hospital for Special Surgery in New York, dur-

ing the first half of the Seventies; rather, they constitute their natural evolution. Based on an analysis of the various series, it has emerged that 90-95% of patients operated on present with survival of the prosthetic implant after 10-15 years. Thus, results are so satisfactory in time that indications for knee replacement have gradually been enlarged, to also include relatively young patients or those with marked anatomical changes. Some aspects, such as the role of the posterior cruciate ligament, resurfacing of the patella, use of a mobile surface, are still quite controversial, while the use of cement continues to represent the gold standard. The main problem, similar to what occurs in the hip, is constituted by polyethylene wear, that is however characterized by specific pathogenetic mechanisms. Thus, research is taking innovative routes with the purpose of allowing for an even longer survival of implants in the near future. The work has been divided into five sections, each including several chapters assigned to renowned specialists, to thus deal in an organic and modern manner with the most significant problems of knee replacement surgery.

TOM SCULCO AND ERMANNO MARTUCCI

Contents

Foreword   5

Introduction   7

Section 1 - Biomechanics   11

Chapter 1   Knee Biomechanics and Prosthetic Design
Timothy M. Wright   13

Chapter 2   Prosthetic Design and Patellofemoral Function
Bruce H. Robie, Daniel E. Rosenthal   27

Section 2 - Surgical Technique   37

Chapter 3   Preoperative Planning and Prosthetic Selection
S. David Stulberg   39

Chapter 4   Surgical Approaches
Ermanno A. Martucci   45

Chapter 5   Soft-Tissue Balancing
Ermanno A. Martucci   53

Chapter 6   Patellofemoral Joint
M.A.R. Freeman, S.K. Kulkarni, J. Poal Manresa   61

Chapter 7   Bone Grafting in Primary and Revision Total Knee Arthroplasty
Thomas P. Sculco   71

Chapter 8   Total Knee Arthroplasty Following High Tibial Osteotomy
Charles L. Nelson, Steven B. Haas   91

Chapter 9   Total Knee Arthroplasty in the Stiff Knee
Thomas P. Sculco, Ermanno A. Martucci   103

Section 3 - Prosthetic selection   111

Chapter 10   Unicompartimental Knee Arthroplasty
Nikolaus M. Boehler   113

Chapter 11   The Posterior Cruciate Ligament and Total Knee Arthroplasty
Richard S. Laskin   121

Chapter 12   Posterior Cruciate Ligament-Substituting Total Knee Arthroplasty: Rationale and Results
Mark W. Pagnano, Giles R. Scuderi, John N. Insall   131

Chapter 13   Meniscal-Bearing Knee Arthroplasty
Frederick F. Buechel   141

Chapter 14   Total Internal Constraint Prosthesis
Giorgio Fontanesi, Roberto Rotini   151

Section 4 - Complications   161

Chapter 15   Wound Complications in Total Knee Arthroplasty
Douglas A. Dennis   163

Chapter 16   Mechanical Loosening of Total Knee Arthroplasty
Paul Lombardi, Alexander Miric, Thomas P. Sculco   171

Chapter 17   Treatment of the Infected Total Knee Arthroplasty
Russell E. Windsor   179

Chapter 18   Periprosthetic Fractures
Francesco Giron, Paolo Aglietti   189

Chapter 19   Prophylaxis of Deep Vein Thrombosis After Total Knee Arthroplasty
Geoffrey H. Westrich, Steven B. Haas   209

Section 5 - Miscellanea   223

Chapter 20   Blood Management in Knee Arthroplasty
Battista Borghi   225

Chapter 21   Rehabilitation Following Total Knee Arthroplasty
Sandy B. Ganz   231

Chapter 22   Revision Total Knee Arthroplasty
Thomas P. Sculco   241

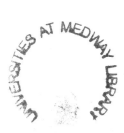

Section 1
BIOMECHANICS

Chapter 1
Knee Biomechanics and Prosthetic Design

Timothy M. Wright
The Hospital for Special Surgery - New York

The design of a total knee replacement must meet several important mechanical goals in order to restore joint function for the lifetime of the patient. The first goal is to provide appropriate kinematics so that the joint will function like a normal knee joint. This objective involves, of course, not only implant design, but also consideration of the soft tissues around the joint. The second goal is to successfully transfer the large loads that cross the knee joint to the surrounding bony structures. A third goal is to provide secure fixation of the implant components. A final goal is to provide long-term wear resistance. Wear debris should not be generated in large enough volumes at large enough rates to cause osteolysis.

The implant designer has two factors with which to work in meeting these goals: the shape of the implant components and the materials from which they are fabricated. Important shape considerations include the geometries of the joint surfaces and the location and shapes of fixation structures, such as pegs, stems, porous coatings, and screws. Important material factors include mechanical and wear properties of the metallic alloys and ultra-high molecular weight polyethylene (UHMWPE).

Unfortunately, the three design goals are not independent. For example, the shapes of the joint surfaces that create the best kinematics for a knee replacement may adversely affect UHMWPE wear. Thus, compromises between these competing goals must be sought. To understand the limitations that these compromises can create on implant performance, the orthopaedic surgeon must consider both the function and structure of the natural joint and the specific aspects of each of the design goals.

The Natural Knee

Functional Considerations

The primary motion of the knee joint is flexion and extension in the sagittal plane. The kinematics of the femur and tibia during this activity are determined primarily by the geometry of the femoral condyles and tibial plateaus, the muscle forces exerted across the joint, and the constraints of the cruciate ligaments. In the sagittal plane, a femoral condyle may be approximated by two radii. One radius forms the anterior portion of the condyle and contacts the tibial plateau at and near extension. A second, smaller radius forms the posterior portion and contacts the plateau in flexion. The tibial plateaus are relatively flat. Based on the bony geometry alone, contact between the condyles and the plateaus would occur over a very small area, producing large contact stresses. Fortunately, the menisci and articular cartilage distribute joint loads more uniformly over a larger area.

As the knee is flexed, the contact areas between the condyles and the tibial plateaus move posteriorly. This rollback motion of the femur with respect to the tibia is controlled by the action of the posterior cruciate ligament (PCL). The posterior translation provided by the rollback assures that the femoral shaft will not impinge on the posterior tibial plateau at large flexion angles and thus provides for a very large range of motion. Rollback also increases the moment arm of the quadriceps with respect to the joint contact point, providing an added mechanical advantage to this muscle in resisting flexion and in extending the knee (14). This advantage is important for functional activities such as walking up and down stairs and rising from a chair.

The motions of the knee in other directions, such as in the medial-lateral plane and in internal and external rotation are smaller. For example, the reaction force between the ground and the foot during the stance phase of walking has both medially and laterally directed components that create varus and valgus moments, respectively, at the knee joint (Fig. 1). The primary mechanism for generating internal moments in the knee to resist these external moments is to redistribute the load between the two plateaus (14, 41). This redistribution is possible because of the compliance of articular cartilage and re-

quires little medial-lateral translation between the joint surfaces. When more load is taken on one plateau relative to the other, the effect is to shift the joint contact point, creating an internal moment that resists the externally applied moment (Fig. 2). Secondary mechanisms for generating additional internal moments to resist varus-valgus moments include voluntary co-contraction of extensor and flexor muscles and stretching of the collateral ligaments (14, 39, 46).

The forces across the knee joint during activities of daily living are estimated to be as high as four times body weight (41). The contact forces are very large because the external loads applied to the leg produce large moments about the knee (Figs. 1 and 2). The muscles that span the knee must provide resisting moments, but are at a mechanical disadvantage compared to the external loads. This is because the moment arms of the muscles with respect to the

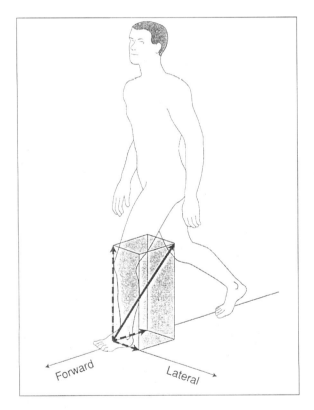

FIG. 1 - The components of the ground reaction force during level gait often have large lever arms about the knee joint. Large moments are created even by small components of the force because of the large lever arm (moment = force x lever arm). These large moments must be resisted internally by the joint contact force and by muscle forces. Because the joint contact point and the muscles have much small lever arms, the contact and muscle forces must be much larger than the ground reaction forces to generate sufficient internal moments and thus insure equilibrium. (Used with permission from Reference 15.)

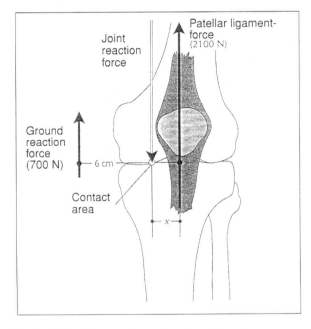

FIG. 2 - When the ground reaction force (Fig. 1) passes to the medial side of the knee, it causes an external varus moment. The magnitude of the moment about the center of the knee (through which the patellar ligament force passes) is 700 N multiplied by 6 cm, or 42 N-m. If the joint reaction load (2800 N) shifts an amount "x" equal to 1.5 cm, the resulting internal valgus moment generated by the reaction load will be 2800 N multiplied by 1.5 cm or 42 N-m. The two moments balance one another and the knee is maintained in equilibrium. (Used with permission from Reference 15.)

joint are much shorter than those of the external loads. Consequently, even small external loads applied at the foot during gait must be resisted by much larger muscle forces to maintain equilibrium. These large muscle forces across the knee in turn produce large contact forces between the femur and the tibia.

The primary motion of the patella with respect to the femur is in the sagittal plane. The motion of the patella is determined by two factors: the geometry of the articulating surfaces of the patella and the trochlear groove and the forces applied to the patella by the quadriceps mechanism. The total resultant force on the distal femur is made up of a component due to patellofemoral contact and a component due to tibiofemoral contact (14). During normal gait, the contact points between the patella and the femur and between the tibia and the femur move, and the positions and magnitudes of the contact forces change. However, the positions and magnitudes of these forces vary in such a way that the direction of the total resultant force on the tibia remains relatively constant. This is consistent with the need for only small variations in surface curvature of the tibial plateau to maintain equilibrium through joint compression loading (15).

Structural Considerations

The primary loads acting on the proximal tibia are the distally directed joint contact loads. These loads are created by the femoral condyles pushing on the tibial plateaus as a result of externally applied loads and muscle contractions. During normal activities, the additional loads caused by stretching of the cruciate and collateral ligaments are quite small compared to the joint contact loads.

Just below the joint surface and subchondral bone, the loads on the tibial plateaus are shared by the cancellous bone and the outer cortical shell. In such composite structures, loads can follow more than one path (for example, load could flow through the cancellous bone, the cortical shell, or some combination of the two). The amount of load following each path is determined from the relative stiffnesses of the components of the composite structure. The component that has the greatest structural stiffness carries the most load.

The apparent density and therefore the stiffness of the cancellous bone in the proximal tibia decrease distally. The opposite is true of the cortical bone in the outer shell; it has the prop-

erties of cancellous bone near the joint line (42), but the stiffness of the outer shell of the tibia increases significantly as the metaphysis is approached. Because the ratio of the loads carried by the cancellous bone and the outer shell is equal to the ratio of their structural stiffnesses, the axial load is carried almost entirely by the cancellous bone proximally near the joint and is gradually transmitted to the cortical bone as the stiffness of the cancellous bone decreases and the stiffness of the outer shell increases.

Cancellous bone properties also vary with position in the transverse plane of the proximal tibia (28). The bone directly beneath the central areas of the plateau that are in contact with the femoral condyles during most activities has the greatest density and therefore the largest elastic modulus and mechanical strength (17). The least dense cancellous bone is found in the central portion between the plateaus. This bone has little stiffness or strength, consistent with the low mechanical demand put on this region of the proximal tibia. The distal femur also consists of cancellous bone within an outer cortical shell. The cancellous bone is most dense near the joint immediately beneath the articular surfaces of the condyles. Both the distribution of density and the orientation of the bone in the distal femur show that the load is transferred from the dense subchondral bone to the cortical bone of the diaphysis over a relatively short metaphyseal region (48).

Design Considerations

Kinematics

In the natural knee, the large range of flexion is achieved through a combination of bony and cartilage geometries, muscle action, and ligamentous constraint. Total knee replacement designs provide flexion-extension motion through the geometry of the femoral condyles and the tibial plateaus in the anteroposterior plane. Virtually all contemporary knees approximate the anteroposterior geometry of each femoral condyle using two radii, a large radius that contacts the plateau near extension and a smaller posterior radius that contacts as the knee flexes. Many current designs use the same two radii in the lateral and medial condyles, so that the component is symmetric about the sagittal plane.

In the medial-lateral direction, many designs have contact geometry consisting of a single radius for each condyle of the femoral component and a single, slightly larger radius for each tibial plateau. Rotational laxity is limited even in the natural knee, so these curved surfaces can be quite, though not completely, conforming in the medial-lateral direction (15). The curved surfaces also provide large contact areas, even when load must be redistributed onto one condyle to resist varus-valgus moments (Fig. 3).

Perhaps the most controversial kinematics concept in knee replacement design has centered on the treatment of the PCL. In the natural knee, posterior translation of the femur on the tibia during flexion is controlled by the PCL, which tethers the femur to the tibia and prevents anterior translation of the femur. Three different approaches for providing posterior translation of the femur have been taken in total knee replacement designs: maintaining the ligament in an effort to allow it to provide the same function as in the natural knee (PCL retaining designs), substituting for the ligament by providing a geometric constraint to anterior translation of the femoral component through a post and cam mechanism (posterior-stabilized designs), and sacrificing the ligament without substitution by providing constraint to translation through the geometry of the articulating surfaces alone.

Proponents of retaining the PCL point to potential advantages such as maintaining more natural kinematics, as well as the proprioception and load transfer capabilities of the PCL (29, 31). However, studies show that the PCL is difficult to balance and often does not remain functional after knee replacement (19, 30). Additional work suggests that the proprioception of a reconstructed knee joint in which the PCL is retained does not differ from that in which the PCL is resected (18).

PCL retention has disadvantages as well. To insure that the ligament functions properly after total knee replacement, the joint line must remain near its preoperative level. If the joint line is not reproduced, the kinematics are altered, the loads across the joint can increase, and the UHMWPE tibial surface can experience increased wear. The same result can occur if too thick a component is used, so that the PCL becomes too tight in flexion, again causing increased contact stresses and UHMWPE wear (31). In knees with varus or valgus deformity, the PCL must be considered a part of the cause of the deformity. PCL retaining knee replacements should not be considered in such cases (37).

A number of PCL retaining designs employ a flat surface on the tibial component in the an-

teroposterior direction to ensure that the contact surfaces do not constrain the posterior translation created by the pull of the ligament. These designs often have flat surfaces in the medial-lateral direction as well. Flat articulating surfaces in both directions allows for large contact areas, thus minimizing stresses and UHMWPE wear in the tibial component. In fact, when joint load is shared by both condyles, these designs have larger contact areas than a more condylar, conforming design and, therefore, lower contact stresses (Fig. 3).

The problem with flat surfaces in both planes occurs when the knee joint must resist external varus and valgus moments (15). In a knee replacement with flat medial-lateral femoral and tibial surfaces, a varus or valgus moment applied across the joint causes the load to be concentrated over a very small area at the

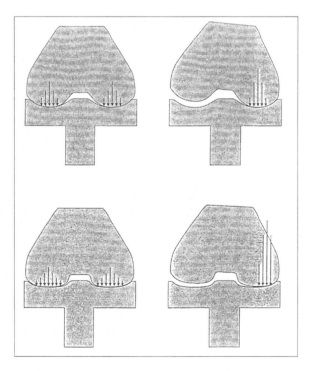

FIG. 3 - When load is shared evenly between both condyles, a condylar design with a single radius of curvature for the femoral and tibial components in the medial-lateral direction has a smaller contact area (top, left) than a flatter design with a larger central radius and small radii at the edge of the flat (bottom, left). But when the load is redistributed to one condyle, the single radius of curvature design maintains a large contact area (top, right), while the flatter design suffers edge loading on a much smaller contact area (bottom, right) causing large contact stresses. (Used with permission from Reference 15.)

outer edge of one plateau (Fig. 3), which, in turn, leads to locally high stresses in the UHMWPE and the underlying cancellous bone. Meeting one design objective to insure appropriate kinematics for the PCL while ignoring the kinematic design objective of adequately resisting varus and valgus moments adversely affects implant performance (49). Significant wear damage is often observed at the edges of UHMWPE components in designs with flat tibial and femoral articulating surfaces (57). The tendency for these components to experience delamination and cracking at the periphery is consistent with the large stresses created as a result of the load concentration. Many contemporary PCL retaining designs no longer have flat contact surfaces, and instead have more curved, condylar surfaces. It is unknown, however, how such surfaces interact with the PCL and, therefore, PCL function in these joints is questionable.

Substituting for the PCL provides both range of motion and joint stability and allows for more conforming surfaces without compromising kinematics. Posterior translation can be achieved by designing the equilibrium position (the "low point") of the tibial articulating surface to be posterior. The posterior position of the femur relative to the tibia can be assured by the incorporation of a cam mechanism (Fig. 4). A disadvantage of posterior-stabilized designs is that they require more resection of femoral bone from the intercondylar notch to make room for the cam mechanism. Sacrificing the PCL without posterior stabilization can be achieved by the same design approach for the articulating surfaces. Most surgeons choose, however, posterior stabilization for the added assurance of rollback and for the added resistance to anterior dislocation.

Differences in performance and clinical outcome of contemporary PCL retaining and PCL substituting designs are generally insignificant. Studies in which direct comparisons between the two types of design were performed in bilateral knee replacement patients found no preference for one type of design over the other (10, 22). Patients with either type of design achieve excellent range of motion (typically greater than 110 degrees). Though patients in whom the PCL is retained are believed to perform stair climbing tasks in a more normal fashion, results from gait analysis studies on this subject are contradictory (35, 52), suggesting that little difference in function exists between patients with the two types of designs.

Load Transfer

Most primary total knee designs are surface replacements. The components of these implants do not rely on intramedullary stems for fixation. Instead, the components are designed to cover the joint surfaces of the bones, thus transferring joint loads directly to the underlying cancellous bone. The designs mimic the way in which loads in the natural joint are borne by subchondral bone. The joint loads are distributed over the cancellous bone in the proximal tibia and the distal femur and gradually transferred to the cortical shell.

Load transfer can be understood by considering three important questions. First, how is the load distributed over the articulating surface? Next, how does the implant change its shape as a result of this load distribution? Finally, how do the joint load distribution and the distortion that occurs in the implant affect the load distribution to the bone-implant interface and the underlying bone?

Load distribution on the articulating surface depends upon the elastic moduli of the contacting materials, the shape of the contacting sur-

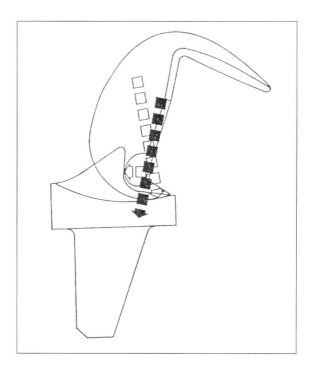

FIG. 4 - Posterior stabilization utilizes a post and cam interaction to substitute for the function of the PCL. (Used with permission from Reference 32.)

faces, and the thickness of the component (3, 15). Consider, for example, a modern condylar total knee replacement (design A) that is 8 mm thick and which is made from conventional UHMWPE with an elastic modulus of 1 gigapascal (Fig. 5). For the purposes of comparison, the relative peak contact stress with the load shared equally between the condyles is assumed to have a value of one for this design.

In a second design (design B), the same surface shapes and the same thickness are used, but the elastic modulus for UHMWPE is doubled to 2 gigapascals (as might be the case with an "enhanced" material such as Hylamer). The contact stress for this design is forty percent higher. Next, consider a third design (design C) in which conventional UHMWPE is used (elastic modulus of one gigapascal) and again the thickness remains unchanged. In this design, however, the shape of the contacting surfaces are made less conforming by increasing the medial-lateral radius of the tibial component from 14 to 16 millimeters. This decrease in conformity increases the peak contact stress by fourteen percent. Finally, consider a design (design D) with the same curvature and elastic modulus as our first example, but with a thinner tibial component of five millimeters. The peak contact stress in this case increases by twenty-nine percent.

Not all knee functions result in equal load sharing between the medial and lateral plateaus, and, therefore, the sensitivity of joint loading to the shapes of the contacting surfaces under

these other conditions must also be considered. For example, functions for which a valgus moment is applied across the knee joint may cause the load to be totally concentrated on the one plateau. If an extreme moment is applied, the medial tibial plateau and the medial femoral condyle will separate, producing a gap. The load distribution induced by such a valgus angulation will again depend on the shapes of the contacting surfaces.

The shape change in the implant caused by the applied loads significantly affects the way in which the loads are transferred to the supporting cancellous bone. With most implant designs, the contacting surfaces between implant and cancellous bone are initially conforming. For loads to be transferred uniformly over as large an area as possible, the prosthesis should change shape as little as possible. The interaction between load, implant shape, and load transfer at the bone-implant interface can be understood by considering two implants, a total condylar plateau and a unicondylar tibial plateau. When the load is applied to one condyle of the total condylar plateau (Fig. 6), contact forces develop at the prosthesis-cancellous bone interface. The area over which the load is distributed at the interface is larger than the area over which the contact force is distributed on the joint surface. The bending moment created by this difference in distribution causes the opposite plateau to deform concave upward. The deformed prosthesis is no longer contiguous with the bony surface. If no means exist for resisting the deformation (such as an interlocking surface on the tibial plateau for cement to penetrate), separation could occur and no load would be transferred. If a means exists (such as cement interlocking), tensile forces will develop at this interface.

For the unicondylar plateau (Fig. 6), the areas over which the load is distributed at the interface and over which the contact force is distributed on the joint surface are more nearly equal. The bending moment is reduced over the case of the condylar plateau, and the tibial plateau transfers load to the bone-implant interface in an almost uniform manner. Unfortunately, the sudden change in load distribution at the edges of the unicondylar plateau creates high shear stresses in the bone. This phenomenon explains the tendency for unicondylar implants to subside (16).

In the natural knee joint, joint loads are distributed to the underlying cancellous bone over a very large area by the stiff subchondral bone.

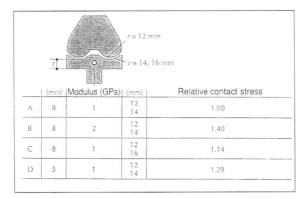

	(mm)	Modulus (GPa)	(mm)	Relative contact stress
A	8	1	12 14	1.00
B	8	2	12 14	1.40
C	8	1	12 16	1.14
D	5	1	12 14	1.29

FIG. 5 - Three factors affect contact stresses in total knee components: the elastic modulus of the UHMWPE (compare A and B), the conformity between the articulating surfaces (compare A and C), and the thickness of the UHMWPE (compare A and D). (Used with permission from Reference 15.)

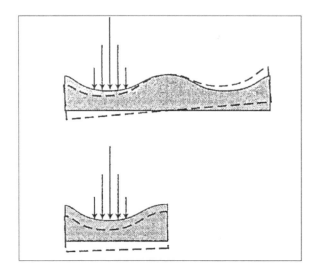

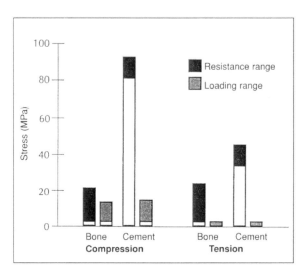

FIG. 6 - When the load is distributed over one condyle of a bicondylar tibial component, significant bending deformations occur, greater than in the unicondylar component which has a much smaller medial-lateral dimension. (Used with permission from Reference 15.)

FIG. 7 - The ranges of compression and tension stresses that cancellous bone and PMMA cement experience due to loading (the Loading ranges) are compared to the strength ranges for the two materials. PMMA strengths are much greater than the stresses they experience; unfortunately, the same is not true for cancellous bone. (Used with permission from Reference 15.)

This bone is removed, however, in most knee replacement surgeries. The remaining cancellous bone is less stiff and less strong than normal subchondral bone and thus becomes the weak link in the bone-implant system. Even when components are fixed to the bone with cement, failure may be most probable in the cancellous bone. For example, large compressive stresses are created in the cement and cancellous bone under the contact area when load is taken by a single condyle. If the contact area is near the edge of one plateau, large tensile stresses are created under the opposite plateau. The maximum stresses in the cement and in the cancellous bone are virtually identical (Fig. 7). Comparing the strengths of the two materials to the stresses that they experience, the stresses in the bone are of the same magnitude as its tensile and compressive strengths. The situation with the bone cement is quite different. Neither load condition produces tensile or compressive stresses that approach the strengths of the cement. Thus, PMMA is an appropriately strong material to insert between the bone and prosthesis.

Most contemporary prostheses have incorporated a metallic tray in the tibial component to distribute the joint loads uniformly over a large area of cancellous bone. The effect of interposing a stiff metallic layer can be seen in

Figure 8, which compares maximum cancellous bone stresses beneath a UHMWPE component and a metal-backed component (3). The metal backing reduces the maximum compressive stresses. The reduction in stresses is marginal when the loads are shared evenly between the plateaus. However, a substantial reduction occurs when the loads are applied to just one plateau. The presence of a metallic peg does not add significantly to the reduction in compressive stress. The plateaus are directly coupled to the underlying dense cancellous bone, whereas the peg is coupled to the more porous, less stiff cancellous bone in the central region of the proximal tibia.

Although the metal backing decreases the maximum compressive stress in the bone, it also increases the maximum tensile stress, especially when the loads are applied asymmetrically (Fig. 8). The opposite plateau of the metal-backed component tends to lift off from the cancellous bone, similar to the situation described above for the plastic plateau (Fig. 6). To prevent this occurrence, tensile strength must be provided at this interface.

The addition of the metal backing can create additional design problems, including providing a secure attachment between the polyethylene insert and the metallic tray and providing sufficient thickness in the insert to ensure low

UHMWPE stresses and thus to avoid wear and surface damage. These problems together with the added cost of a metallic tray have caused some surgeons to advocate the use of all-polyethylene tibial components for primary total knee arthroplasties with good ligamentous stability. These reconstructions can be accomplished to insure primarily symmetric loading for which a metal backing provides little advantage in terms of load transfer. Considering the small differences in long term survival of metal-backed and all-polyethylene condylar designs in primary knee replacements, even in young patients (20), all-polyethylene tibial components would appear warranted in elderly, low demand patients.

Though this discussion of load transfer has focused on the tibial component, the same biomechanical considerations apply to femoral and patellar components (48). Load transfer for these two types of implants has not been explored extensively, probably because fewer clinical problems are related to load transfer to these bones.

Fixation

PMMA bone cement remains the "gold standard" for fixing total knee components to the surrounding bone. Loosening of cemented components is a rare complication in most large clinical series (24). Loosening occurs less frequently than with total hip femoral components followed for comparable periods of time. Some

surgeons remain reluctant to use cemented prostheses in young active patients, however. Press-fit and porous-coated total knee replacements have been introduced with the aim of achieving stable biologic fixation without cement.

Design goals for cementless fixation are much less clear than for cement fixation. The relationship between the way loads are transferred in the initial period after implantation and the subsequent extent and distribution of tissue ingrowth is often unpredictable, as is the subsequent remodeling that might occur in the surrounding bone. Stable initial fixation must be achieved for adequate tissue ingrowth to occur. Devices to provide this initial fixation include screws and pegs. Regardless of technique, a fibrous layer may form at the interface between the porous layer and the bone because of the repetitive motions that can occur at this interface.

Whether fabricated from UHMWPE or metal, the pegs employed in many contemporary cementless designs can be thought of as supplemental fixation. When pegs are centrally located between the plateaus, they are coupled to more porous, less stiff cancellous bone. Little load sharing occurs between peg and bone (Fig. 8). However, the pegs do provide additional resistance to shear and torsional loads between the implant and the bone. They can also supply redundant fixation if loosening occurs under the plateaus of the component. Small pegs have also been incorporated into porous-coated prostheses to provide supplemental fixation. However, preferential ingrowth of bone occurs into these pegs at the expense of adequate ingrowth into the rest of the undersurface of the plateau (44), and thus fixation can be jeopardized.

Press-fit knee prostheses have incorporated UHMWPE pegs with numerous protruding flanges (40). The pegs are intended to become mechanically interlocked with the trabeculae of the cancellous bone as they are inserted into undersized drill holes beneath the plateaus. Adaptive bone changes around the press-fit component, including bone ingrowth into the spaces between the UHMWPE flanges, have been demonstrated with this type of fixation. Despite the fact that excellent long-term fixation has been achieved in these types of prostheses (36), this type of press-fit design has not gained wide acceptance, perhaps because of concern over wear between the UHMWPE pegs and the cancellous bone.

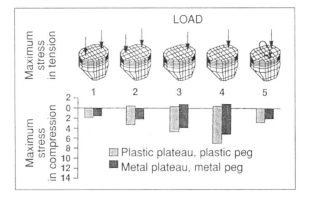

FIG. 8 - Maximum stresses in cancellous bone are plotted for several loading conditions and for all-polyethylene and metal-backed plateaus. (Used with permission from Reference 6.)

Wear

Wear of the articulating surfaces of UHMW-PE components in total knee replacements is inevitable. The large contact stresses experienced by the material even in highly conforming designs are sufficient to cause wear damage (2, 4). Surface damage in turn generates polyethylene debris that accumulates in the soft tissues. Though osteolytic changes leading to loosening seem more rare in total knee replacements than in total hip replacements (56), minimizing the stresses responsible for the generation of this debris through the choice of geometry and UHMWPE material properties must remain a design goal in total knee arthroplasty.

The types of wear observed in total knee replacements are different from that seen in total hip replacements. In total hips, abrasive and adhesive wear dominate, causing burnishing and scratching of the UHMWPE surface. In total knees, pitting and delamination are more often observed. These damage modes can release large amounts of debris, though the particle size is larger (47). This may be why osteolytic lesions and biologic reaction to debris is less severe than in total hips (56). The mechanism for pitting and delamination in tibial components is fatigue. As the contact area moves over the tibial component during functional loading of the knee, large repetitive stresses occur which cause cracks to initiate and propagate from surface or subsurface defects (5, 9).

Considerable insight to the wear problem in total knee replacements has been gained from static analyses of the stresses that are most likely associated with crack propagation (2, 4, 5). For example, such analyses have shown that the magnitudes and locations of the maximum principal stresses and the maximum shear stress are affected by the conformity of articulating surfaces, by the thickness of the component, and by the elastic modulus of the UHMWPE. These are the same design factors that were found to be important when considering load transfer (Fig. 5).

More recently, dynamic analyses of the contact problem have demonstrated that substantial residual stresses also result from the moving contact area (23, 33). Contact stresses are very high, often exceeding the yield stress of the material in regions at or near the articulating surface. The residual stresses that remain in a region of the material after the contact area passes add to the overall stresses when the contact area again passes over the region. The added stress makes the surface even more prone to fatigue failure.

Conformity between the femoral and tibial components affects both the contact area (and therefore the stresses associated with wear) and the constraint. For example, total condylar type implants utilize two radii for the tibial component, one in the anteroposterior direction and one in the medial-lateral direction, and three radii for the femoral component, two in the anteroposterior direction (one for flexion and one at and near extension) and one in the medial-lateral direction. The conformity could be increased in either direction by matching the tibial and femoral radii more closely (2). The stress is relatively insensitive, however, to conformity changes in the anteroposterior direction (Fig. 9). This is fortunate, because conformity choices in this direction are more important in terms of providing appropriate flexion-extension motion to the knee replacement than in terms of wear.

Conformity changes in the medial-lateral direction significantly affect both contact stress and constraint. If the femoral and tibial radii were made the same, the contact area would be maximized and the stress would be reduced considerably (Fig. 9). This is the same situation as described earlier for PCL sparing designs in which the femoral and tibial components were made flat in the medial-lateral direction; in that case, the radii were both equal to infinity. These surfaces presented no rotational constraint, but caused unacceptable edge loading under varus and valgus moments (Fig. 3). Making the radii the same for a condylar implant, however, would effectively eliminate rotational laxity because of the constraint between the two curved surfaces. Thus, the surrounding soft tissue structures would be unable to share torsional loads about the knee joint. The torsional load would be taken entirely by the prosthesis with increased stresses placed on the fixation interfaces and increased likelihood for loosening.

Appropriate condylar design, therefore, requires a compromise between two objectives: minimizing contact stresses and minimizing fixation surface stresses. Conforming surfaces provide rotational constraint that is inversely proportional to the radius. Smaller radii provide more constraint, while larger radii (i.e., flatter surfaces) have less resistance to rotation. The choice of the appropriate radii can be examined by plotting the results of analytical studies on a graph of the tibial medial-lateral radius plotted against the femoral medial-lateral radius (Fig.

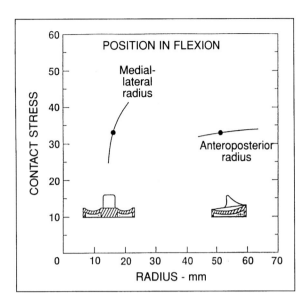

FIG. 9 - Contact stress plotted against the radius of the tibial surface for a total knee replacement. Keeping the femoral radius constant, changes in the medial-lateral radius affect contact stress much more than changes in the anteroposterior radius. (Used with permission from Reference 6.)

10). An analysis of contact stresses leads to a set of lines depicting constant maximum contact stress. A second analysis leads to a set of lines representing constant rotational resistance under joint compressive load. In this manner, the surgeon or designer can choose a desired rotational resistance and determine the radii with the least contact stress (15).

An alternative to the compromise between contact and constraint that exists for fixed bearing designs is to use a movable bearing. In movable bearing designs, the movement needed for function is separated from the movement between the articulating surfaces. Movable bearing designs have the potential advantage of allowing natural movement by minimizing constraint between UHMWPE inserts and an underlying metallic tray, while at the same time allowing for a high degree of conformity at both the articulating and movable surfaces (13). Compromise from complete conformity of the articulating surfaces is necessary, however, to prevent too large a posterior displacement of the bearings in flexion (43).

Though movable bearing designs have shown good long-term results (12), they have disadvantages as well. The potential exists, for example, that the highly conforming movable

surfaces will suffer abrasive and adhesive wear much like total hips, leading to small particles and the potential for osteolysis. A more prevalent disadvantage, however, is the high incidence of dislocations and bearing fractures, ranging between two and nine percent (7, 34, 51).

The thickness of the UHMWPE portion of the tibial component is another important factor affecting stresses associated with wear (2, 4). As UHMWPE thickness increases, the stresses associated with pitting and delamination decrease and become less sensitive to thickness (Fig. 11). For thick components (> 8 mm), stresses show little sensitivity to UHMWPE thickness. Further increases (for example, from 8 to 12 mm) create only small decreases in stress (of about fifteen percent). For thinner components, however, a similar change in thickness (for example, from 4 to 8 mm) creates a very large decrease in stress (about thirty-five percent). Based on these results, it is commonly recommended that a minimum UHMWPE thickness of 8 to 10 mm be maintained for tibial components, though thickness is sometimes limited to somewhat smaller values in metal-backed components.

The elastic modulus of UHMWPE is an important factor in wear because it is the material property that most influences the contact stress in metal-on-plastic knee joint replacements. The elastic modulus of a metallic alloy such as

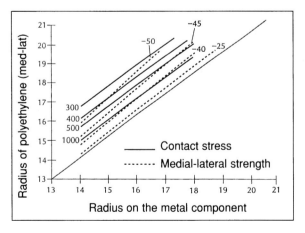

FIG. 10 - The compromise between contact and constraint can be examined from this analysis of a condylar type knee in which the contact stress and the constraining medial-lateral force are plotted as a function of the medial-lateral radii of the contacting tibial and femoral components. (Used with permission from Reference 15.)

cobalt-chrome-molybdenum alloy is two hundred times that of UHMWPE, so that the femoral component is a rigid indenter compared to the UHMWPE tibial component. Therefore, the UHMWPE controls the stresses created by contact between the two components. Unfortunately, efforts to strengthen polyethylene so as to make it more resistant to failure usually have been accompanied by significant increases in elastic modulus. The addition of carbon fibers, for example, caused a doubling of the modulus from 1 to 2 GPa. This increase produced contact stress variations of greater than one to two (55) and generally poorer wear behavior (53, 58). Careful analysis is required, therefore, to determine if increase in contact stress due to increased modulus overshadows any strength advantage of a stronger, higher modulus UHMWPE. An obvious material design goal is to disconnect modulus and strength variations to make stronger, lower modulus polyethylene.

UHMWPE properties can also be altered by radiation sterilization and exposure to oxidative environments (11, 38, 57). Molecular chain length can be decreased and cross-links between chains can be increased, causing the density and the elastic modulus to increase. The change in properties varies according to the depth beneath the articulating surface, often peaking below the surface in the region where maximum shear stresses in knee components are predicted to be quite high. The increased modulus results in even higher stresses and decreased wear resist-

ance. Degradation has been implicated in severe wear of total knee components (49, 56, 57), though no clear correlation between degradation, increased wear, and clinical performance has been established, primarily because of the number of other uncontrolled factors that affect wear and performance.

A number of material factors influence degradation, including method of manufacturing and resin type. Recently, analyses of retrieved UHMWPE tibial components have shown that the particular combination of molding and 1900 resin was essentially resistant to oxidative degradation after as much as nine years of shelf aging or eleven years of clinical use, while degradation can be quite prevalent in as little as four years in other resins used to machine (rather than mold) tibial components (25, 26). The increased degradation resistance has been used to explain the lack of wear on a flat, non-constrained, PCL sparing knee design whose tibial component was manufactured by molding 1900 resin (45).

Additional Design Considerations for Revision Knee Replacement

Fixation

Revision surgery often raises additional concerns for fixation because of loss of bone stock, ligamentous instability, or a periarticular fracture. Failure of the previous prosthesis often leaves a bony defect in the proximal tibia, for example, which raises two important questions. First, what is the best method for filling the defect and reconstituting the load transfer pathway from the implant to the tibial cortex? Second, what if any additional fixation should be considered because of the defect?

Bone defects may be filled with bone graft, bone cement, or metal. The biological solution using graft is by far optimal, provided that the defect is shaped so that the graft material can be contained and will not be required to play an immediate load-bearing role. PMMA cement has the advantage of filling the defect intimately and creating a mechanical bond to the surrounding bone, but has the disadvantage of minimal strength (Fig. 7) for such a structural role. Metallic implants are an effective alternative (3). With careful preparation of the remaining bone to match the implant geometry, the metal provides an immediate stiff and strong load path. For this reason, most contemporary knee

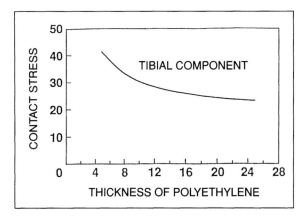

FIG. 11 - Contact stress plotted as a function of UHMWPE thickness for a condylar type knee replacement. (Used with permission from Reference 6.)

replacement systems incorporate wedges and inserts that can be attached to the tibial and femoral components at surgery.

Additional fixation is indicated in revision cases. Often an intramedullary stem is used with both the femoral and tibial components. Stems have been fixed to the surrounding cortex with cement in constrained type condylar implants with long-term clinical success (21). Stems have also been advocated for use with a press fit into the bone (1, 7). The press-fit stem is intended to share bending loads with the cortical bone in the metaphysis, but to allow axial compressive loads to be transferred through the epiphyseal cancellous bone. Often flutes are incorporated along the stem to cut into the endosteal cortical surface so that torsional loads can be transmitted directly to the diaphysis.

The clinical success of press-fit stems has been controversial. Some clinicians have found a high rate of aseptic loosening with the use of a constrained tibial insert and an uncemented stem (50), while others have not (27). Aggressive reaming, bone quality, and the previous presence of infection have been indicated as mitigating circumstances in poor results with uncemented stems. Clear guidelines for the optimal diameter and length of stem and for the appropriate fit into the medullary canal are needed, however, and additional research should provide justification for the use of press-fit stems. Again, most contemporary knee systems provide the ability to attach intramedullary stems at the time of surgery.

Constraint

The design goals for the total joint replacement of a knee with inadequate or absent collateral ligament constraints must extend to provision of adequate joint stability under the internal and external rotations and the varus and valgus movements encountered during daily activities. Many of the early hinged designs of total knee replacements routinely sacrificed the collateral ligaments. Ligament function was replaced with a linked component. One reason often cited for the poor clinical results achieved with these prostheses is the rigidity of the metal-to-metal hinge, which transferred much of the torsional load directly to the interfaces between the bone, cement, and prosthesis. This problem led to a high complication rate, including loosening and implant failures.

Hinged designs have advanced considerably from these earlier times, incorporating metal-on-polyethylene bushings and "sloppy" hinge design intended to provide a small amount of rotational and varus-valgus laxity.

A more common method for providing constraint is the use of a constrained condylar knee replacement. Constraint is provided by a polyethylene central spine on the tibial insert that fits into a mating intercondylar box on the femoral component (21). Varus-valgus and rotational constraints occur by contact between the medial and lateral surfaces of the polyethylene spine and the corresponding surfaces of the metallic intercondylar box.

The mechanical performance of constrained condylar designs has only recently been investigated (54). Analysis of retrieved implants was combined with mechanical tests on new components to determine design factors that might influence performance. Retrieved components often showed permanent medial-lateral deformation of the spine, consistent with large varus and valgus bending moments being resisted by these structures. Retrieval analysis revealed that patients damaged the spines under both varus and valgus loads, even though their clinical deformities were in a single direction. The correlation between wear damage observed on the surfaces of the spines and permanent deformation underscores the destruction that UHMWPE experiences when it serves as a structural constraint during knee motion and raises the design question as to the appropriate compromise between polyethylene damage and adequate constraint.

Mechanical testing of constrained condylar implants in which the spine was loaded in bending demonstrated that the varus-valgus constraint was dictated by local UHMWPE deformation and not by the metallic reinforcing post, even though posts are widely used clinically. The type of locking mechanism between the tibial insert and the underlying metallic tray significantly affected the stiffness of the spine and, therefore, the constraint provided by the spine. A less secure locking mechanism added to the overall deflection as the insert deformed within the tray.

Despite the clinical success of constrained condylar implants (21), these studies emphasize that this type of constraint cannot provide all of the varus-valgus stability to the knee. The surgeon must strive to balance the soft tissues so that these structures continue to contribute to the stability of the joint.

References

1) Albrektsson BE, Ryd L, Carlsson LV, et al: The Effect of a Stem on the Tibial Component of Knee Arthroplasty: A Roentgen Stereophotogrammetric Study of Uncemented Tibial Components in the Freeman-Samuelson Knee Arthroplasty. J Bone Joint Surg 72B:252-258, 1990.

2) Bartel DL, Bicknell VL, Wright TM: The Effect of Conformity, Thickness, and Material on Stresses in UHMWPE Components for Total Joint Replacement. J Bone Joint Surg 68A:1041-1051, 1986.

3) Bartel DL, Burstein AH, Santavicca EA, Insall JN: Performance of the Tibial Component in Total Knee Replacement: Conventional and Revision Design. J Bone Joint Surg 64A:1026-1033, 1982.

4) Bartel DL, Rawlinson JJ, Burstein AH, Ranawat CS, Flynn WF Jr. Stresses in Polyethylene components of Contempprary Total Knee Replacements. Clin Orthop 317:76-82, 1995.

5) Bartel DL, Rimnac CM, Wright TM: Evaluation and Design of the Articular Surface. In Controversies of Total Knee Arthroplasty (ed by V Goldberg), pp 61-73, Raven New York, 1991.

6) Bartel DL, Wright TM: Design of Total Knee Replacements. In Total Joint Replacement (ed by W Petty), pp 467-481, WB Saunders, Philadelphia, 1991.

7) Bert JM: Dislocation/Subluxation of Meniscal Bearing Elements After New Jersey Low-Contact Stress Total Knee Arthroplasty. Clin Orthop, 252:211, 1990.

8) Bertin KC, Freeman MAR, Samuelson KM, Ratcliffe SS, Todd RC: Stemmed Revision Arthroplasty for Aseptic Loosening of Total Knee Replacement. J Bone Joint Surg 67B:242-248, 1985.

9) Blunn GW, Walker PS, Joshi A, Hardinge K: The Dominance of Cyclic Sliding in Producing Wear in Total Knee Replacements. Clin Orthop 273:253-260, 1991.

10) Bolanos AA, et al: Posterior Stabilized Total Knee Prosthesis Versus Posterior cruciate Ligament Retaining Prosthesis: A Comprehensive Comparison. Presented at 63rd Ann Mtg of AAOS, Atlanta, GA, Feb. 23, 1996.

11) Bastrom MP, Bennett AP, Rimnac CM, Wright TM: The Natural History of Ultra High Molecular Weight Polyethylene. Clin Orthop 309:20-28, 1994.

12) Buechel FF, Pappas MJ: New jersey Low-Contact-Stress Knee Replacement System: Ten year Evaluation of Meniscal Bearings. Orthop Clinics North America, 20(2):147-177, 1989.

13) Buechel FF, Pappas MJ: The New jersey Low-Contact-Stress Knee Replacement System: Biomachanical Rationale and Review of the First 123 Cemented Cases. Arch Orthop Trauma Surg 105:197-204, 1986.

14) Burstein AH. Wright TM: Biomachanics. In Surgery of the Knee, 2nd Ed (ed by JN Insall), pp 43-62, Churchill Livingstone, New York, NY, 1993.

15) Burstein AH, Wright TM: Fundamentals of Orthopaedic Biomechanics. Williams & Wilkins, Baltimore, 1994.

16) Cameron HU, Hunter GA: Failure in Total Knee Arthroplasty: Mechanisms, Revisions, and Results. Clin Orthop 170:141-146, 1982.

17) Carter DR; Hayes WC: The Compressive Behavior of Bone as a Two-Phase Porous Structure. J Bone Joint Surg 59A:954-962, 1977.

18) Cash RM, Gonzalez MH, Garst J, Barmada R, Stern SH: Proprioception after arthroplasty: Role of the Posterior cruciate Ligament. Clin Orthop 331:172-178, 1996.

19) Corces A, Lotke PA, Williams JL: Strain Characteristics of the Posterior cruciate Ligament in Total Knee Replacement. Orthop Trans 13:527-528, 1989.

20) Diduch DR, Insall JN, Scott Wn, Scuderi GR, Font-Rodriguez D: Total Knee Replacement in Young, Active Patients: Long-Term Follow-Up and Functional Outcome. J Bone Joint Surg 79A:575-582, 1997.

21) Donaldson WF III, Sculco TP, Insall JN, et al: Total Condylar III Knee Prosthesis: Long term Follow-up Study. Clin Orthop 226:21-28, 1988.

22) Dorr LD, Ochsner JL, Gronley J, Perry J: Functional Comparison of Posterior Cruciate-Retained Versus cruciate-Sacrificed Total Knee Arthroplasty. Clin Orthop 236:36-43, 1988.

23) Estupiñan JA, Bartel Dl, Wright TM: Surface residual Tensile Stress After Cyclic Loading of UHMWPE by a Rigid Indenter. Trans Ortho Res Soc 21:48, 1996.

24) Font-Rodriguez D, Scuderi GR, Insall JN: Survivorship of Cemented Total Knee Arthroplasty. Clin orthop 345:79-86, 1997.

25) Furman BD, Awad Jn, Chastain KE, Li S: Material and Performance Differences Between Retrieved Machined and Moldel Insall/Burstein type Total Knee Arthroplasties. Trans Ortho Res Soc 22:643, 1997.

26) Furman BD, Ritter MA, Perone JB, Furman GL, Li S: Effect of Resin Type and Manufacturing method on UHMW-PE Oxidation and Quality at Long Aging and Implant Times. Trans Ortho Res Soc 22:92, 1997.

27) Haas SB, Insall JN; Montgomery W III, Windsor RE: Revision Total Knee Arthroplasty with Use of Modular components With Stem Inserted Without Cement. J Bone Surg 77A:1700-1707, 1995.

28) Hayes WC, Swenson lW, Schurman DJ: Axisymmetric Finite element Analysis of the lateral Tibial Plateau. J Biomech 11:21-33, 1978.

29) Hungerford Ds, Kenna RV: Preliminary Experience with a Total Knee Prostehesis with porous Coating Used Without Cement. Clin Orthop 176:95-107, 1983.

30) Incaro SJ, Johnson CC, Beynnon BD, Howe JG: Posterior Cruciate Ligament Strain Biomechanics in Total Knee Arthroplasty. Clin Orthop 309:88-93, 1994.

31) Insall JN: Surgery of the Knee, pp 750-753, Churchill Livingstone, New York, 1993.

32) Insall J, Lachiewicz PF, Burstein AH: The Posterior Stabilized Condylar Prosthesis: A Modification of the Total Condylar Design. J Bone Joint Surg 64A:1317-1323, 1982.

33) Ishikawa H, Fujiki H, Yasuda K: Contact analysis of ultra high molecular weight polyethylene articular plate in artificial knee joint during gait movement. J Biomech Engr 118:377-386, 1996.

34) Jordan LR, Olivo JL, Voorhorst PE: Survivorship Analysis of Cementless Meniscal Bearing Total Knee Arthroplasty, Clin Orthop 338:119-123, 1997.

35) Kelman GJ, Biden EN, Wyatt MP, Ritter MA, Colwell CW, jr: Laboratory Analysis of a Posterior Cruciate-Sparing Total Knee Arthroplasty in Stair Ascent and Descent. Clin Orthop 248:21-26, 1989.

36) Laskin RS: Total Knee Arthroplasty Using an Uncemented, Polyethylene Tibial Implant: A seven-Year Follow-Up Study. Clin Orthop 288:270-276, 1993.

37) Laskin RS: Total Knee Replacement with Posterior Cruciate Ligament Retention in Patients with a Fixed Varus Deformity. Clin Orthop 331:29-34, 1996.

38) Li S, Burstein AH: Ultra-High Molecular Weight Polyethylene: The Material and Its Use in Total Joint Implants. . J Bone Joint Surg 76A:1080-1090, 1994.

39) Mikosz RP, Andriacchi TP: Anatomy and Biomechanics of the Knee. In Orthopaedic knowledge Update: Hip and Knee Re-

construction (ed by JJ Callaghan, et al), pp 227-240, American Academy of Orthopaedic Surgeons, Rosemont, IL, 1995.

40) Moreland JR, Thomas RJ, Freeman MAR: ICLH Replacement of the Knee: 1977 and 1978. Clin Orthop 145:47-59, 1979.

41) Morrison JB: Mechanics of the Knee Joint. J Biomech 3:51-61, 1970.

42) Murray RP, Hayes WC, Edwuards WT, Harry JD: Mechanical Properties of the Subchondral Plate and the metaphyseal Shell. Trans Ortho Res Soc 9:197, 1984.

43) Pappas MJ, Buechel FF: On the Use of a Constant Radius Femoral Component in Meniscal Bearing Knee Replacement. J Orthop Rheumatology 7:27-29, 1994.

44) Ranawat CS, Johanson NA, Rimnac CM, Wright TM, Schwartz RE: Retrieval Analysis of Porous-Coated Components for Total Knee Replacement: A Report of Two Cases. Clin Orthop 209:244-248, 1986.

45) Ritter MA, Worland R, Saliski J, et al: Flat, Nonconstrained, Compression Molded Polythylene Total Knee replacement. Clin Orthop 321:79-85, 1995.

46) Schipplein OD, Andriacchi TP: Interction Between Active and Passive Stabilizers During Level Walking. J Orthop Res 9:113-119, 1991.

47) Shanbhag AS, Bailey HO, Eror NG, Woo SLY, Rubash HE: Characterization and Comparison of UHMWPE Wear Debris Retrieved from Total Hip and Total Knee Arthroplasties. Trans Orthop Res Soc 21:467, 1996.

48) Tissakht M, Ahmed AM, , Chan KC: Calculated Stress-Shielding in the Distal Femur after Total Knee Replacement Corresponds to the Reported Location of Bone Loss. J Orthop Res 14:778-785, 1996.

49) Tsao A, Mintz L, McCrae CR, Stulberg SD, Wright TM: Severe Polyethylene Failure in PCA Total Knee Arthroplasties. J Bone Joint Surg 75A:19-26, 1993.

50) Vince KG, Long W: Revision Kmee Arthroplasty: The Limits of Press Fit Medullary Fixation. Clin Orthop 317:172-177, 1995.

51) Weaver JK, Derkash RS, Greemwald AS: Difficulties with Bearing Dislocation and Breakage Using a Movable Bearing Total Knee Replacement System. Clin Orthop, 290:244-252, 1993.

52) Wilson SA, McCann PD, Gotlin RSm, Ramakrishanan HK, Wootten ME, Insall JN: Comprehensive Gait Analysis in Posterior.Stabilized Knee Arthroplasty. J Arthroplasty 11:359-367, 1996.

53) Wright TM, Astion DJ, Banssal M, et al: Failure of Carbon Fiber-Reinforced Polyethylene Total Knee Components: Report of Two Cases. J Bone Joint Surg 70A:926-932, 1988.

54) Wright TM, Daellenback K, Rosenthal D, Robie B, Bolanos A: Mechanical Performance Of Constrained Total Knees. Annals Biomed Eng 25 (Suppl 1):S-73, 1997.

55) Wright TM, Fukubayashi T, Burstein AH: The Effect of Carbon Fiber Reinforcement on Contact Area, Contact Pressure and Time Dependent Deformation in Polyethylene Tibial Components. J Biomed Mat Res 15:719-730, 1981.

56) Wright TM, Goodman SB: Implant Wear: The Future of Total Joint Replacement. American Academy of Orthopaedic Surgeons, Rosemont, IL, 1996.

57) Wright TM, et al: Wear of Polyethylene in Total Joint Replacements. Observations from Retrieved PCA Knee Implants. Clin Orthop 276:126-134, 1992.

58) Wright TM, Rimnac CM, Faris PM, Bansal M: Analysis of Surface Damage Occurring in Carbon Fiber-Reinforced and Plain Polyethylene Tibial Components from Posterior Stabilized Type Total Knee Replacement. J Bone Joint Surg 70A:1312-1319, 1988.

Chapter 2
Prosthetic Design and Patellofemoral Function

Bruce H. Robie, Daniel E. Rosenthal

The Hospital for Special Surgery - New York

Introduction

In the early 1970's, devices like the duo-condylar knee were used to treat tibiofemoral arthritis, leaving the patellofemoral joint intact (22). Later that decade, the duopatellar and the total condylar knees (25, 14) replaced the patellofemoral joint as well as the tibiofemoral joint. Initially, these knee replacements were used both with and without patellar resurfacing. However, long-term follow-up of patients who did not receive a patellar replacement found a high incidence of reoperation to replace the patella articulation and relieve pain (15). This finding led to standard tricompartmental total knee arthroplasty.

Two decades later, surgeons are again considering whether patellar replacement is advised as part of knee arthroplasty (3). Why the reconsideration? Because the patellofemoral joint is the most likely cause of complications in knee arthroplasty (5, 16). Insall (16) found patellofemoral complications represented eighty-five percent of device-related complications. The complications relating to the patellofemoral joint include: subluxation, dislocation, patella fracture, patellar component fracture, excessive wear of the patellar component, soft tissue catching (so called clunk) and general anterior knee pain.

While patellofemoral complications are multifactorial in origin, mechanical factors can be associated with each complication. Mechanics is the study of an object's motion and the loads applied to it. Subluxation and dislocation are examples of abnormal motion, due to forces that overcome the constraints of the patellofemoral articulation. Fractures result when loads exceed a structure's strength and damage either the bone or the implant. Wear results from a combination of forces and motions. Soft-tissue catching results from forces acting on soft tissue to limit motion. Therefore, the purpose of this chapter is to review the mechanics of the patellofemoral joint and the aspects of implant design that relate to patellofemoral function.

Relevant Anatomy

The motion of the patella is partially governed by the articulation between the patella and distal femur. There have been a series of studies recently looking at the anatomy of the distal femur. These studies use the mechanical axis of the femur to help describe the relevant femoral anatomy. The mechanical axis is defined as a line drawn between the center of the femoral head to the origin of the posterior cruciate ligament on the distal femur. Yoshioka (31) found that the anatomic axis of the femur is an average of five degrees off of the mechanical axis, with a standard deviation of approximately one degree (Fig. 1). Statistically, the range between three and seven degrees represents ninety-five percent of the population and this ninety-five percent descriptor will be used throughout the chapter to represent ranges.

In 1996, Eckhoff (7) examined the relationship between the mechanical axis, the anatomic axis and what was described as the sulcus axis. The sulcus axis was defined as the plane passing through the low points of the sulcus when the femur was held while resting the posterior condyles and the greater trochanter on a flat surface (Fig. 1). Eckhoff reported that the sulcus

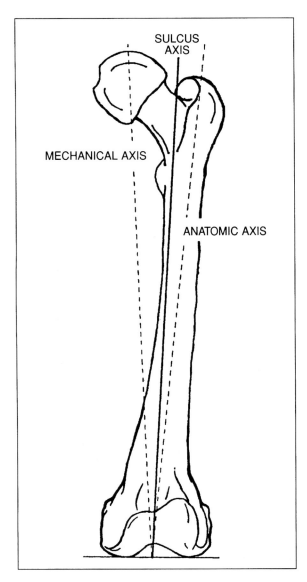

FIG. 1 - The mechanical axis is defined as a line drawn between the center of the femoral head to the origin of the posterior cruciate ligament on the distal femur. The sulcus axis is defined as the plane passing through the low points of the sulcus when the femur is held while resting the posterior condyles and the greater trochanter on a flat surface. (Used with permission from Reference 7.)

danese Nubia. Bones from a single genetic group would be expected to have less variation than bones from a multicultural population.

These results suggest that the patella would follow the sulcus axis in a plane slightly oblique to the anatomic axis of the femur. This can be translated into medial-lateral motion of the patella as the knee moves from extension to flexion. At full extension, the patella sits at its most proximal position in the sulcus. Since the sulcus axis is in varus (medial) to the anatomic axis, the patella will be at its most medial, relative to a coordinate system aligned with the anatomic axis of the femur. As the knee moves into flexion, the patella articulates further distally in the sulcus, resulting in increasing lateralization of the patella.

However, the forces that drive the location of the patella must also be considered. Studies of soft-tissue alignment have been conducted. Insall (13) studied chondromalacia patellae and defined the Q angle to represent the alignment of the quadriceps with the patellar ligament. Patients with poor alignment (Q angle greater than 20 degrees) were likely to suffer from diffuse aching anterior knee pain, made worse by stair climbing - a symptom similar to many total knee patients with patellofemoral complications.

As measured, the Q angle assumes that the quadriceps pulls along the anatomic axis of the femur. But the origin of all of the quadriceps muscles does not lie in the midplane of the thigh. So, it is not certain that the direction of pull of the quadriceps is directly along the anatomical axis, especially in instances when not all of the four muscles are active. Unfortunately, there is no study that looks at muscle origins relative to the anatomy of the distal femur to help explain the patellar motion and loads.

Huberti and Hayes (12) examined the effect of changing the Q angle on patellofemoral contact areas, pressures and forces. Changes in the Q angle are qualitatively similar to firing of selective quadriceps. For example, if just the vastus lateralis were fired, the pull of the vastus would be lateral to the anatomic axis, similar to increasing the Q angle. Huberti and Hayes found that increasing the Q angle led to increased maximum pressures and in many cases, an increase in contact areas on the lateral facet. This was not, however, a uniform finding as only six of the twelve specimens showed an increase in the lateral facet contact area. An equal number of specimens showed a pattern where contact areas shift away from the ridge separat-

axis was approximately two degrees (range: zero to four degrees) varus relative to the anatomic axis and three and one-half degrees valgus to the mechanical axis (range: 2.6 to 4.6). These results are consistent with Yoshioka in that the mechanical axis was approximately five degrees off of the anatomic axis. However, there were relatively small variations in this study. This is likely due to the source of the specimens: Su-ing the two facets. Similarly wide variations in results will be seen in many of the other studies discussed in this Chapter. The patellofemoral joint seems to be uniquely tuned to each individual.

Natural Patellar Mechanics

The mechanical behavior of the patella has been extensively studied, in both natural and replaced conditions. These studies are typically *in vitro* experiments (1, 6, 10, 12, 17, 18, 19, 20, 21, 24, 26, 27, 28, 30) although there have also been a few studies using computer models (4, 11). No *in vivo* studies have examined patellar motion.

The methodology of the *in vitro* experiments was similar. Usually, a cadaveric specimen was placed in an apparatus, such as that shown in Figure 2. A weight at the hip joint tended to flex the knee. This force was resisted by a sheathed cable attached to the quadriceps. Force changes in the cable resulted in different flexion-extension positions. The ankle was allowed only to rotate. An alternative test apparatus allowed the ankle free motion and fixed the femur (17). Motions of the patella were measured using a variety of techniques, including Roentgen Stereophotogrammetric Analysis (RSA) (28), x-rays

(30), light-emitting diodes (LED's) used with image capturing (1), custom measurement instruments (19) and magnetic field sensors (6).

Natural Patellar Motion

There have been a series of reports describing the natural motion of the patella. They cover a variety of topics, but discussion here will be limited to three motions. These are medial-lateral motion, tilt and flexion-extension. Medial-lateral motion is defined as the translations perpendicular to either the anatomic or mechanical axis. Tilt is defined as a rotation about the long axis of the patellar ligament, with medial tilt defined as rotation that forces the medial facet of the patella towards the medial condyle of the femur (28). Flexion-extension is defined as rotation of the patella seen in a sagittal view. It can be measured relative to the long axis of the femur or relative to the long axis of the tibia.

The qualitative findings regarding patellar motion are similar among the different studies. The first common finding is the patella moved slightly medial and then laterally as flexion increased (19, 28). The medial shift occurred within the first thirty to sixty degrees of flexion. By sixty degrees of flexion, the patella again returned to a neutral alignment. Beyond sixty degrees it was lateral. Figure 3, from Nagamine (19), shows their data for medial-lateral position.

The second common finding is the significant variation from specimen to specimen, so

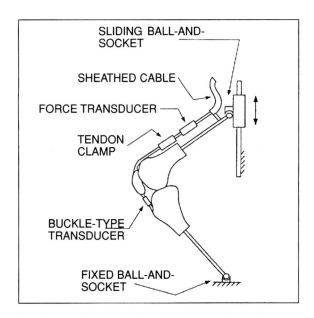

Fig. 2 - Typical test setup for in vitro patellofemoral experiments. (Used with permission from Reference 26.)

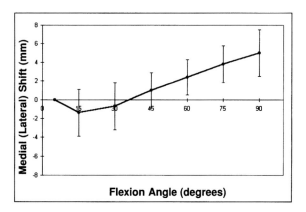

Fig. 3 - Medial-lateral translation of the patella during flexion. A small medial shift occurs during early flexion with a larger lateral shift occurring in late flexion. (Used with permission from Reference 19.)

the standard deviations for a group of subjects can be very large, meaning that the natural range is wide. Nagamine had a standard deviation of two mm on medial-lateral position, so that the range of normal variation was eight mm wide. For example, at seventy-five degrees of flexion, the patella should be 3 3/4 mm lateral to the anatomic axis, but the range would be between 1/4 mm medial to almost 8 mm lateral. To provide some context for this variation, consider the dimensions of a mid-sized femur. If the overall medial-lateral width is approximately 65 mm, the anterior width is approximately 50 mm. So the natural variation in medial-lateral position represents about one sixth of the anterior width. While this variation seems large, it would be even larger if the authors had not removed data from two other samples because they were 'abnormal.'

The patella has a slight tendency to tilt medially then laterally with increasing flexion, but the variation among specimens overwhelms the typical behavior. Figure 4, from Van Kampen and Huiskes (28), shows the tilt for four different specimens. For these specimens, at a single position like seventy-five degrees, the patellae tilted anywhere from four degrees medial to twelve degrees lateral. Nagamine found a standard deviation of approximately five degrees in tilt at seventy-five degrees of flexion. This results in a range of twenty degrees of tilt. This is similar to Van Kampen and Huiskes' findings of a range of sixteen degrees.

The flexion-extension rotation of the patella lags the flexion-extension of the knee, in a con-

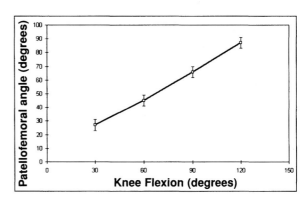

FIG. 5 - The flexion-extension rotation of the patella for 10 in vitro specimens. The data show a consistent trend of patella flexion approximately 2/3 of knee flexion. (Used with permission from Reference 18.)

sistent way. Figure 5, from Lee (18), shows flexion-extension of the patella versus knee flexion angle. For every thirty degrees of knee flexion, there was about twenty degrees of patellofemoral flexion. The difference between knee flexion and patellofemoral flexion defines the relative motion between the femur and patella. The graph also shows that there was little variation between specimens, relative to the magnitudes of the angles measured. This is in striking difference to the results for medial-lateral motion or tilt.

Natural Patellar Loads

Patellar loads have been examined using similar apparati to those already described. Both indirect and direct measurements of load have been used. Indirect measurements include force in the quadriceps (17) and patellar contact areas (10). Loads have also been measured directly using pressure sensitive film (12) and load cells (21, 26).

The load on the patella increases as knee flexion increases up to ninety degrees. Huberti and Hayes (12) estimated that the load could range from 500 N at near extension to a maximum force on the patella of 4600 N in ninety degrees of flexion. This force was equivalent to approximately 6.5 times body weight. Under less than maximal loading conditions, they also found that there was significant variation in the force necessary to maintain a specific flexion position. For example, at ninety degrees of flexion, the mean contact force was 1500 N, but the range was between 900 N and 2200 N. This

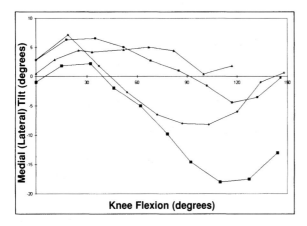

FIG. 4 - Medial-lateral tilt of the patella during flexion for four in vitro specimens. The data show a large variation in tilt between specimens. (Used with permission from Reference 28.)

again points out the large variation in the natural patellofemoral joint.

Beyond ninety degrees, the force on the patella diminishes. Two factors influence this diminution. The first is contact between the quadriceps tendon and femur. Huberti and Hayes estimated that one-third of the patellar contact force was transmitted to the femur through the quadriceps tendon at one hundred twenty degrees of knee flexion. This contact reduced the force on the patella. The second reason for the reduction of the force on the patella relates to the overall body mechanics. Imagine a person squatting with their knees flexed at ninety degrees. The mass of the trunk exerts a force on the femoral head of the femur. This mass induces a flexion moment at the knee. This trunk moment is equal to the mass of the trunk multiplied by the length of the femur (its moment arm). The trunk moment is resisted by the quadriceps. At ninety degrees, the moment arm for the trunk mass is at its maximum. Additional flexion begins to bring the trunk mass closer, in a horizontal direction, to the knee. At 120 degrees, the moment arm of the trunk mass is reduced by 13%. The quadriceps needs to carry less force to resist the moment due to the trunk mass. This reduces the force on the patella.

The area in contact between the patella and femur moves proximally on the patella with increasing flexion. Goodfellow (10) showed that the contact was at the distal pole of the patella when the knee approached full extension (Fig. 6). As knee flexion increased towards ninety degrees, the contact area moved superiorly. By ninety degrees, it reached the superior pole of the patella. Beyond ninety degrees, the odd facet contacted on the medial side of the patella and the lateral facet contacted laterally, but the ridge dividing the medial and lateral facet was not in contact. This was in contrast with contact between twenty and ninety degrees of flexion, where contact was a band with roughly equivalent areas on both the medial and lateral facets of the patella and included the ridge dividing the two facets.

There is an underlying assumption to all of these *in vitro* load studies. Each study severed the quadriceps and tied weights to the quadriceps mechanism so as to model its behavior. The amount of weight used was set based on obtaining equilibrium. That is, if too little weight was attached, the knee would continue to flex. If too much weight was attached, the knee would extend. The proper amount of weight maintained the knee at a specific flexion angle, and

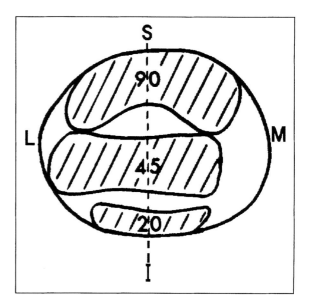

FIG. 6 - Contact areas on the patella at 20, 45 and 90 degrees of flexion. S, I, L, M, represent superior, inferior, lateral, and medial, respectively. The contact moves from the inferior pole of the patella in early flexion to the superior pole of the patella during late flexion (Used with permission from Reference 10.)

differed from one flexion position to another. Modeling the quadriceps tension with weights presumes that the force necessary to achieve equilibrium can be generated naturally by the quadriceps. This assumption is rarely checked for the specific positions studied.

Design Goals Based On Natural Mechanics

Based on the preceding review, design goals can be established for the mechanical behavior of a patellofemoral joint and the patellar component of a total knee replacement.

1) The total knee should allow the patellar component to move laterally with increasing flexion.

2) The total knee should allow the patellar component to track in a eight mm wide band in the medial-lateral direction.

3) The total knee should allow twenty degrees of patellar tilt.

4) The patellar component and its articulation with the femoral component should tolerate increasing loads up to ninety degrees of knee flexion, where forces could reach 4600 N.

5) The total knee should allow the patellar component to flex and extend relative to the

femoral component, while contact moves smoothly from inferior to superior on the patellar component as knee flexion increases, without changing the contact area significantly.

Implant Design and Mechanics

Both the implant designer and the surgeon implanting the total knee significantly affect patellofemoral function. The implant designer determines the features necessary to achieve the design goals. These features include the angle of the femoral sulcus relative to the distal femur, the height of the lateral anterior condyle that has been used to limit subluxation and dislocation, the shape of the patellar articulation (domed, sombrero, anatomic, etc.), the conformity between the femoral and patellar components, the depth of the sulcus on the femoral component and the method of fixation of the patellar component. The surgeon controls implant position and orientation. The surgeon determines proximal-distal and medial-lateral position of the femoral component, as well as the extent of external rotation. Additionally, the surgeon determines the medial-lateral position of the patellar component relative to the patella. Decisions made by the surgeon can compensate for implant design limitations or, conversely, can exacerbate design limitations.

The remainder of this chapter will review each of the items identified above, in light of the stated design goals, consider published research on the specific topic and come to conclusions regarding the value of the particular item. Many of the surgical positioning issues have been evaluated using *in vitro* tests similar to those described in the section on natural mechanics. Additionally, there are a few *in vitro* studies examining some of the features controlled by the designer. Finally, there are long-term clinical follow-up studies that support or refute specific design features.

Angling the femoral sulcus relative to the distal femur has not been shown to ensure more natural patellofemoral tracking nor to reduce shear forces that could induce subluxation or dislocation. Evidence of this conclusion is found in both Chew (6) and Petersilge (21). Chew compared a design with a symmetric sulcus, where the sulcus was perpendicular to the distal condyles, and an asymmetric design, where the sulcus was not perpendicular to the distal condyles. The symmetric sulcus design was the PFC Sigma (Johnson & Johnson); the

asymmetric sulcus design was the Genesis II (Smith and Nephew). Measuring patellar tracking, they found no significant differences between these two sulci designs.

An angled sulcus provides relatively little lateralization of the patella. For example, a three degree sulcus angle would match that measured by Eckhoff (7) and would only shift the top of the sulcus approximately three mm laterally. This proximal shift allows the patella to track laterally only in extension, but the patella naturally tracks most laterally in ninety degrees of flexion, where the sulcus provides little lateral tracking. Figure 7 shows that by 50 degrees of flexion, the patella is tracking near the bottom of the anterior flange where an angled sulcus would result in minimal lateralization. Since an angled sulcus does not encourage natural patellar tracking, there does not seem to be a clinical benefit to this design feature.

Petersilge compared the patellar forces resulting from a symmetric flange with those from an asymmetric flange. One would expect that a design with greater medial-lateral shear force on the patella would be at increased risk for subluxation or dislocation. They found that the medial-lateral shear force on a symmetric design was not significantly different from that on an asymmetric design. They did find significant

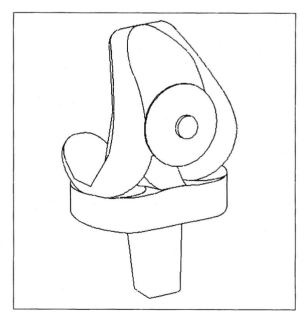

FIG. 7 - A typical total knee replacement in 50 degrees of flexion. Note that the patella is positioned at the distal end of the sulcus.

differences in the superior-inferior shear, but the clinical implications of this result are not clear.

Lateral buildup of the anterior condyle does not provide necessary restriction to prevent subluxation or dislocation. Theiss (27) compared the clinical patellofemoral complication rates between two designs, one which had a lateral buildup (MG I - Zimmer) and one that did not (PFC - Johnson & Johnson). The knee without the lateral buildup had no dislocations or subluxations, whereas the knee with the lateral buildup had a combined subluxation and dislocation rate of eight percent. Again, this is not surprising since the buildup is near the top of the flange and not in a region of high loads on the patella. Since there are other designs, such as the Ortholoc (Wright Medical Technology) with lateral buildups and low subluxation and dislocation rates (29), it does not appear that the buildup has any deleterious effect. This result is also supported by the work of Yoshii (30) and of Chew (6).

The shape of the patellar articulation (domed, sombrero, anatomic, etc.) does have potentially significant implications on patellofemoral function. The design goals state that the implant must allow for twenty degrees of tilt and flexion-extension of the patellar component relative to the femoral component. These required biplane rotations limit the geometry of the patellar articulation. To accommodate these rotations, a doubly curved surface is necessary, with one curve in the medial-lateral direction and another in the superior-inferior direction. The domed patellar articulation fulfills these requirements as do other doubly curved components. All other designs, including the sombrero and anatomic designs, are inappropriate because either tilt or flexion-extension cause edge loading on the rim of the component. Since this plastic is relatively thin, it puts the patellar component at risk for failure due to wear or fracture. The mobile bearing provides rotational adjustment, but not tilt or flexion-extension of the component. Since its articulation is fundamentally the same as non-domed patellae, it is also sensitive to tilt.

Conformity between the femoral and patellar components influences the joint's ability to tolerate natural variations in motion and also wear of the patellar component. Unfortunately, these are competing objectives. To tolerate natural variations in motion, there must be some nonconformity. Nonconformity allows the patella to move in a medial-lateral direction as needed to establish an equilibrium of forces. Once a limit on medial-lateral motion is reached, then additional motion occurs from tilt or anterior displacement. This additional motion further translates the tendon and ligament attachments. If this additional motion is insufficient to equilibrate the forces on the patella, then subluxation or dislocation occurs. So motion is the means by which shear forces on the patella are avoided. Limiting the motion by increasing the conformity will increase the risk of subluxation or dislocation.

In contrast, the potential for wear increases with decreasing conformity. As conformity decreases, the contact stresses in the polyethylene increase, similar to tibiofemoral contact stresses described in Chapter 1. Increases in the contact stresses put the patellar component at greater risk for wear or long term failure.

But the conflict between motion and conformity is not new. Ever since the Total Condylar I, there has been concern with patellar complications. With fifteen year follow-up, the results from the Total Condylar I showed that the percentage of knees revised for patellofemoral complications was 1% (23). The lack of failures in this and other series suggests that it is possible to compromise between motion and conformity. Alternatively, designs that constrain the patella will most certainly fail, as will those that are completely unconstrained.

Perhaps the most important variable at the control of the implant designer is the depth of the femoral sulcus. Both Petersilge (21) and Yoshii (30) showed that small increases in the depth of the sulcus result in better patellofemoral behavior. Yoshii examined the effect of a one mm increase in depth and found that it provided more natural motion of the patella. Petersilge showed that a two mm deeper sulcus reduced the forces on the patella in comparison to implants with shallower sulci.

There are three concerns with the research on sulcus depth. The first is the measurement of sulcus depth. Neither of these authors describe how the depth was measured. Given that the sulcus is curved, there are multiple places and orientations for possible measurement. Therefore, describing differences between two knees based on a single number is nearly meaningless.

The second concern is that 'depth' represents a shift below the most proud surface of the femoral component. As such, it has much to do with that most proud surface. As an example, compare the Insall-Burstein II knee (Zimmer, Cremascoli) with the '913' knee ('913' - Cre-

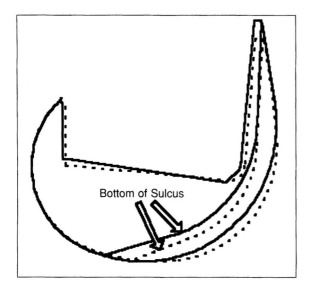

Fig. 8 - Sagittal profiles of the '913' (solid line) and Insall-Burstein II (dashed line). Note the Insall-Burstein II has more material in the antero-distal corner of the femur, in comparison to the '913'. The depth of the sulcus is the same for both knees.

mascoli, Optetrak - Exactech, Advance - Wright Medical Technology). Both are shown in Figure 8. The sagittal profiles of the two knees are different, with the Insall-Burstein II having more material in the antero-distal corner of the femur, in comparison to the '913.' Yet the depth of the sulcus is the same for both knees. Unpublished experience at the Hospital for Special Surgery suggests that the number of patellofemoral complications are much reduced in the '913' in comparison to the IB II. This result would not be expected based on the depth measurement.

Depth has been used as a simple parameter to represent the patellofemoral function of a design. However, an appropriate parameter must be related to knee equilibrium. Knee equilibrium is a function of many parameters including the trunk moment, the force in the quadriceps, the contact between the femur and tibia, the position and orientation of the patellar ligament, and the contact between the patella and femur. In turn, these are influenced by friction, muscle generating capacity, passive stretch of the muscles and tendons and the joint kinematics. Therefore, it seems inappropriate to use depth as a sole comparitor between implant designs. Unfortunately, there is no other single parameter at this time that can better represent knee equilibrium and patellofemoral function. So surgeons must evaluate the influence of the

patellofemoral kinematics on knee equilibrium.

The third concern is that too much depth also will have detrimental consequences. Remember that the force in the patellar tendon results in an extension moment to counter the moment created by the mass of the trunk. If the depth of the sulcus is deepened excessively, the moment arm of the tendon will diminish and a greater quadriceps force will be necessary to hold the joint in a fixed position.

The last design feature that must be addressed is the fixation of the patellar component. Cemented dome all-polyethylene patellar components are more reliable than metal backed components and metal backing offers no mechanical advantage to the surgeon. The long history of cemented all-polyethylene buttons shows that they do not loosen, nor do they contribute so much debris as to risk loosening due to osteolysis (9, 23). They accommodate non-conformity by creeping in ways to reduce the contact stress on the polyethylene. Metal backing was proposed to enhance fixation. Since there have been so few failures of cemented all-poly patellar components, this reason is without merit. Additionally, the first generation of metal backed patellae had catastrophic failures associated with them, including dissociation of the plastic from the metal and fracture of the plastic component (2).

In summary, the design issues of concern to the surgeon should be the interaction between the patellofemoral kinematics and knee equilibrium, including the 'depth' of the sulcus, the use of spherical or doubly curved patellar articulations and the use of a cemented all-polyethylene component.

In contrast, there is much that a surgeon can do by positioning to enhance patellofemoral function. Appropriate proximal-distal and medial-lateral position of the femoral component, as well as the extent of external rotation have been shown to improve the performance of the patellofemoral joint. Additionally, the medialization of the patellar component relative to the patella has been shown to better replicate natural kinematics and forces. The surgeon must also correctly reproduce the thickness of the patella to avoid increasing patellar forces.

In 1986, Figgie (8) showed that femoral components put in proximally were at significantly greater risk for patellofemoral complications. This was a retrospective clinical study based on a review of one hundred sixteen total knee replacements in one hundred one patients. Patients whose implant joint line was within eight mm of the natural joint line had no complaints of patellofemoral pain or other mechanical symptoms. In contrast, ten percent of those whose joint line was shifted proximally by more than eight mm were revised for patellofemoral symptoms.

Lateralization of the femoral component and medialization of the patellar component have both been shown to result in more natural patellar kinematics. Rhoads (24) found that a five mm lateral shift of the femoral component was preferable to either a neutral position or a medial shift of five mm. This was not, however, statistically significant. Possible reasons for this are the number of specimens tested (seven) and the amount of variation that is typically seen in studies of the patella. Yoshii (30) showed that medialization of the patellar component by ten mm resulted in more natural patellar kinematics than when the patella was placed centrally on the cut surface. Both lateralization of the femoral component and medialization of the patellar component allow the patella to track laterally in flexion.

How far should the patellofemoral joint be shifted laterally? The data from Nagamine (19) on natural motion suggests, on average, that a shift of four to five mm is necessary at ninety degrees of flexion. But the variation among subjects suggests that some will need only a couple of mm shift, whereas others will need nearly a centimeter shift. This guidance matches with the results of Rhoads and Yoshii. Since the amount of medial-lateral shift is specific to each patient, evaluation of the medial-lateral position of the patellofemoral joint on each patient is important. The most lateral position of the patella occurs at ninety degrees of flexion. This is also where the load reaches its maximum. So the evaluation of medial-lateral positioning of the components should occur at ninety degrees of flexion.

External rotation of the femoral component has also been shown to result in more natural patellofemoral kinematics. Rhoads showed that a ten degree external rotation resulted in relatively natural kinematics up to 100 degrees of flexion. Beyond 100 degrees, external rotation caused medial displacement of the patella relative to the femur. Using similar techniques, Anouchi (1) showed that a five degree external rotation resulted in more natural kinematics as

compared to neutral or internal rotation of the femoral component. The kinematics beyond ninety degrees were not studied. Based on these results, it is not possible to recommend a specific amount of external rotation. Some slight amount of external rotation is necessary, but excessive external rotation could lead to problems in patients who achieve flexion beyond ninety degrees.

The forces on the patella increase when the reconstructed patella is thicker than the natural patella. In an *in vitro* model, Oishi (20) found that an increase in patellar thickness of only two mm resulted in a significant increase in shear forces on the patella. Clinically, this is supported by findings of a higher incidence of patella fracture with thicker patellar components (16). The sensitivity of load to changes in patellar thickness is similar to the sensitivity of load to changes in sulcus depth. Even small increases in thickness or small decreases in depth force the patella to move anteriorly resulting in higher loads.

Conclusions

The achievement of proper mechanical patellofemoral function relies on both the surgeon and the implant designer. To allow the patella to track laterally with increasing flexion, the surgeon must position the femoral component in a slightly lateral position while medializing the patellar component. To allow the patella to function naturally in a variety of patients, the implant designer must allow for some nonconformity between the articulation of the patellar component and the femoral component. To allow for appropriate patellar tilt and flexion-extension of the patellar component, a domed or doubly curved patellar articulation should be used. To ensure that the loads on the patella are not increased following total joint replacement, the patellofemoral kinematics and sulcus depth must be set appropriately by the implant designer. The surgeon must also accurately reconstruct the thickness of the patella. To tolerate the high *in vivo* loads, a cemented all-polyethylene patellar component is recommended. Following these guidelines will increase the likelihood of successfully reconstructing this most individualized of joints.

References

1) Anouchi YS, Whiteside LA, Kaiser AD, Milliano MT: The Effects of Axial Rotational Alignment of the Femoral Component of Knee Stability and Patellar Tracking in Total Knee Arthroplasty Demonstrated on Autopsy Specimens. Clin Orthop 287:170-177, 1993.

2) Bayley IC, Scott RD, Ewald FC, Holmes GB Jr: Failure of the Metal-Backed Patellar Component After Total Knee Replacement. J Bone Joint Surg 70A:668-674, 1988.

3) Barrack RL, Wolfe MW, Waldman DA, Milicic M, Bertot AJ, Myers L: Resurfacing of the Patella in Total Knee Arthroplasty. J Bone Joint Surg 79A:1121-1131, 1997.

4) Blaankevoort L, Kuiper JH, Huiskes R, Grootenboer HJ: Articular Contact in a Three-dimensional Model of the Knee. J Biomech 24:1019-1031, 1991.

5) Brick GW, Scott RD: The Patellofemoral Component of Total Knee Arthroplasty. Clin Orthop 231:163-178, 1988.

6) Chew ITH, Stewart NJ, Hanssen AD, Luo ZP, Rand JA, An KN: Differences in Patellar Tracking and Knee Kinematics Among Three Different Total Knee Designs. Clin Orthop 345:87-98, 1997.

7) Eckhoff DG, Burke BJ, Dwyer TF, Pring ME, Spitzer VM, VanGerwen DP: Sulcus Morphology of the Distal Femur. Clin Orthop 331:23-28, 1996.

8) Figgie HE III, Goldberg VM, Heiple KG, Moller HS III, Gordon NH: The Influence of Tibial-Patellofemoral Location on Function of the Knee in Patients with the Posterior Stabilized Condylar Knee Prosthesis. J Bone Joint Surg 68A:1035-1040, 1986.

9) Font-Rodriguez DE, Scuderi GR, Insall JN: Survivorship of Cemented Total Knee Arthroplasty. Clin Orthop 345:79-86, 1997.

10) Goodfellow J, Hungerford DS, Zindel M: Patello-femoral Joint Mechanics and Pathology. J Bone Joint Surg 58B:287-290, 1976.

11) Heegard J, Leyvraz PF, Curnier A, Rakotomanana L, Huiskes R: The Biomechanics of the Human Patella During Passive Knee Flexion. J Biomechanics 28:1265-1279, 1995.

12) Huberti HH, Hayes WC: Patellofemoral Contact Pressures: The Influence of Q-Angle and Tendofemoral Contact. J Bone Joint Surg 66A:715-724, 1984.

13) Insall J, Falvo KA, Wise DW: Chondromalacia Patellae. J Bone Surg 58A:1-8, 1976.

14) Insall J, Ranawat CS, Scott WN, Walker P: Total Condylar Knee Replacement: Preliminary Report. Clin. Orthop. 120:149-154, 1976.

15) Insall J, Scott WN, Ranawat CS: The Total Condylar Knee Prosthesis. J Bone Joint Surg 61A:173-180, 1979.

16) Insall JN; Lachiewicz PF, Burstein AH: The Posterior Stabilized Condylar Prosthesis. J Bone Joint Surg 64A:1317-1323, 1982.

17) Kaufer H: Mechanical Function of the Patella. J Bone Joint Surg 53A:1551-1560, 1971.

18) Lee TQ, Gerken AP, Glaser FE, Kim WC, Anzel SH: Patello-femoral Joint Kinematics and Contact Pressures in Total Knee Arthroplasty. Clin Orthop 340:257-266, 1997.

19) Nagamine R, Otani T, White SE, McCarthy DS, Whiteside LA: Patellar Tracking Measurement in the Normal Knee. J Orthop Res 13:115-122, 1995.

20) Oishi CS, Kaufman KR, Irby SE, Colwell CW Jr: Effects of Patellar Thickness on Compression and Shear Forces in Total Knee Arthroplasty. Clin Orthop 331:283-290, 1996.

21) Petersilge WJ, Oishi CS, Kaufman KR, Irby SE, Coldwell CW Jr: The Effect of Trochlear Design on Patellofemoral Shear and Compressive Forces in Total Knee Arthroplasty. Clin Orthop 309:124-130, 1994.

22) Ranawat CS, Insall J, Shine J: Duo-Condylar Knee Arthroplasty. Clin Orthop 120:76-82, 1976.

23) Ranawat CS, Flynn WF Jr, Saddler S, Hansraj KK, Maynard MJ: Long Term Results of Total Condylar Knee Arthroplasty. Clin Orthop 286:94-102, 1993.

24) Rhoads DD, Noble PC, Reuben JD, Tullos HS: The effect of Femoral Component Position on the Kinematics of Total Knee Arthroplasty. Clin Orthop 286:122-129, 1993.

25) Scott RD: Duopatellar Total Knee Replacement: The Brigham Experience. Orth. Clin North Am, 13:89-102, 1982.

26) Singerman R, Berilla J, Davy DT: Direct In Vitro Determination of the Patellofemoral contact Force for Normal Knees. J Biomechanical Eng 117:8-14, 1995.

27) Theiss SM, Kitziger KJ, Lotke PS, Lotke PA: Component Design Affecting Patellofemoral Complications After Total Knee Arthroplasty. Clin Orthop 326:183-187, 1996.

28) Van Kampen A, Huiskes R: The Three-Dimensional Tracking Pattern of the Human Patella J Orthop Res, 8:372-382, 1990.

29) Whiteside LA: Cementless Total Knee Replacement: Nine-to 11Year Results and 10-year Survivorship Analysis. Clin Orthop 309:185-192, 1994.

30) Yoshii I, Whiteside LA, Anouchi YS: The Effect of Patellar Button Placement and Femoral Component Design on Patellar Tracking in Total Knee Arthroplasty. Clin Orthop 275:211-219, 1992.

31) Yoshioka Y, Siu D, Cooke TD: The Anatomy and Functional Axes of the Femur. J Bone Joint Surg 69A:873-880, 1987.

Section 2
SURGICAL TECHNIQUE

Chapter 3
Preoperative Planning and Prosthetic Selection

S. David Stulberg
Northwestern Hospital - Chicago

As is true for all surgical procedures, a careful and complete preoperative preparation is essential to the ultimate success of a total knee replacement. Most orthopaedic surgeons are aware of this fact and have at least a vague idea of what they must do to prepare for an upcoming total knee procedure. However, if the total knee procedure is to be successfully and safely carried out, preoperative preparation must also be carried out by the patient and his or her family and by the hospital at which the procedure is to be performed The surgeon is responsible for initiating and guiding this preparation by the patient and the hospital. The surgeon must recognize and acknowledge the importance of this preparation and should be prepared to assure that the patient and hospital are as ready for the upcoming total knee arthroplasty as he or she is. In this chapter, I will discuss the preparation that the surgeon, patient and hospital should carry out prior to the performance of a primary or revision total knee arthroplasty

A) Preparation by the Surgeon

A surgeon and his or her staff can best get ready for an upcoming total knee procedure if he or she organizes the preparation process into four areas: 1) patient issues, 2) exposure issues, 3) equipment issues, and 4) reimbursement issues. The preparation process will be much easier if the surgeon and his or her staff has formalized preoperative preparation in each of these areas. A surgeon who does joint replacement surgery should develop a series of checklists that guide the preoperative preparation process.

1) Patient Issues

Every patient undergoing a total knee replacement must have a careful general medical evaluation, including laboratory tests. Although the nature and extent of this evaluation may vary from surgeon to surgeon and hospital to hospital, the purpose of the medical evaluation is to assure to the greatest extent possible that the patient is medically capable of safely having a total knee procedure. This medical examination should be performed one to four weeks before the proposed surgery. If the initial evaluation indicates the need for further tests or treatment, enough time should exist for these to be carried out. Patients, like physicians, find last minute delays in surgery which result from the need for further testing or treatment to be frustrating, aggravating, costly and emotionally unsettling. Most patients and their families have organized their personal and employment schedules in anticipation that the surgery will be carried out as scheduled. They expect their surgeon to organize the preoperative evaluation to minimize the likelihood of such delays. It can be anticipated that older patients may require tests in addition to those routinely obtained prior to total knee replacement surgery. For example, a coronary artery stress test may be found to be necessary once an intial medical evaluation is performed. Patients with a history, signs or symptoms of peripheral vascular disease (venous or arterial) or carotid artery disease may require special vascular studies. Surgeons can increase the likelihood of anticipating the need for special studies if they obtain a systematic history of a patient's past medical care during the initial orthopaedic evaluation. If the orthopaedic surgeon requires, as I usually do, that older patients whose medical care has been provided by physicians not associated with the hospital at which the total knee surgery is to be performed be evaluated by a medical physician who can be available if needed after the surgery, it may be particularly likely that more than the routine medical and laboratory evaluations will be needed. In such situations it is not uncommon to discover previously unsuspected medical or dental conditions that require treatment prior to the performance of the knee replacement.

The type of procedure that is performed influences the type of medical and laboratory preoperative evaluation that is carried out. For example, simultaneously performed bilateral total knee replacements may be associated with an increased risk of cardiac, respiratory and neurologic complications. Patients that require bilateral knee replacements who have a history suggestive of significant cardiac, respiratory or cerebral vascular disease need particularly careful preoperative evaluation. The evaluation of these higher risk patients will help the surgeon determine whether the bilateral procedures should be performed simultaneously, i.e., during one anesthetic, or sequentially, i.e., during separate anesthetics, perhaps weeks apart. Other examples of total knee procedures that might require laboratory tests that are not routine are: 1) revision procedures, which may require an aspiration of the knee prior to surgery, or 2) knees with severe fixed flexion contractures or fixed valgus deformities which may require particularly careful evaluation of the peripheral neurovascular status of the affected extremity.

It is particularly important that the orthopaedic surgeon determine clearly whether and how **musculoskeletal** conditions other than the affected knee may impact the outcome of the proposed total knee procedure. Such conditions are frequently present in the population of patients that require knee replacement surgery. The orthopaedic surgeon is in the best position to identify and prepare for these conditions. Examples of such musculoskeletal conditions include: 1) a history of back disease, which may require an alteration in the routine postoperative knee rehabilitation program; 2) a history of severe arthritis of the feet, ankle or hips, which may require alterations in the routine postoperative rehabilitation program; 3) upper extremity arthritis, which may require special supportive aids after surgery; 4) a history of gouty arthritis or pseudogout, which may flare-up following surgery; 5) rheumatoid arthritis, which may require special management of medication and therapy

in the perioperative period; and 6) a history of non-rheumatoid inflammatory arthritis which may require medication postoperatively to control generalized musculoskeletal symtoms. This medication may interfere with anti-thrombolic agents such as warfarin or low molecular weight heparin. A plan for successfully controlling such symptoms safely should be in place prior to the performance of the total knee proceduere.

It is essential that the orthopaedic surgeon obtain appropriate preoperative musculoskeletal radiographic studies. Routine primary total knee replacements usually require: 1) a full-length, standing x-ray of both lower extremities (this study should include the hip, knee and ankle joint); 2) a lateral view of the knee to be operated upon; 3) a sky-line view of both patellae. The full-length standing radiograph reveals the extent of angular deformity and bone loss present which allows the surgeon to more accurately anticipate his or her prosthetic and bone graft needs. The lateral view reveals the extent of posterior femoral and tibial osteophyte formation. This information alerts the surgeon to the need for the removal of these osteophytes, which may be difficult to see during the performance of a routine total knee procedure. An awareness of the need to remove these osteophytes may lead the surgeon to perform a more extensive than usual exposure of the posterior surfaces of the femur and tibia. The extensive removal of osteophytes may also require the use of a relatively constrained prosthesis system, which the surgeon must arrange to have available. The lateral view also reveals the position of the patella relative to the femur. This information may be important for avoiding patellar-tibial impingement or quadriceps tensioning and alignment problems. The patellar view is particularly important. The surgeon should know preoperatively if the patellae are subluxated or tilted. Such patellae are more likely to require the performance of a lateral retinacular release. If a skyline view indicates that the patellae are subluxated or tilted, the surgeon will need to take special care that at the conclusion of the total knee replacement the quadriceps mechanism tracks properly. This is particularly true for knees which have preoperative fixed valgus, external rotation deformities. The orthopaedic surgeon preparing for a revision should realize that the routine (and even the special x-ray views discussed below) preoperative radiographic studies are not reliable for accurately assessing component alignment, especially rotational alignment. Thus, the surgeon should not depend upon preoperative radiographs for determining whether or not a particular implant that appears well-fixed will require removal for malpositioning.

Some surgeons routinely obtain, preoperatively, standing x-rays with the knee flexed 30-45 degrees. Although this x-ray view often gives information about the extent of the degenerative disease, it does not often influence intraoperative decisions during the performance of a tri-compartmental total knee arthroplasty. However, if a uni-compartmental procedure is being contemplated, the flexion, weight-bearing view may provide the surgeon with information that would assist in the determination of the appropriateness of this procedure. A uni-compartmental arthroplasty may be less appropriate if the weight-bearing, flexion view reveals much more extensive articular cartilage damage than was suspected on the conventional standing x-ray. Some surgeons also preoperatively obtain varus-valgus stress views and/or single-leg standing views. These x-rays may give a more accurate representation of the lateral stability of the knee than conventional standing x-rays. Thus, they may be important in determining the appropriateness of a uni-compartmental arthroplasty. Moreover, such views may alert the surgeon to the need for a more constrained implant system than he or she may routinely use. However, the intraoperative assessment of stability, made after the bone cuts have been completed and trial reduction carried out, is a much more accurate determination than a radiographic estimation with stress x-rays or single leg stance films. It is for this reason, as is discussed below, that the surgeon should use one of the modern implant systems which permit that the extent of constraint be determined intraoperatively. These systems include devices of varying constraint the bone cuts for which are interchangeable.

Most revision procedures do not require x-rays in addition to those needed for primary replacements. **Serial** x-rays are the most important and helpful radiographic studies that a surgeon can use when preparing for a revision total knee replacement. A vigorous effort should be made to obtain as many prior radiographs, including the x-rays taken before the first total knee replacement, as possible. Serial radiographs can give very valuable information about the **stability** of the implants. A change in implant position over time is the most definitive evidence of loosening. Progression in the size and character of interface radiolucencies is also strong evidence of implant instability. Serial x-rays also provide very important information about the quality and extent of the **bone stock** near the total knee implants. For

example, the presence and extent of femoral osteolysis can often best be determined by examining serial routine lateral radiographs. This information is essential in planning for possible revision of a femoral component. Standing serial radiographs may be helpful in establishing the presence and extent of **polyethylene wear**. Progressive joint space narrowing is a sign of such wear. Standing serial radiographs are often the best way of establishing progressive **femoral-tibial subluxation**. This subluxation may be the result of implant malposition, progressive ligament laxity, polyethylene wear or a combination of these causes. Its presence will influence the revision procedure that is performed. Similarly, serial sky-line views of the patella may reveal progressive **patellar instability**. It may be important for the type of revision that is performed to distinguish progressive patellar instability, as observed on serial x-rays, from instability that was present immediately following, or proceeding, the primary total knee procedure. Thus, it is difficult to overemphasize the usefulness of serial radiographs. Every effort should be made to obtain these studies.

In certain situations, special radiographic procedures may be required for the performance of primary, and, particularly, revision total knee replacements. Interface radiographs, i.e., x-rays taken with the beam of the x-ray at a right angle to the interface between implant and bone, can be very helpful in assessing the extent of fixation of an uncemented implant. They can also be helpful in the evaluation of a painful, cementless prosthesis that appears to be well-aligned and fixed on routine radiographs. However, a surgeon should remember that radiographs can not be relied upon to depict accurately the state of fixation of total knee implants. Fixation is much more accurately determined intraoperatively. A surgeon should be prepared for the possibility that implants that appear well-fixed, even on interface views, may be loose. If long tibial and/or femoral stems are likely to be used, it is wise to have long lateral radiographs of the tibia and femur to be sure that the shape of these bones will accomodate stems of unusual length. Although bone scans, white blood cell scans and indium scans may be helpful in occasional **hip** replacement revisions for distinguishing septic from aseptic mechanical loosening, these studies are rarely necessary for total knee revisions, including those performed for sepsis. Computed Tomographic (CT) Scans are only needed in situations where the anatomy is so unusual that a surgeon suspects he or she may need a custom implant.

By identifying and dealing with the necessary preoperative **patient** issues, the orthopaedic surgeon can acquire all of the information that is needed to maximize the likelihood that the total knee procedure will be performed safely and successfully.

2) Exposure Issues

Most primary and many revision knee replacement procedures can be carried out through surgical exposures that do not require special preoperative planning However, in certain situations it is essential that the surgeon carry out such planning. If a patient has had previous significant knee procedures, particularly if these procedures have been associated with postoperative infections, special surgical exposures may be required and must be planned for. If a patient has a severe preoperative deformity, e.g., flexion contracture, special measures for handling the skin and soft tissues about the knee may be necessary. If a patient has extraordinarily obese legs or an unusual distribution of fat about the knee, the exposure may require special instruments, leg holders or tourniquets. Unusual exposures or skin conditions may require the assistance of a plastic surgeon, e.g., for the insertion and management of a tissue expander or transfer of a muscle flap. Such assistance must be anticipated and arranged for prior to surgery. The success or failure of a knee replacement procedure can be determined at the time of exposure. It is essential that patients requiring special exposure considerations be identified preoperatively.

3) Equipment Issues

When surgeons think about the need for preoperative planning for a total knee procedure, they are often apt to equate that planning with the need to be sure that the correct implants and instruments are available. Although this is a critical part of the preoperative planning process, it should be, for the vast majority of primary knee replacements and most revision replacements, relatively easy to carry out successfully. However, in order to assure that this part of the planning process is consistently successful, it is important that the surgeon use an appropriate total knee replacement system. Most modern knee replacement systems provide the surgeon with a large number of options for treating conditions that are encountered during surgery. For example, most systems have a wide range of implant sizes. Thus, a surgeon should not have to routinely template x-rays preoperatively to determine the size of implant that he or she is likely to use. Moreover, the intraoperative methods commonly used to determine correct implant size are much more accurate than templating on routinely obtained preoperative x-rays. In addition, many implant systems currently allow the surgeon to select the extent of constraint desireable during the performance of the procedure. Some systems also allow the surgeon to attach intramedullary rods of varying length and diameter and augmentation blocks of various sizes to the femoral and tibial components used in the performance of a primary replacement. The instrumentation of these systems makes the use of these rods and augmentation blocks a natural extension of the primary knee replacement technique.

Although the large majority of primary total knee replacements can be successfully performed with a standard, well-designed nonmodular cruciate retaining or sacrificing implant system, a small proportion of primary cases (perhaps 5 %) will require more than the usual constraint, longer than usual intramedullary rods or augmentation blocks. Frequently, these cases can not be anticipated prior to surgery, even when careful, complete preoperative planning has been performed, e.g., severe osteopenia requiring prophylactic intramedullary rods. Some of these cases result from conditions that are produced in the operating room, e.g., femoral condylar fracture or collateral ligament laceration. Moreover, when these conditions are encountered in the operating room-successful treatment is often relatively easy if modular implant systems are available and extremely difficult if they are not. In summary, modular total knee systems may be expensive for a hospital or implant distributor to provide. However, any orthopaedic surgeon who does more than an occasional, uncomplicated total knee procedure should work with his or her hospital administration to assure that an adequate implant system is available for all total knee replacement procedures. The cost of having such systems routinely available within the hospital may be less than the cost of bringing such systems in on a loaner basis. The surgeon should encourage the hospital and implant distributor to examine this issue carefully.

It is particularly important that an orthopaedic surgeon have appropriate implants, instruments and grafting materials available for a **revision** total knee replacement procedure. A number of modular knee implant systems offer the range of implant sizes, intramedullary rod lengths and sizes and augmentation shapes to make possible the performance of the large proportion of revision procedures. Thus, the surgeon planning the performance of a revision replacement should become familiar with the options that various modular systems offer and be sure that these options are adequate for the procedure being contemplated.

In particular, it is important that the surgeon have available an implant system that provides adequate **constraint**. It is not uncommon to find during the performance of a revision procedure that the usual methods for obtaining adequate soft tissue balance are insufficient for providing acceptable stability.

In such situations, very constrained, non-linked devices, e.g., a CCK type of implant, or even linked devices may be necessary.

Some revisions require the replacement of a single component, e.g., the tibia, or part of a component, e.g., the modular tibial insert. If the surgeon anticipates that only a portion of an implant system will require replacement, he or she must be sure to establish, preoperatively, the 1) manufacturer, 2) model, and 3) size of the prothesis. Because specific implant systems may be modified over the years, e.g., the polyethylene capture mechanism may be changed, it is important that the surgeon know in what year the prosthesis was inserted. It is also possible that special instrumentation is required to insert these components. This must be determined preoperatively. In order to obtain this information it may be necessary to have available a copy of the patient's previous operative reports and portions of the hospital record from that previous procedure.

The performance of a complex primary or revision knee replacement procedure may require special instruments. For example, if a knee replacement procedure is to be performed on an extremity that already has a total hip replacement, extramedullary femoral alignment guides may be required. If prostheses and cement must be removed, special tools for accomplishing this will be necessary. Osteotomes, gigli saws, power-driven burrs, or metal cutters, and implant extraction devices may all be required. Implants with long, cemented intramedullary stems are particularly difficult to remove safely. Careful preoperative preparation is essential if such devices require removal.

4) Reimbursement Issues

Identifying the agency responsible for payment of a total knee procedure, identifying the services covered by that agency and obtaining permission to carry out the procedure can be a time consuming and frustrating activity for the surgeon and his staff. Private insurance companies and government agencies vary widely with regard to the type and extent of financial support they provide for total knee replacement care. The type of preoperative evaluation permitted, the type of procedure covered, the extent of hospitalization allowed and the amount and location of postoperative care covered varies substantially among insurers. Unusual preoperative tests, e.g., cardiac stress tests or CT scans, may not be routinely covered. The use of unusual implants or equipment may require special preoperative authorization from an insurance carrier. Insurers may not pay for the evaluation of new devices, anesthetics or thromboembolic agents. Permission for an in-patient stay beyond a specified number of days may require that special arrangements are made preoperatively. The extent and type of postoperative care permitted by government or private insurers is particularly variable.

Surgeons who perform total knee replacement surgery must anticipate that a significant effort will be required by their staffs to arrange for insurance coverage. The safety and quality of the procedure requires that these arrangements be carried out successfully. Adequate time and support must be given for these arrangements to be made.

B) Preparation by the Hospital

It is also in the hospital's interest to be sure that the proposed total knee procedure is accomplished safely, successfully and cost-efficiently. Surgeons who perform total knee surgery should work with their hospitals to put in place preoperative programs that assure such an outcome. For example, the hospital can assist in the preoperative evaluation of a total knee patient by assuring that the preoperative tests are performed efficiently and accurately. Moreover, it is the hospital's responsibility to be sure that the results of tests that are performed are completely and accurately available to the surgeon and internist in a timely fashion. It is essential to the safe and successful performance of a total knee replacement that appropriate anesthesia be given. The hospital should provide an area where an anesthesiologist can carefully evaluate a patient's anesthetic needs and desires. Patients are very concerned about the anesthetic that they will receive. Total knee patients, in particular, may be appropriate candidates for regional anesthesia. It is important that an anesthesiologist have an opportunity to explain the risks and benefits of the various anesthetic options. Moreover, patients are very concerned about the way in which pain will be treated postoperatively. An anesthesiologist is a good and often very reassuring source of information about this very important subject.

A hospital, like a surgeon, wishes to attract and satisfy patients. The way in which a total knee patient is treated by the hospital in the preoperative period can greatly affect the attitude the patient has about his or her upcoming surgery. One of the most effective methods for preparing a patient for such surgery is to provide detailed information about the upcoming surgery. This information can be provided in written material, in a video or in a preoperative visit to the hospital. A particularly helpful method for providing information to a patient and his family is by means of a preoperative teaching class. Participants in this class can include nurses from the surgical floor, physical therapists, occupational therapists, insurance and home health advisors and representatives from the operating room. These classes allow the hospital personnel to learn of a patient's particular needs and wants. Such classes are particularly helpful in educating a patient's family about its role in the upcoming surgery.

Hospitals, like surgeons, are under increasing pressure to reduce the costs of total knee replacement surgery. This pressure will result in continually shorter lengths of hospital stay and reduced in-hospital services (such as physical therapy). Patients and their families will be unhappy and frustrated by these decreased services and will be concerned about the effect of these reductions on the quality of their care. Patients and their families are most likely to understand and cooperate with these decreases in lengths of stay and services if they feel that the hospital and physician understand and are responsive to their concerns. Providing patients with information about their upcoming surgery helps demonstrate that concern. Preoperative classes provided by the hospital allow this concern to be expressed in

a direct and personalized way. Such classes also allow patients and their families to meet the individuals, including nurses, therapists, discharge planners and insurance coordinators, with whom they will be interacting during their hospital stay. This familiarity with the staff will help put patients and their families more at ease about their upcoming surgery. Equally importantly, the hospital staff will be able to emphsize to the members of a patient's family the importance of their participation in a total knee replacement patient's care. Succesfully enlisting family support is one of the most effective ways of making cost reduction measures, such as shortened lengths of stay, acceptable to patients.

C) Preparation by the Patient and Family

A total knee replacement will be successful only if the patient and his or her family do their part. A patient and his or her family must prepare for the surgery and take an active role in the recovery. This is most likely to occur if the surgeon properly educates the patient and family preoperatively. The prospective total knee replacement patient should be familiar with and carry out preoperatively the exercises that will be required following surgery. The patient and family should be aware of the importance of preventing infection and have eliminated any possible causes of infection, e.g., dental, urinary tract, biliary tract. The patient and family should have a clear concept of what the posthospital experience will be like so that appropriate home arrangements and family schedules can be organized. Patients who are employed must make appropriate arrangements for returning to work. As government and private insurers reduce financial support for the postoperative care of total knee replacement patients, the burden for providing this care will fall increasingly on the patient, his or her family and friends. The surgeon must make the patient aware of the importance of this care and assist in preparing for it.

Careful preoperative planning, guided by the surgeon and carried out by the patient, his or her family, the hospital and the surgeon, is essential for assuring that the surgeon will perform the procedure correctly and the patient will participate appropriately in his or her recovery.

Chapter 4
Surgical Approaches

Ermanno A. Martucci
Rizzoli Orthopaedic Institute - Bologna

Modern reconstructive surgery of the knee is the consequence of about 25 years of experience. The continuous progress made in the different fields of surgery, the design of prosthetic components, and the technology of biomaterials have, in fact, led to excellent clinical and radiographic medium-term results. Like for any surgical procedure, exposure of the anatomical structures in knee replacement surgery must be sufficiently wide, taking into consideration the fact that the periarticular tissues must be "treated" with great accuracy. In fact, the knee is relatively superficial as compared to the hip, which is the other joint most commonly submitted to reconstructive surgery; consequently, the tissues surrounding it are characterized by minor extension, Thus, when this type of surgery is approached, the risk of skin complications, particularly necrosis, must not be overlooked, as they may influence the very survival of the prosthetic implant itself. The incision must be sufficiently long, and at any rate easily extendable in a proximal and distal direction, to allow for the adequate visualization of the anatomical structures involved, but also to avoid excessive tension on the soft tissues. Particular care must be taken when there are previous skin incisions. Transverse ones made, for example, in meniscectomy or tibial osteotomy, are safely transected at a right angle. Vertical ones must possibly be incorporated in the new incision; if the contrary should occur, the latter must be sufficiently distant (at least 7 cm) from the previous one. When multiple longitudinal parallel incisions are present, the lateral one is to be preferred. In patients with multiple scars and adherent skin a "sham" incision is a good option; if after 3 weeks normal healing occurs, the definitive knee arthroplasty procedure may be performed. Furthermore, when planning the skin incision, the surgeon must not overlook the fact that a new operation may be required in the future.

The incision used most frequently is vertical and median (9). Few surgeons prefer the medial parapatellar one, while the lateral parapatellar one is only used for valgus knee (10) (Fig. 1). Transcutaneous measurements of the tension of the oxygen taken before and after making different incisions on the skin of the knee have shown reduced values of the lateral skin margin. Thus, by moving the incision medially, the size of the lateral flap increases, and its oxygenation is further compromised. Furthermore, it is important not to overlook the fact that the lymphatic drainage in the knee has a mediolateral direction.

"Standard" Approach

The skin incision begins about 7 cm proximal to the patella and ends medial to the tibial tubercle. Dissection is made deeper through the subcutaneous tissue until the thin pre-patellar fascia is revealed. After it is incised, proceeding in a craniocaudal direction, the adipose tissue appears, covering the quadriceps tendon and the medial capsule. Thus, a medial plane develops posterior to the prepatellar fascia, revealing the extensor apparatus and the retinaculum. It may be useful to apply two stitches at the medial margin of the fascia to be used as retractors on the medial flap, to keep the improper use of metal instruments from separating the subcutaneous tissue of the fascia, thus injuring the perforating arterioles on which the plexus localized in the derma depends, which is responsible for hematic irroration of the skin.

Standard arthrotomy is parapatellar and slightly curved: the incision initiates proximally within

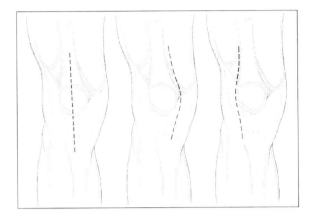

FIG. 1 - The median incision is generally used in knee arthroplasty, the parapatellar, medial or lateral, more rarely.

the context of the quadriceps tendon, 1 cm from the vastus medialis; it is prolonged distally along the internal margin of the patella, leaving at least 5 mm of retinaculum and capsule to allow for excellent reconstruction, and of the patellar tendon, about 1 cm away, ending in the site corresponding to the tibial tubercle (8) (Fig. 2A).

Insall (8) instead proposed a medial rectilinear arthrotomy: the incision initiates at the apex of the quadriceps tendon, to continue distally along the medial third of the patella and the medial margin of the patellar tendon. The expansion of the quadriceps is detached from the anterior aspect of the patella until it reaches the medial border, so that

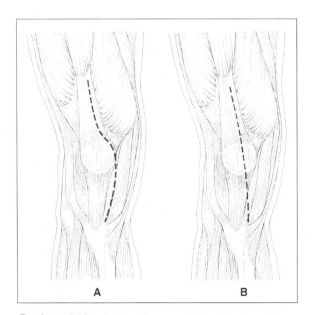

FIG. 2 - (A-B) Standard median parapatellar arthrotomy (A), according to Insall (B).

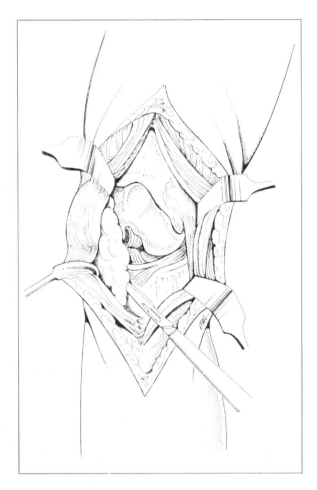

FIG. 3 - The fat pad is detached from the capsule and the ligamentum patellae is sectioned.

the synovial membrane may thus be incised (Fig. 2B). The medial tibial plateau is exposed subperiosteally. Once the knife has been inserted at the level of the bursa localized posterior to the Hoffa body, the latter is detached from the anterolateral capsule, and the ligamentum patellae is sectioned to facilitate dislocation of the patella (Fig. 3). The knee is thus flexed, carefully and gradually extrarotating the tibia to avoid sudden tension on the patellar tendon. A retractor is applied, and the patella is dislocated laterally, the femoropatellar ligament is incised, and the menisci are excised, thus obtaining adequate exposure of the tibial joint surface.

"Midvastus" and "Trivector" Approaches

These approaches were proposed with the purpose of obtaining greater stability of the femoropatellar joint, and more rapid functional recovery of the extensor mechanism. A median skin incision is used for both.

In "midvastus" approach (4) (Fig. 4), after sectioning the prepatellar fascia, dissection is continued medially in order to adequately expose the vastus medialis and the retinaculum. In the area corresponding to the proximal pole of the patella, with the knee flexed or extended, the fibers of the vastus medialis are dissociated, following their direction for a length of about 5 cm; furthermore, the aponeurosis that covers the deep side is incised.

Subsequently, a medial arthrotomy is carried out, and disinsertion of the vastus internus from the patellar margin is associated. Suturing is carried out keeping the knee in flexion to restore correct tension to the extensor apparatus.

"Trivector" approach is thus defined because the trivectorial structure of the quadriceps mechanism is saved (1). Keeping the knee at 90° of flexion, after carrying out parapatellar arthrotomy about 1 cm from the medial margin of the patella, the incision is prolonged in a proximal direction through the fibers of the vastus medialis, following

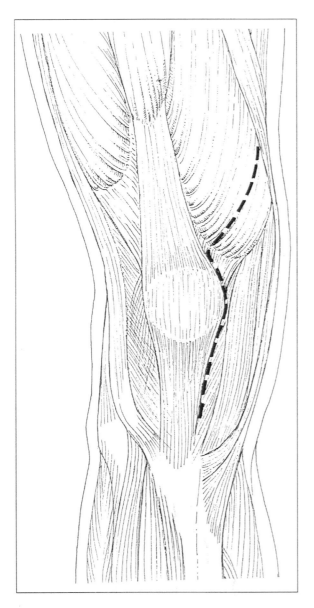

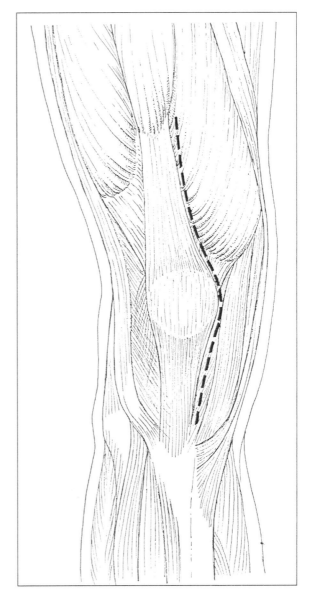

FIG. 4 - Midvastus approach requires dissociation of the fibers of the vastus medialis for a length of 4-5 cm, and incision of the deep muscular aponeurosis.

FIG. 5 - In Trivector approach, the vastus medialis is sectioned parallel to the margin of the quadriceps tendon, that thus remains whole.

a vertical line about 6 cm long starting from the proximal pole of the patella, 1 cm away from the quadriceps tendon (Fig. 5).

It is evident how in both "midvastus" and "trivector" approaches the extensor apparatus is left intact, with consequent positive repercussions on patellar tracking. Furthermore, the former may be said to have supplementary advantages, such as less bleeding and reduced scar tissue formation, dissection being carried out between and not through the fibers of the vastus medialis. Contraindications to their use are: flexion less than

80°, obesity of the patient, previous tibial osteotomy, considerably hypertrophic arthritis.

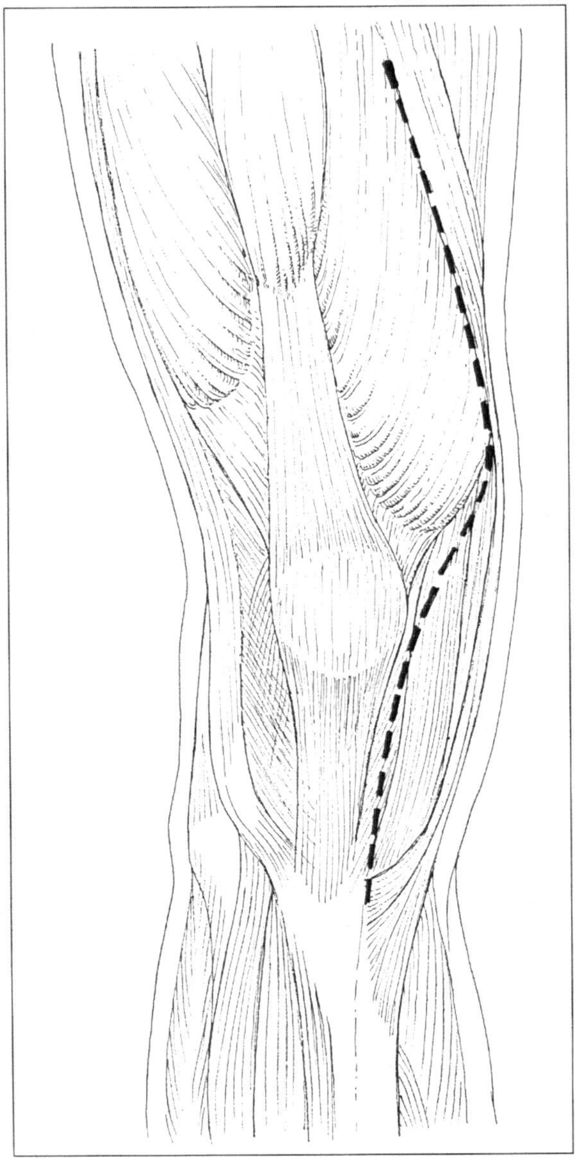

"Subvastus" (Southern) Approach

Described for the first time in 1929 (5), it has recently been resorted to for primary reconstructive surgery of the knee (7). It differs from the standard anteromedial approach because it does not pass through the quadriceps tendon, but rather dorsal to the inferior margin of the vastus medialis (Fig. 6). Thus, the extensor apparatus and hematic irroration of the patella remain unviolated. Other advantages are: more anatomical patellar tracking, postoperative pain is less intense, reduced incidence of skin complications, more rapid recovery of extensor capacity. Absolute contraindications, instead, are the obesity of the patient, and previous tibial osteotomy or arthrotomy; in conditions such as these, dislocation of the patella is

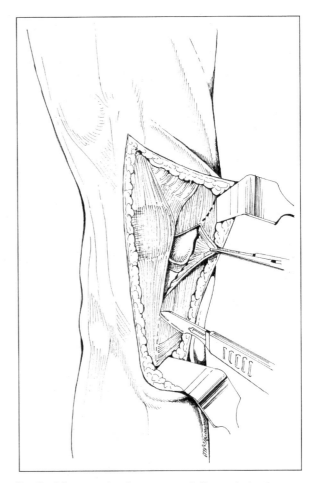

FIG. 6 - The subvastus approach saves the vastus medialis that is detached from the intermuscular septum.

FIG. 7 - After retracting the vastus medialis anteriorly, the capsule is incised in an inverted L.

considerably difficult. The skin incision is anterior and median, with the knee flexed at 90°: it begins 8 cm transverse to the patella and ends 1 cm distal to the tibial tubercle, slightly medialized in relation to the latter. The fascia is opened following the same line as the skin incision, to then detach it in a craniocaudal direction from the thin perimuscular fascia of the vastus internus. After the posterior margin of this muscle has been determined, it is bluntly detached from the intermuscular septum and from the periosteum for a distance of about 10 cm proximal to the tubercle of the adductors. The muscle belly is retracted anteriorly, and its tendinous insertion is identified and sectioned transversally on the medial capsule. After completing arthrotomy in a routine manner, the patella is dislocated.

Complications may include the formation of a hematoma below the vastus medialis, related to dissection of the intermuscular septum, and the occurrence of ischemia of the vastus medialis when the extensor apparatus is dislocated laterally.

Lateral Approach

It has been proposed for reconstructive surgery of valgus knee, assuming that medial peripatellar arthrotomy may involve a few drawbacks, particularly in the extensor apparatus (12). Thus, lateral approach would be favored, essentially because it is directly involved by the periarticular components of the most injured compartment. Moreover, as release of the lateral retinaculum is one of the procedures routinely carried out, by performing lateral arthrotomy "ab initio," hematic irroration of the patella is only partially compromised, the medial vascular supply being saved (11). A slightly curved median skin incision is made, or a lateral one, following the Q angle. Medial dissection is absolutely to be avoided. To carry out lateral arthrotomy, the incision initiates proximal to the lateral margin of the quadriceps tendon, it proceeds distally along the medial border of Gerdy's tubercle, to end 2 cm lateral and 3 distal to the tibial tubercle, within the context of the fascia covering the anterior muscle group (Fig. 8). Forcing the knee extended in varus, the amount of retraction of the iliotibial band must be evaluated, with the purpose of immediately releasing it. The fat pad and the capsule are mobilized: during suturing, they are often required to fill the gap of the lateral retinaculum that remains after correction of the deformity. The tibial tubercle is osteotomized and

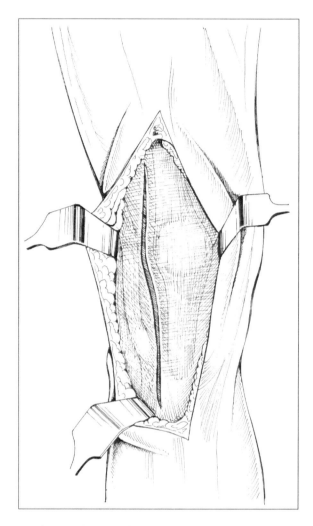

Fig. 8 - Lateral parapatellar arthrotomy in the valgus knee.

the patella is everted, dislocating the extensor apparatus medially. Ensuing tibial intrarotation allows for the easy exploration of the posterolateral structures. To expose the medial compartment, the tibia must be brought back to neutral rotation.

Exposure of the "Difficult Knee"

When the knee is stiff or there is marked contraction in flexion, alternative surgical methods may be required to be able to dislocate the extensor apparatus and thus obtain excellent exposure of the joint. Some authors (6, 9, 13) suggest intervening on the proximal portion of the extensor apparatus, others (13, 14, 15, 16) instead on the distal portion by osteotomy of the tibial tubercle. Consequently, these methods may be used to mobilize the patella laterally and, depending on the cases, caudally and cranially.

Turndown Procedures

The original technique described by Coonse and Adams (2) includes "upside-down Y" incision with the apex at the proximal end of the quadriceps tendon and the distal base (Fig. 9). It was then modified by Insall so as to be used at any given moment during arthroplasty simply as a variation in standard medial parapatellar arthrotomy (9, 13). When the surgeon is not capable of adequately dislocating the patella and visualizing the joint, a second incision may be made on the quadriceps tendon that begins from the proximal apex of the former with an angle of about 45°, and is prolonged distally as far as the context of the vastus lateralis, attempting to save the lateral superior genicular artery (Fig. 10). The patella with the quadriceps tendon is then reflected distally and laterally allowing access to the knee joint. Closure is done with the knee at 30°.

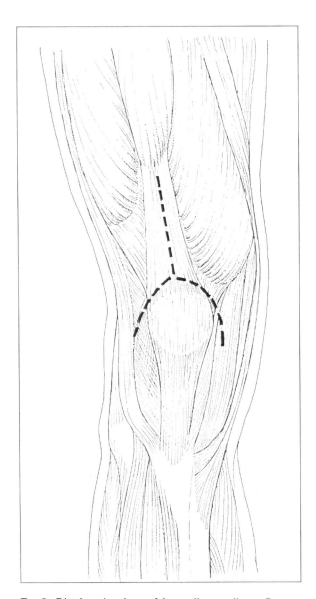

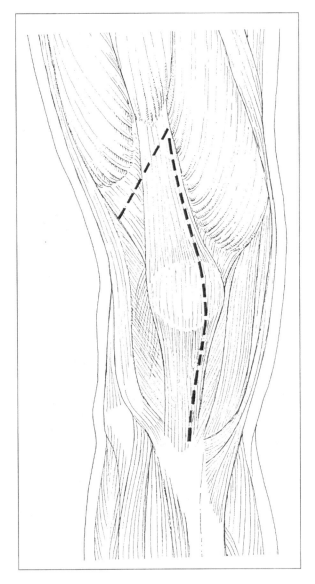

FIG. 9 - Distal turning-down of the patella according to Coonse-Adams.

FIG. 10 - Distal turning-down of the extensor apparatus according to Insall.

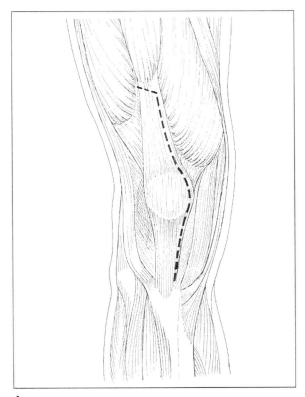

A

B

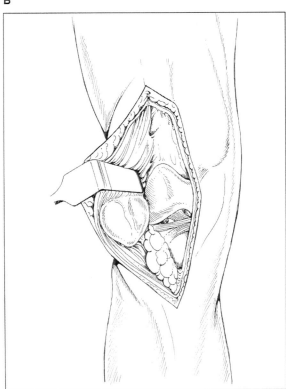

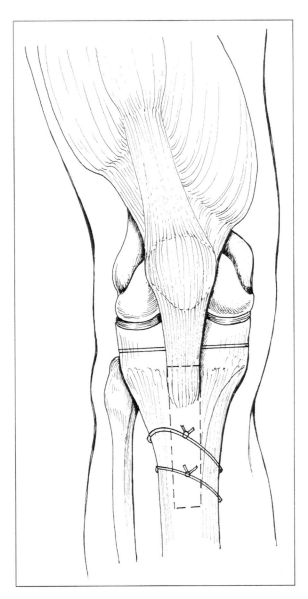

Fig. 12 - Osteotomy of the tibial tubercle allows for wide exposure of the joint by proximal turning down of the extensor apparatus. After implanting the prosthesis the tibial tubercle is stabilized, preferably with 2-3 metal wires.

Fig. 11 (A-B) - The rectus snip allows for lateral mobilization of the extensor apparatus.

The main drawbacks to using this method are fibrosis of the quadriceps mechanism and possible ischemia of the patella.

The Quadriceps Snip

This constitutes a subsequent modification of the method previously described, aimed at reducing the occurrence of fibrotic phenomena in the extensor apparatus (6).

After performing medial arthrotomy and longitudinal incision of the quadriceps tendon, this may be prolonged in a cranial and lateral direction at 45° with the fibers of vastus lateralis, so that the tendon of the rectus femoris is sectioned (Fig. 11). When necessary, at a subsequent stage, release of the lateral retinaculum may also be carried out. Closure is performed with a side-to-side anastomosis throughout the length of the capsular incision.

Osteotomy of the Tibial Tubercle

It is used in place of the previous techniques to avoid the risk of possible insufficiency of the extensor apparatus (13, 14, 15, 16). It is of essential importance that with osteotomy a segment of the anterior tibial crest be obtained that is sufficiently long (8 cm) and thick (1 cm at least in the more proximal portion). Lateral muscle insertion must be respected to be able to have an osteomuscular flap that is well-vascularized. After performing osteotomy with an oscillating saw, the bone segment is mobilized externally together with the entire extensor apparatus.

At the end of the implant procedure, it is brought back to its site and stabilized using 2 or 3 metal wires angulated caudally at 45° (Fig. 12). In case of patella baja the tibial tubercle is reinserted as proximally as possible.

This method is contraindicated when severe osteopenia is present.

References

1) Bramlett K. W.: Trivector Retaining Arthrotomy For Total Knee Arthroplasty- Orthop. Trans., 17, 1174, 1993
2) Coonse K, Adams J. D.: A New Operative Approach To The Knee Joint-Surg. Gynecol. Obstet., 77, 344. 1943
3) Dolin M. G.: Osteotomy Of The Tibial Tubercle In Total Knee Replacementj.Bone Joint Surg., 65-A, 704,1983
4) Engh G. A., Holt B.T., Parks N-L.: A Midvastus Muscle-Splitting Approach For Total Knee Arthroplasty-J. Arthr., 12,3, 322, 1997
5) Erkes F.: Weitere Erfahrungen Mit Phisiologischer Schnittfuhrung Zur Eroffnung Des Kniegelenks-Bruns Beitr Zur Klin Chir, 147, 221, 1929
6) Garvin K. L., Scuderi G., Insall J. N.: Evolution Of The Quadriceps Snip-Clin. Orthop., 321, 131, 1995
7) Hoffmann A. A., Plaster R. L., Murdock L. E.: Subvastus (Southern) Approach For Primary Total Knee Arthroplasty-Clin. Orthop., 269, 70, 1991
8) Insall J. N.: A Midline Approach To The Knee-J. Bone Joint Surg., 53-A, 1584, 1971
9) Insall J. N.: Surgical Approaches-In: Surgery Of The Knee-Churchill- Livingstone, New York, 1993, Pag. 137-
10) Johnson D. P.: Midline Or Parapatellar Incision For Knee Arthroplasty- J. Bone Joint Surg. ,70-B,656,1988
11) Kayler D. E., Lyttle D.: Surgical Interruption Of Patellar Blood Supply By Total Knee Arthroplasty-Clin. Orthop., 229, 221 1988
12) Keblish P. A.: The Lateral Approach To The Valgus Knee-Surgical Technique And Analysis Of 53 Cases With Over Two-Year Follow-Up Evaluation-Clin. Orthop., 271, 52, 1991
13) Scott R. D., Siliski J. M.: The Use Of A Modified V-Y Quadricepsplasty During Total Knee Replacement To Gain Exposure And Improve Flexion In The Ankylosed Knee-Orthopaedics, 8, 1, 45 1985
14) Whiteside L. A., Ohl M. D.: Tibial Tubercle Osteotomy For Exposure Of The Difficult Total Knee Arthroplasty-Clin. Orthop., 260, 6, 1990
15) Whiteside L. A.: Exposure In Difficult Total Knee Arthroplasty Using Tibial Tubercle Osteotomy-Clin. Orthop., 321, 32, 1995
16) Wolff A. M., Hungerford D. S., Krackow K. A., Jacobs M. A.: Osteotomy Of Tibial Tubercle During Total Knee Replacement- A Report Of Twenty-Six Cases-J. Bone Joint Surg., 71-A, 848, 1989

Chapter 5
Soft-Tissue Balancing

Ermanno A. Martucci

Rizzoli Orthopaedic Institute - Bologna

The knee is the joint most affected by arthritis, which causes degenerative changes not only in the osteocartilaginous tissue but also in the surrounding capsuloligamentous structures. In fact, these undergo compromise of the collagen fibers with a reduction in glycosaminoglycans and water content (2). If we use the femorotibial angle delimited by the anatomical axis as a reference parameter, the knee is defined varus when this angle is ≥ 0° with the apex directed laterally, valgus when the angle is ≥ 10° with a medial apex, neutral if the angle is included between 1° and 9° with the apex turned in a medial direction (13). Deformity of the knee is generally the result of abnormal skeletal structure and capsuloligamentous imbalance. Corresponding to the knee, the periarticular tissues constitute a sort of envelope, whose circumference is partially interrupted by the presence of the patella. The occurrence of osteocartilaginous pathology results in contracture, that is, anatomofunctional adaptation, of some of the capsuloligamentous formations that make up this envelope. Depending on the localization of the osteocartilaginous defect, which is generally asymmetrical, contracture may involve the medial, lateral and/or posterior compartment of the knee, thus producing a deformity in varus, valgus, and flexion, respectively. In gonarthrosis, the osteocartilaginous defect is usually medial (Fig. 1). To redistribute the mechanical stress on a wider surface, osteophytic formations develop to a greater or lesser extent. This triggers shortening of the medial collateral ligament and, because of the high compressive forces on the medial compartment, lengthening of the lateral collateral ligament may also take place. In this manner, contracture in varus originates, representing the most common deformity. With very minor frequency, and more often in rheumatoid arthritis, the lateral compartment becomes involved. The consequent deformity in valgus is also characterized by extrarotation of the tibial axis due to involvement of the iliotibial band. Contracture in flexion, finally, represents one of the most severe and complex deformities; it may be presented in an isolated form or, more often, associated with one of the anatomopathologic conditions previously described. The ligamentous imbalance that characterizes each deformity is substantially corrected by means of the "release" of the retracted structures, that is, those corresponding to the concave side. Subsequent to surgery, they are reinserted on the skeletal surface at a different level, conditioned by the new femorotibial angle and the spacing effect of the prosthetic components. Correction of the joint deformity is obtained by using the method constituted by the "tensioning" of the ligamentous structures (7), and by carrying out bone resections of a thickness equal to that of the prosthetic components to be implanted. At the end of surgery, the ligamentous formations must have a correct tension in complete extension and at 90° of flexion, the femorotibial angle must be 5°-7°, and the patella must track centrally. Joint excursion should reach 140° of flexion, initiating from the condition of extension; nonetheless, it is significantly influenced by preoperative mobility.

Anatomy

The structures of the medial compartment are distributed in three superimposed planes (19)

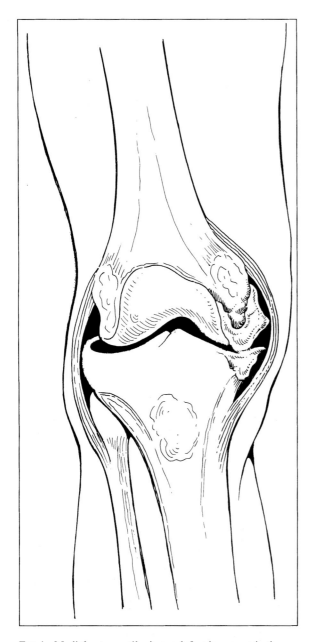

FIG. 1 - Medial osteocartilaginous defect is present in the varus knee. The osteophytes tighten the medial collateral ligament, that gradually tends to shorten. Their excision is essential to obtain excellent ligament balancing.

(Fig. 2). The most superficial one corresponds to the crural fascia, that covers the sartorius muscle and the two ends of the gastrocnemius, joining anteriorly and distally with the periosteum of the tibia; the intermediate one is represented by the superficial collateral ligament. Between these two layers are the tendons of the semitendinosus and the gracilis. The deeper one is constituted by the joint capsule and the deep collateral ligament. The insertions of the semimembranosus muscle are joined with the deep and intermediate layer. Three different planes may also be distinguished in the lateral compartment (16) (Fig. 3). The superficial one includes the iliotibial band and the femoral biceps, the intermediate one the retinaculum of the quadriceps and the collateral, meniscus patellar, and femoral patellar ligaments. Finally, the deep one corresponds to the capsule and to the arcuate and fabelloperoneal ligaments. The posterior compartment contains the posterior cruciate ligament, the capsule, and the flexor muscles of the foot.

Varus Knee

Varus knee is the condition that most frequently requires arthroplasty (8, 10, 14, 18). It is the result of anomalous forces that produce medial femorotibial compression, thus causing collapse of the tibial plateau and, at times, subsequently of the condyle of femur. Bone defect is generally associated with retraction of the medial, deep and superficial collateral ligaments, of the posteromedial capsule, of the tendons of the pes anserinus and of the semimembranosus muscle. The cruciate ligaments, instead, because of their central position, tend to keep their normal length. Later on, there may be lengthening of the external collateral ligament, and in more severe cases this may be associated with lateral translation of the tibia. Release of the retracted soft medial parts is done preliminarily, also to allow for adequate exposure of the joint surfaces. After removing the medial and lateral menisci, as well as the tibial meniscal ligament, keeping the tibia in external rotation, the deep medial collateral ligament is disinserted by subperiosteal approach, and proceeding in a posterior direction, the tendons of the semimembranosus and of the capsule are also disinserted. This allows for easy anterior subluxation of the tibia and consequent visualization of the entire joint surface (Figs. 4-5). In more severe deformities, it may be necessary to detach the periosteum distally, thus disinserting the tendons of the pes anserinus, and at times also posteriorly, consequently including the fascia of the soleus and of the popliteus. Instead, disinsertion at the tibial level of the superficial medial collateral ligament and of the medial end of the gastrocnemius is quite infrequent. After completing exposure of the joint,

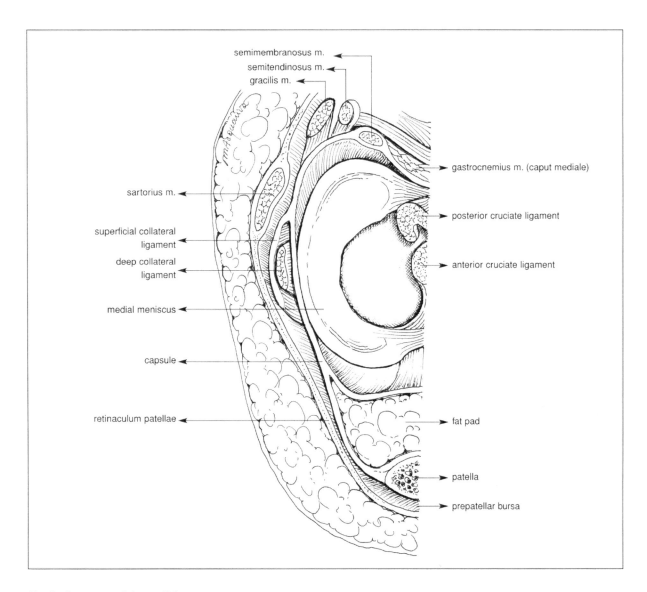

FIG. 2 - Structures of the medial compartment.

it is important to remove all of the osteophytes including the posterior tibial ones, and this will be followed by bone resections. In the knee that is more than 20° varus, preservation of the posterior cruciate ligament may constitute a severe obstacle for the restoration of correct alignment of the limb, also because it is believed that it is involved in the degenerative process that has affected the joint (3). In cases such as these, it may be useful to excise it, and to thus use a prosthetic system with posterior stability. It is recommended that bone resections be carried out using the uninjured or less compromised joint surface as a reference, that is, the lateral one correspon-

ding to the femur and, above all, to the tibia. In this manner, the joint level remains substantially unchanged, and, furthermore, balancing of the ligamentous structures is simplified, as they will have to be of the same length in the medial and lateral compartments. The final proof of alignment and joint stability, in extension and at 90° of flexion, must be obtained after applying the trial prosthetic components. The joint must adequately resist stress in valgus; however, a medial opening of the rima up to 2-4 mm is acceptable. Release of the retracted structures is thus completed during this phase, so that the flexion and extension gaps are perfectly equal and rec-

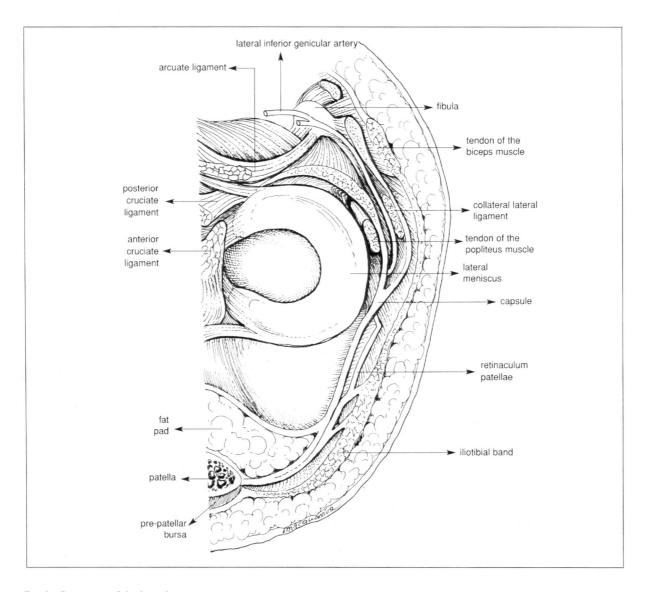

FIG. 3 - Structures of the lateral compartment.

tangular. When contracture in flexion is present, the posterior capsule must be detached from the femoral condyles, removing any posterior osteophytes (Fig. 6); in some cases, it is necessary to re-cut the distal femur to broaden the extension space. Surgeons who use prosthetic systems that include preservation of the posterior cruciate ligament must very carefully evaluate its tension after positioning the trial prosthesis. If it seems to be too tight (the tibial prosthetic component tends to lift anteriorly; there is excessive femoral roll-back), it will have to be released at the tibial and/or femoral insertion (15) (Fig. 7). Lengthening may compromise integrity of the

ligament: in this case, it is best to remove it, and implant a posterior-stabilized prosthesis.

Recently an alternative surgical technique was proposed for severe deformity in varus-flexion (5), that consists in performing osteotomy of the medial epicondyle, after exposing the joint surfaces through the usual anterior access.

Maintaining the knee at 90° of flexion, the medial epicondyle is osteotomized, obtaining a bone fragment that is at least 1 cm thick with the osteotome positioned parallel to the femoral diaphysis. After mobilizing the epicondyle in a distal direction, access to the posterior capsule of the knee is easily gained, disinserting it to

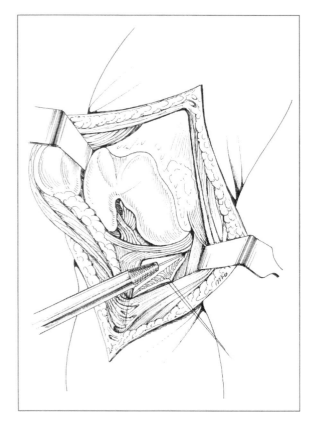 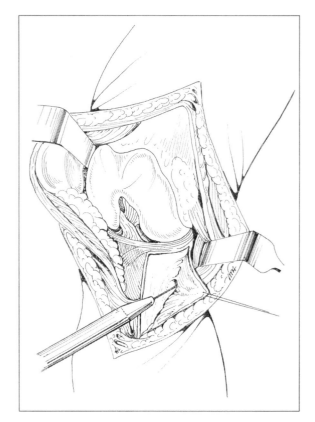

FIG. 4 - FIG. 5 - Exposure of the proximal tibia requires disinsertion of the retinaculum and of the capsule, at times also of the semimembranosus. In more severe forms of varus knee, release of the pes anserinus and at times also of the superficial medial collateral ligament is indispensable.

correct contracture in flexion; at the end of the implant, it is reinserted by non-resorbable transskeletal suturing. This method would have the advantage of avoiding release of the capsuloligamentous formation, that is generally rather wide in severe deformities.

Valgus Knee

Valgus deformity of the knee generally accompanies hypoplasia of the lateral femoral condyle, that is articulated with the posterior portion of the corresponding tibial plateau. In fact, we frequently intraoperatively observe loss of bone substance in the area corresponding to the posterior distal surface of the femoral condyle and of the posterolateral joint surface of the tibia. Bone defect means progressive retraction of the external collateral ligament, which is at a maximum in the position of complete extension, and less marked in

flexion, of the iliotibial band, influencing external rotation of the tibia, of the lateral and posterior capsule, of the popliteus, and at times also of the femoral biceps and of the lateral end of the gastrocnemius. Lengthening of variable extent of the medial collateral ligament is associated further on (1, 4, 9, 11, 12, 17). This complex deformity is prevalently observed in patients affected with rheumatoid arthritis. The basic principles that guide surgical strategy are similar to those used in the case of varus knee, nonetheless, the presence of the external popliteal sciatic nerve requires greater care. Release of the retracted lateral soft tissues is carried out proximally, at the femoral insertion, but it must be monitored at every step as over-release may cause joint instability, particularly in flexion, as well as neurapraxia. After performing internal arthrotomy, the capsule is disinserted medially, avoiding, however, going beyond the median line of the tibial plateau, to avoid injuring the stabilizing medial struc-

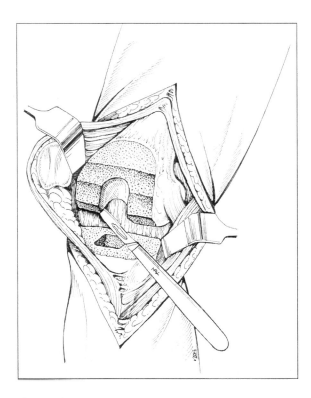

FIG. 6 - If deformity in flexion persists, the capsule will have to be detached from the posterior femoral condyles.

tures. After anteriorly retracting the patellar tendon, the anterior aspect of the lateral tibial plateau is exposed, the patella is thus dislocated and the knee is flexed, resulting in external rotation. The fat pad is at least partially ex-

cised, the femoral patellar ligament is sectioned to reduce tension on the extensor apparatus, and the anterior capsule and iliotibial band are disinserted in the area corresponding to Gerdy's tubercle. To make sure that there are no residual fibers on the latter, the knee is extended, it is stressed in varus, and at the same time, the iliotibial band is palpated deep at the lateral retinaculum. Different methods are described, such as transverse section of the band, at the level of the joint rima or proximal to the patella, or its lengthening by multiple transverse punctures (Fig. 8). In deformities that measure less than 15°, release of the band is generally sufficient to obtain complete correction of the malalignment. It is useful to complete detachment of the joint capsule by proceeding from Gerdy's tubercle as far as the insertion site of the posterior cruciate ligament on the posterior surface of the tibia. Subsequently, bone resection is performed. Postoperative alignment of the prosthetized knee must have a valgus measuring 2°-7°. Nonetheless, while for varus knee an angle measuring 5°-7° is advised, in the valgus knee a smaller angle must be searched for, from 2° to 5°, to contrast the tendency of the deformity to recur, clearly acknowledging that tibial resection must in any case be absolutely perpendicular to the mechanical axis. After applying the trial prosthetic components, in addition to alignment, joint stability in complete extension and in flexion must be evaluated. The most difficult knees are those in which there is consider-

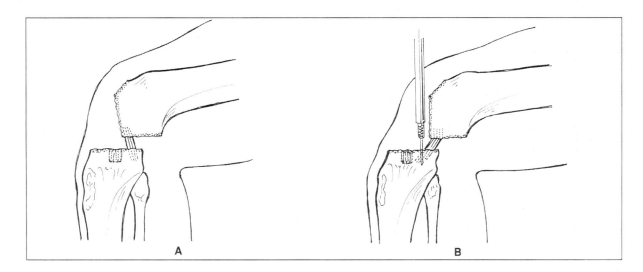

FIG. 7 (A-B) - Release of the posterior cruciate ligament is carried out at the tibial insertion, after evaluating tension by applying the trial prosthetic components.

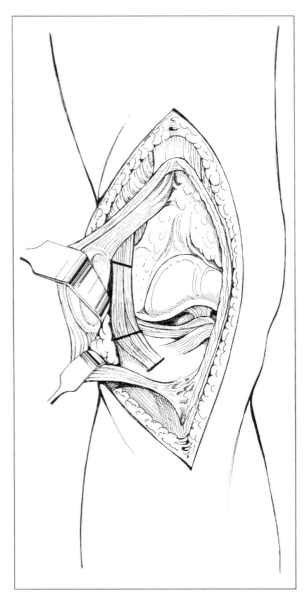

FIG. 8 - The iliotibial band is commonly disinserted at Gerdy's tubercle. As an alternative, it may be sectioned transversally, or lengthened using the method of multiple punctures.

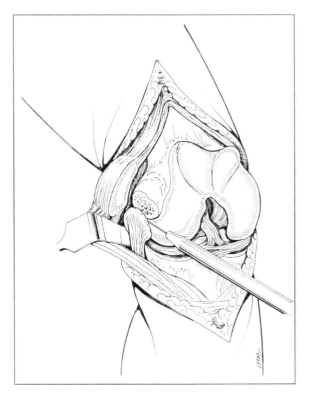

FIG. 9 - Release of the external collateral ligament is carried out at the femoral insertion.

able medial laxity, revealed by stress in valgus, as well as retraction of the lateral structures. In cases such as these, excision of the posterior cruciate ligament is recommended, the presence of which would obstruct correction of the deformity, as well as release of the external collateral ligament in the area corresponding to the femoral insertion (Fig. 9), or its lengthening by multiple transverse punctures technique, to avoid the risk of lateral in-

stability in flexion. More rarely, the tendon of the popliteus must be disinserted, that would mean rotatory instability, and the lateral gastrocnemius must also be disinserted. In fact, it is very important to recall that one must preserve at least one or two lateral stabilizers of the knee to avoid the occurrence of a condition of instability caused by over-release. This would mean resorting to a constrained, CCK type, or "hinge" prosthesis. In younger and more active patients with marked laxity of the medial collateral ligament tensioning may be carried out by using the method described by Krackow (7).

Particular care must be aimed at the search for correct alignment of the patella, as quite frequently in the prosthetized valgus knee it tends to dislocate because of the lateral direction of the resultant force of the extensor apparatus. After applying the trial prosthetic components, patellar tracking is observed, particularly between 60 and 90° of flexion, without applying any external pressure (no thumb

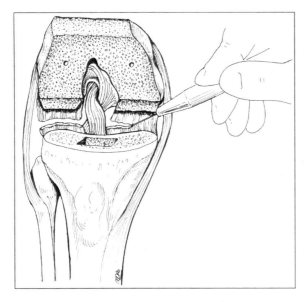

FIG. 10 - When severe flexion is present, it is best to section the posterior capsule, and possibly re-cut the distal femoral condyles.

rule). If the patella does not come into contact with the medial femoral condyle, or if it actually tends to dislocate laterally, after verifying and eventually correcting the position of the trial prosthesis, release of the external retinaculum must be performed, using the in-out technique or vice versa, about 2 cm from the patellar margin, possibly saving the lateral superior genicular artery that runs transversally at the superior pole of the patella. When severe contracture in flexion is present, an attempt is made to correct it by incising the posterior capsule and removing the posterior osteophytes (6) (Fig. 10). At times, however, to adequately broaden the extension space, a recut of the distal femur will be required. In prosthetic surgery of the valgus knee, it is usually not necessary to preliminarily isolate the external popliteal sciatic nerve: nonetheless, during the twenty-four hours subsequent to surgery, it is best to keep the knee in moderate flexion so as to reduce tension on the nervous trunk.

References

1) Aglietti P., Giron F.,Buzzi R.: Ligament balancing in the valgus knee. In: Current concepts in primary and revision total knee arthroplasty. Lippincott-Raven, Philadelphia, 1996.,

2) Akeson W., et al.: Effects of immobilization on joints. Clin Orthop., 219, 28, 1987

3) Alexiades M., et al.: A histologic study of posterior cruciate ligament in the arthritic knee. Am. J. Knee Surg, 2, 153, 1989.

4) Buechel F.F.: A sequential three-step lateral release for correcting fixed valgus knee deformies during total knee arthroplasty. Clin Orthop., 260, 170, 1990

5) Engh G.A., Ammeen D.J.: The clinical results of medial epicondylar osteotomy to correct severe varus deformity with total knee arthroplasty. AAOS, Anaheim, 1999.

6) Firestone T.P., et al.: The management of fixed flexion contractures during total knee arthroplasty. Clin Orthop., 284, 221, 1992

7) Freeman M.A.R.: Arthritis of the knee. Clinical features and surgical management. Springer-Verlag, New York, 1980

8) Krackow K.A.: The technique of total knee arthroplasty. Mosby, St Louis, 1990

9) Krackow K.A. et al.: Primary total knee arthroplasty in patients with fixed valgus deformity. Clin Orthop., 273, 9, 1991

10) Laskin R.S., Schob C.J.: Medial capsular recession for severe deformities and arthroplasty. Am. J. Knee Surg, 2, 153, 1989

11) Laurencin C.T., et al.: Total knee replacement in severe valgus deformity. Am. J. Knee Surg., 5, 135, 1992

12) Miyasaka, Ranawat C.S. Mullaji A: 10 to 20 years follow up of total knee arthroplasty for valgus deformities. Clin Orthop., 345, 29, 1997

13) Moreland J.R., Bassett L.W. Hanker G.J.: Radiographic analysis of the axial alignment of the lower extremity. J. Bone J. Surg., 69-A, 745, 1987

14) Ranawat C.S.: Total condylar knee arthroplasty. Technique, results and complications. Springer-Verlag, New York, 1985

15) Ritter M.A Faris P.M., Keating E.M..: Posterior cruciate ligament balancing during total knee arthroplasty. J.Arthroplasty, 3, 323 1988

16) Seebacher J.R., et al.: The structure of the postero-lateral aspect of the knee. J. Bone J. Surg., 64-A, 536, 1982

17) Stern S.H., Moeckel B.H., Insall J.:Total knee arthroplasty in valgus knee. Clin Orthop., 273, 5, 1991

18) Teeny S.M., et al.: Primary total knee arthroplasty in patients with severe varus deformity. Clin Orthop., 273, 19, 1991

19) Warren L.F., Marshall J.L: The supporting structures and layers on the medial side of the knee. J. Bone J.Surg., 61-A, 56, 1979.

Chapter 6
Patellofemoral Joint

M.A.R. Freeman, S.K. Kulkarni, J. Poal-Manresa

The Royal London Hospital - London

In 1994 Rand (1) reviewed the patello-femoral joint in total knee arthroplasty with special reference to the complications and clinical results. The present chapter builds on Rand's contribution but with an emphasis upon the natural patellofemoral anatomy and its implication for prosthetic design. Thus, this chapter should be read in conjunction with that of Rand. Inevitably the arguments put forward here, being the views of the author, are to some extent incorporated in the author's publications and prosthesis.

Patellofemoral complications have occurred in all forms of TKR whether the patellar articular surface is replaced or not: indeed at one time such complications represented the largest group of postoperative problems following this operation. The nature of these complications (i.e., subluxation, wear, loosening, pain and the "patellar clung") were such as to suggest an aetiology based upon the magnitude of patellofemoral stresses and the nature of patellar tracking after TKR. In this chapter these issues are addressed with special reference to the anatomy of the natural and replaced trochlear and patellar surfaces. It will be argued that the former merits particular attention. Various angles and linear dimensions will be given for the natural patellofemoral joint. Only a single value without limits of variation and without the qualification "approximately" will be quoted for the sake of brevity and simplicity. In practice it is hard to measure any dimension or angle on an irregular curved structure such as the distal femur. Add to that the variation between specimens (2) and the uncertainty over reference lines to which to relate a measurement (3), and it becomes obvious that engineering accuracy is unattainable.

1. The Anatomy

1.1 The Trochlea as Viewed from the Side

0-90° Flexion: Viewed from the side, the trochlea represents a 70° arc of a circle recessed into the antero-distal femur (Fig. 1) and has a radius of about 21 mm (4, 5). The effect of this femoral geometry upon the relative position of the tibia and patella during flexion is shown in Figure 2. Note in this figure that the femur is shown as rotating around a fixed axis relative to the as described by Hollister et al. (6) represented by the posterior portion of the condyles. Thus no femoral "roll-back" has occurred. Nevertheless the patella moves backwards relative to the tibia (causing an increased inclination of the ligamentum patellae) during flexion because the floor of the trochlea is further from the centre of rotation of the femur as measured anterio-posteriorly than it is as measured proximally-distally (Figs. 1 and 2).

The motion of the patella is governed by the floor, not by the shoulders, of the trochlea: indeed the latter are non-articular. Thus, the natural patella moves (relative to the femur) around a circular arc from about 10° to 100° of flexion (i.e., "a" in Figure 1) whilst at the same time becoming more posterior relative to the tibia.

Since the patella moves around a circular surface, it would seem reasonable to provide a similar motion pattern in the replaced knee rather than the non-circular track with an antero-distal prominence that is in fact the usual geometry. It is intuitively obvious that tibifemoral function would be interfered with if the tibial surface of the femur were non-circular, having a rounded "corner" at about 45° flexion. Equally, a round-

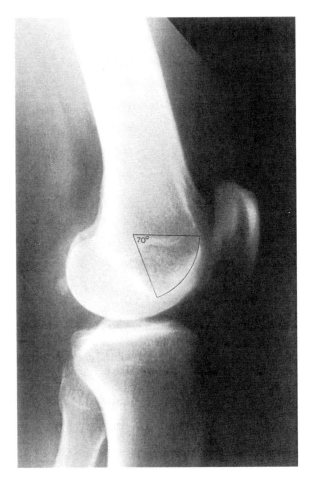

FIG. 1 - A lateral radiograph of the femur. The trochlea (outlined) represents a 70° arc of a circle recessed into the antero-distal femur.

ed "corner" in the patellar surface might also be expected to interfere with function. Why then have almost all femoral components from the Total Condylar prosthesis onwards been designed to have such a step in their trochlear surface?

The first prostheses of the condylar type for the replacement of the tibiofemoral joint (e.g., the Freeman-Swanson and the Geomedic prostheses) were not provided with an anterior patellar flange since patellar replacement was not planned as part of the operation. When (in the Total Condylar prosthesis) an anterior flange was provided, anterior and posterior chamfer cuts of equal size were made in the femur for reasons which are not now clear (to the present author). Possibly they derived from the approximately symmetrical lateral appearance of the

"external" surfaces of the femur (Fig. 1). In contrast to the femoral "external" surfaces, the femoral articular surfaces are strongly asymmetrical, the recessed position of the patellar surface contrasting with the prominence of the posterior tibial surface. This articular asymmetry can only be fully accommodated in a femoral prosthesis if very asymmetric chamfer cuts are made, to the point where all the chamfer is anterior and little or none is posterior. Such an arrangement, and only such an arrangement, allows the articular surface of the prosthetic trochlea to occupy the same recessed position in the femur as did the natural trochlea. This in turn allows the patella to track normally as viewed from the side, in contrast to the "conventional" arrangement which forces the patella to travel over a "corner," the anterior-distal prominence of which tenses the retinaculae. If anything, this "corner" is accentuated by the presence of the femoral "box" in posterior-stabilized implants, thus perhaps in part accounting for the "patellar clunk" syndrome. That a "corner," in contrast to a smoother radiused trochlear surface, does indeed contribute to patellar symptoms is suggested by the outcome of a clinical comparison of the two (7, 8) whilst Petersilge et al. (9) concluded, on experimental grounds, that a deep, smoothly radiused trochlea would probably reduce surface wear and cold flow in the patella prosthesis. Andriacchi et al. (10) have shown clinically that such a trochlea, as contrasted with one having a "corner," produces a more normal gait on stairs.

To summarise the discussion with regard to patellar tracking as viewed from the side, it is now argued that the floor of the prosthetic trochlea should be circular and recessed to an anatomical extent into the femur so as to restore the patellofemoral joint line (a feature not to be confused with the height of the patella in relation to the tibiofemoral joint line). This necessitates a deep anterior chamfer (passing just below the floor of the natural trochlea) and (optimally) no posterior chamfer.

0-110° Flexion: In relatively deep flexion, the extensor mechanism may be heavily loaded. It therefore seems appropriate to extend the floor of the prosthetic trochlea posteriorly into the intercondylar notch so that the patella contacts the floor at least to 110°. If the patella does not do so, a fibrous nodule may form distal to the patella opposite the intercondylar notch (contributing to the "patellar clunk" syndrome) and increased patellar articular contact stresses in flexion might contribute to wear.

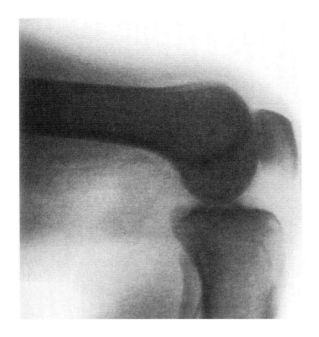

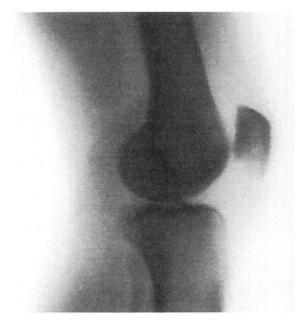

B

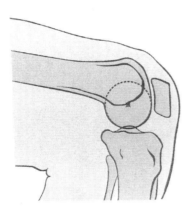

C

D

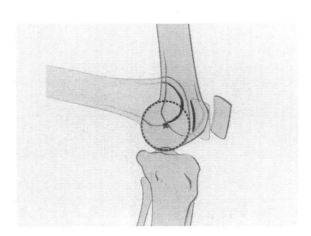

E

FIG. 2 - A fluoroscopic lateral radiograph of the weight bearing knee flexed to 90° (A) and, after "step-up," in extension (B). The outlines of these radiographs are shown separately in Figures 2 (C and D) and overlaid in Figure 2 (E).

Note that the posterior circular segments of the femoral condyles rotate round a stationary axis represented by the centre of this circle. The trochlea is further from this axis in anteroposterior direction than it is proximally-distally. Thus the trochlea, and with it the patella, moves backwards relative to the tibia from 0° to 90° in the absence of femoral roll-back.

Clearly the floor of the trochlea cannot be extended posteriorly in prostheses which retain the ACL, nor in those which are posteriorly stabilized (because the tibial stabilizer peg interferes with the floor of the trochlea in extension). These considerations argue for ACL resection and posterior stabilization by means other than the conventional tibial peg and femoral rod-contained-in-a-box.

1.2 The Trochlea as Viewed from the Front

A description of the anatomy of the trochlea and of patellar tracking as viewed from the front, is difficult to provide in words or pictorially because of the change in anatomical plane which occurs as the patella tracks from the anterior to the distal surface of the femur. It is further complicated by the use of different reference axes, for example "proximal-distal," "mechanical," "anatomical," "transepicondylar" etc. Finally there is some disagreement as to nature of the anatomy, however it is described. In what follows, terms have been used which relate to the two views of the knee obtained during knee replacement since these will be familiar to readers of this chapter. These views are: a view of the anterior aspect of the femur and tibia in the extended knee, and a view of the distal femur and anterior tibia in the knee flexed to 90°. For descriptions of the distal femoral anatomy and of patellar tracking the reader is referred to Yoshioka et al. (11), Freeman et al. (4), Elias et al. (5), Poilvache et al. (3), Feinstein et al. (2). Sakai et al. (12), Siu et al. (13) and Eckhoff et al. (14). These authors are not all in full agreement but the description which follows is presented, for the sake of clarity, without dwelling on the controversies. Although it is, strictly speaking, outside the scope of this Chapter, the work of Hollister et al. (6) dealing with the location of the axis of tibiofemoral flexion/extension and its relationship to the transepicondylar line represents essential reading for an understanding of knee motion.

0°-10°: In full extension (i.e., in many knees, strictly speaking, hyperextension) the lower pole of the (normal) patella lies just proximal to the trochlea (13) when the quadriceps muscle contracts. Thus the patellar articular cartilage is in contact with the synovial membrane covering the distal femur, not with articular cartilage. Laterally the distal pole is in contact with the non-articular, anterior prominence of the lateral femoral condyle. When the quadriceps relax, the patella moves a few millimetres distally and as

flexion begins the patella progressively contacts the trochlea, its course being determined by the floor of the sulcus.

If anterior, lateral femoral condyle in the natural knee is less than normally prominent, the patella may not be guided into the trochlea during the first 10° of flexion resulting in recurrent dislocation of the (natural) patella (15). Thus if the anterior flange of a prosthesis is short with a shallow, broad trochlea, the patella, as in the natural knee with recurrent patellar subluxation (15), may never track accurately within the sulcus. This defect may be ameliorated, but it is not fundamentally solved, by placing the femoral component in a few degrees of external rotation on the femur.

These facts suggest that the anterior flange of a femoral prosthesis should extend sufficiently proximal to replace not only the true anterior articular surface of the femur but also (1) to cover the distal synovial-covered 2 cm of the shaft and (2) to replace the anterior non-articular and articular lateral femoral condyle with a prosthetic condyle of adequate height. In this way, a patellar prosthesis will never lose contact with its metallic counter-surface and the patella itself will always be constrained laterally. Theiss et al. (7), on the basis of a comparison of the incidence of patellar symptoms in two prostheses, have confirmed that these features are indeed clinically important.

Because the anterior section of the trochlea is shallow and short, it is difficult to give a meaningful description of the orientation of its floor. Not surprisingly, therefore, opinion differs as to whether the patella tracks distally and medially (the classical view based on the Q-angle) or distally and laterally (2, 13) over this part of its course. In the author's experience at operation and on x-ray, it would seem that any medial or lateral displacement that may occur in the natural patella is minimal. In the replaced patellofemoral joint, patellar tracking is controlled (especially if the anterior flange and its lateral wall are high as described above) by the design of the sulcus. Whether the sulcus is aligned to the hip or more laterally does not seem to affect the outcome clinically but a 7° angulation proximally and laterally may be desirable since it has been shown to reduce medio-lateral shear by 10% experimentally (9).

Whichever way the anterior floor of the sulcus (and thus patellar tracking) inclines, it is important to note that the sulcus, throughout its extent, is displaced about 5 mm lateral to the midline (14), thus helping to align the patellar track to the tibial tubercle. Were femoral components to reproduce this feature of the normal anatomy, the prosthetic tibial eminence would also have to be displaced laterally necessitating left- and right-sided polyethylene inserts. The advantage would be to "straighten out" the patellar track as viewed from the front and thus presumably to reduce the tendency for lateral patellar subluxation.

10°-45°: As the patella moves around the (circular) antero-distal aspect of the trochlea, it lies in a sulcus, the lateral wall of which is higher and steeper than the medial wall (about 1 cm vs a few mm). This, together with the fact that there is an angle, the Q-angle, of about 14° (12) between the anatomical axis of the femoral shaft and the ligamentum patellae, suggests that the quadriceps exerts a component of force directed laterally.

Whatever the force exerted on the natural patella, in this section of the arc, the bone shafts at most 1mm laterally as the knee flexes in vitro (12). This observation fits with the finding that the trochlear sulcus is here perpendicular to the transepicondylar axis (2), (which in turn approximately corresponds to the axis of tibiofemoral flexion/extension (6)).

45°-90°: If the knee is flexed to 90° and viewed from the anterior aspect of the tibia, it can be seen that the trochlear sulcus in the distal femur runs posteriorly and laterally towards the tibial tubercle. The angle between the sulcus and perpendicular to the transepicondylar axis has been measured to be 11° (2). This results in a lateral shift of the patella in vitro of about 5 mm from 45° to 90° (12).

Not only does the patella shift laterally from 45° to 90°, but also (as mentioned above) the sulcus and with it the patella is located 5 mm lateral to the midline of the knee, not centrally (14).

90° to full-flexion: The floor of the sulcus ends at about 100° flexion (13) and thereafter the patella articulates with the medial and lateral femoral condyles. However in the prosthetic knee the floor of the trochlea can (and, in the author's view, should for reasons outline above) be continued for at least another 20° provided that (1) the ACL is divided and (2) a "conventional" posterior-stabilizing mechanism is avoided since the femoral box of the latter, like the ACL, conficts distally/posteriorly with the base of such an extended sulcus (and indeed, in the case of the box, with a sulcus of anatomical length).

In summary: at 10° flexion the patella enters a groove on the femur (the trochlea) which is circular as viewed from the side having a radius of about 20-25 mm an extent of about 110°. This groove is off-set laterally from the femoral midline by 5 mm and is bounded by a relatively high (10 mm), steep, lateral wall. On one view of this anatomy, the groove "wraps round" the antero-lateral femoral condyle so that the patella at first moves perpendicularly or even medially relative to the transepicondylar axis. On an alternative view, the patella track may incline 15° from medial to lateral thus being aligned with the more distal part of the sulcus. From 45° to 90°, the patella follows the sulcus, so that its track deviates about 10° in a lateral direction as flexion increases. As in extension the sulcus and with it the patella is located 5 mm lateral to the midline of the knee.

2. Implications for Prosthetic Design

2.1 The Femur

The implications of this view of the functional anatomy for the design of the anterior flange of a femoral prosthesis have already been summarised: it should extend 2 cm proximal to the anterior femoral articular surface and be furnished with a prominent lateral shoulder. It would be desirable to extend the base of the sulcus in a posterior direction to about 110° and to displace the sulcus laterally (which would in turn require left- and right-sided tibial components). Such a design change would "straighten out" the lateral wall of the sulcus and could, if carried onto the anterior surface, eliminate the Q-angle. Viewed from the side, the floor of the prosthetic trochlea should be circular and placed so as to lie within the femur in the position once occupied by the floor of the natural trochlea.

These design objectives can be achieved, partially, by externally rotating contemporary symmetrical femoral prostheses. However this reduces the apparent height and increases the obliquity of the lateral wall of the sulcus. (It also increases the posterior projection of the lateral femoral condyle, the implications of which are outside the scope of this Chapter). It would seem preferable to design left- and right-sided femoral (and perhaps tibial) components so as to replicate the normal anatomy.

2.2 The Effect of Tibial Rotation upon Patella Alignment

It is currently fashionable to advocate the provision of a range of tibial rotation in flexion in the replaced knee (although there is little evidence that a knee replaced with a rotating prosthesis in fact itself rotates, because of soft tissue constraints). If such knees do rotate externally. Patellofemoral problems might be exacerbated because of the lateral displacement of the tibial tubercle that would ensue. Thus with regard to the patellofemoral joint, it may be desirable to avoid, rather than to seek, tibial ER in flexion. Whatever the situation with regard to rotation movement of the tibia, the rotational placement of the tibial component should be a matter of surgical concern especially if rotation is not built into the prosthesis: placement of the prosthesis in excessive internal rotation relative to the bone should be avoided.

2.3 The Articular Surface of the Patella

If the patella surface is not replaced, it has been reported that up to 15% of knees will have persistent anterior pain (16). Others have reported that the results are the same with and without replacement (17). Although rarely sufficient to require revision surgery, "patellar" symptoms may be sufficient to spoil an otherwise satisfactory result. Although at first sight it seems obvious that anterior pain arises from the unreplaced surface of the patella, it will be noted that: apparently normal patellae may be associated (especially in young woman) with anterior pain; and that at worst 85% of unreplaced patellae in TKR are painless, as are many severely arthrosic unreplaced patellae in the elderly. In short the relationship between anterior knee pain and the patella is unclear. Possibly, improvement in patellofemoral tracking by attention to the design of the trochlea as outlined above might reduce its incidence after TKR. Perhaps also it will in the future be possible to determine which knees are at risk of pain pre-operatively. As the situation stands today however it is the author's view that all patellae should be replaced provided that the bone is thick enough to do so and that the associated complications do not outweigh the advantage of pain-relief. However, it is self-evident that pain-relief without replacement would be the ideal.

Replacement may be carried out either by resecting the back of the patella and then implanting an all-HDP prosthesis, fixed with cement and 3 pegs (i.e., an "onlay") or by drilling a hole in the patella into which the prosthesis is inserted (i.e., an "inlay"). In the latter case the implant need be no more than 20 mm in diameter provided the design of the trochlea and intercondylar

notch are appropriate. Such an implant might be cemented or uncemented, and, since adequate thickness is assured, it could be metal-backed or all-HDP. The author's preference is for the recessed technique using an all-HDP implant.

Whichever way the bone is replaced, the resultant patella-plus-prosthesis complex should not be over-tick (although how important this is if the trochlea is adequately recessed is not clear).

The articular surface of the implant may be dome- or saddle-shaped. The former provides only line contact and thus is more highly stressed (18). Theoretically it may be less stable laterally than a saddle-shaped implant. The latter provides area contact (provided the trochlea is of a single radius) but is must be implanted in the correct rotational position (a technique which is simple when understood).

It has objected to the use of fixed saddle-shaped patellar components that the natural patella rotates during flexion and that therefore, since a saddle-shaped prosthesis would be rotationally constrained, rotation might loosen the patellar component. In fact, patellar rotation amounts to only about 1° over the first 90° of flexion (12) so that this objection, although valid in theory, is probably not important in practice and certainly has not resulted in loosening in the author's experience (4).

In the natural knee there is a composite structure made up of the patella, the patellar ligament and the fat pad, and the tibial intercondylar eminence which form an approximately vertical "ridge," circular as viewed from the side, projecting backwards into the trochlea and femoral intercondylar notch (Fig. 5). The corresponding structures in the replaced knee should, if they are to reproduce the normal anatomy, also form a similar "tibiopatellar eminence." This implies a saddle-shaped patella prosthesis and a tibial intercondylar eminence of the same shape.

In the author's view the saddle-shaped implant is theoretically preferable but the more usual dome-shaped prosthesis has in practice functioned well.

2.4 Summary

Historically, attention has been paid particularly to the patella when considering the patellofemoral joint. It is here argued, however, that most femoral prostheses have a trochlear surface of the wrong shape located wrongly in the femur. The features which should be incorporated in a prosthetic trochlea were first argued by Freeman et al. (4), the underlying anatomy being discussed by Elias et al. (5). A number of studies published in 1995 and 1996, referred to above, have confirmed and expanded the views set out in these two papers. This chapter represents a synthesis of this literature, particularly regarding the trochlea, which in the author's view should be embodied in femoral prosthetic design in the future. The trochlea should be circular as viewed from the side, extend from 0° to 110° and be recessed with the femur. Its lateral wall should extend to contact the patella in full extension and should be high, relatively steep and straight as viewed from the front and distally. A patellar implant may be optional. If used, it should be saddle-shaped and inlaid with the patella.

3. A Personal Clinical Experience with an "Anatomical" Patellofemoral Joint in TKR

Perhaps the most stringent test of the validity of the design arguments expressed above would be provided by determining using such a configuration for a minimum of 10 years either without replacement or with an HDP uncemented patellar component. (An HDP uncemented patellar replacement will better reveal the intrinsic stability of the fixation than would a cemented implant, whilst if patellar component rotation is really a clinical problem, it will be manifest as osteolysis induced by wear debris because HDP is in contact with the patella).

The Freeman/Samuelson prosthesis (Sulzer Orthopaedics Ltd., Switzerland) is an example of such an implant save that distally the trochlear sulcus is central and the medial wall is equal in height to the lateral (Fig. 6). The patellar component is inset into the patella and is saddle-shaped to provide area contact with the floor and the lateral wall of the trochlea.

By comparing the results of a replaced patella with those achieved without replacement it is possible to draw tentative conclusions as to the extent to which the results are due to the design of the trochlea (common to both) or to the patellar prosthesis.

3.1 Materials and Method

To obtain the patients necessary for a comparison between replaced and unreplaced patellae with a minimum follow-up of ten years, uninfected knees replaced in two hospital ("A" and "B") were reviewed. At hospital "A" essentially all knees replaced during the relevant period were treated with patella replacement using an uncemented polyethylene component. A few knees were replaced using cement simply to validate the cement technique. In contrast, at hospital "B" essentially all knees were treated without patella replacement but again a few knees were treated by replacement with and without cement, again to validate the technique.

A total of 124 knees treated with uncemented patella replacement entered the study with a minimum potential follow up of 10 years at hospital "A" and 143 without patella replacement at hospital "B." During the period of the study uncemented press-fit techniques were used for tibial and femoral replacement at both hospitals. These techniques provided unsatisfactory fixation and were abandoned; 16 of the 124 knees originally entered at hospital "A" were revised for tibiofemoral loosening and 15 were similarly revised at the hospital "B." In none of these knees was the patella the cause of revision. One additional knee was revised at hospital "A" for persistent pain. Ten patients died at hospital "A" and 8 at hospital "B" during the period of the study. Two knees were lost from the patients at hospital "A" and 4 at hospital "B". Thus 96 patients remained for evaluation 10 years after replacement at hospital "A" and 115 at the hospital "B."

The demographic data for these two groups are shown in Table 1. It will be seen that the composition both with respect to diagnosis, gender and age were similar in the two hospitals.

3.2 Result

At review 10-15 years after replacement 2 knees, one replaced and one unreplaced, had developed severe anterior knee pain. Although an-

Table 1

Demographic Data		
	Replaced	Unreplaced
RA.OA	34:62	36:79
Male: Female	31:62	25:90
Age 30-59: > 60	20:76	34:81

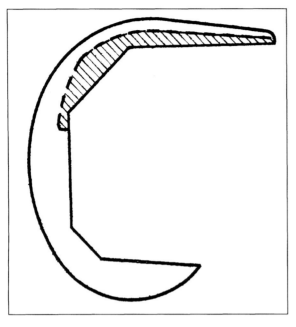

A

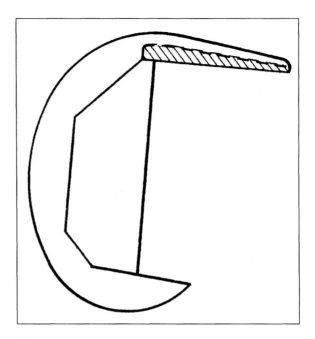

B

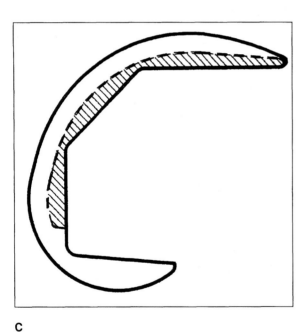

C

Fig. 3

A - The short trochlear surface, with a "corner," present in many prostheses.
B - The effect of a posterior stabilizing mechanism on the trochlear surface.
C - The trochlear surface proposed in this chapter. The surface has a single radius, is recessed antero-distally and is extended over the femoral intercondylar notch.

terior knee pain may be due to factors other than the extensor mechanism, this pain was regarded as being patellofemoral in origin. In the one replaced knee the pain was present at rest and x-rays were unremarkable. No firm diagnosis was made and no treatment given. In the unreplaced knee the patella was treated by replacement but the pain persisted. Nineteen patients, 7 in the replaced group (7.2%) and 12 in the unreplaced group (10,4%), had mild anterior knee pain not requiring analgesia. Although the incidence was slightly higher in the unreplaced group, this difference was not statistically significant.

The preoperative range of flexion in the replaced group was 85° and increased to 98°. In the unreplaced group, the preoperative range was 100° and remained unchanged at 99°.

We were unable to determine reliably the degree of patella tilt that might have been present in the replaced group since the radio-opaque markers in the patella prosthesis did not allow accurate measurements of this abnormality to be made. The prosthesis itself was radiolucent and since no cement was used it was difficult to judge its exact attitude. For similar reasons, tier was difficult to estimate in the unreplaced group. One patella was not in contact with the floor of the trochlea groove in the replaced group and 2 were not in contact with the floor of the groove in the unreplaced group. No patellae were dislocated from the groove.

There was one patella fracture at 12 years in the replaced group and 3 between years 1 and 4 in the unreplaced group. All these fractures were treated conservatively, resulting in intact extensor mechanisms.

Radiologically it was possible to measure forward migration of the patella component relative to the anterior patella cortex in a lateral x-ray. One prosthesis, which also displayed lysis and was thus radiologically loose, was seen to have migrated forwards. The patient was symptomless and is being treated by observation. In the unreplaced group there was lateral sclerosis suggestive of increased lateral patellofemoral contact pressure in 12. We had the impression in both groups that there was some osteopenia on the medial side of some patellae in both groups and similarly a suggestion of "traction osteophytes" developing on the lateral side in both groups. Neither of these impressions could be quantified and they did not appear to be associated with symptoms nor with mal-tracking.

There were no revisions for patellofemoral complications in the replaced group. One patella (already mentioned) was resurfaced for pain which was not relieved by surgery in the unreplaced group.

The survival of the patella prosthesis on a best case scenario was 100%. On a worst case scenario, in which lost patients were regarded as having failed, the survival at 10 years was 96% (95% confidence interval: 92-100% standard error 2%).

3.3 Comment

These results suggest that the addition of a patella prosthesis results in no material complications even if the prosthesis is uncemented. Had these prostheses rotated to any substantial extent over the 10 year period of this review, we would have expected osteolysis in the patella in more than 1%. Having said that the results of patella replacement are benign, it is clear that the results of leaving the patella unreplaced are essentially the same. This suggests, but does not prove, that the design of the trochlea is the key feature which resulted in satisfactory results in these two cohorts of patients rather than the presence of a patella prosthesis in half of them.

This result is similar to that recently reported by Barrack et al. (19) using the MGII prosthesis in which the trochlea surface is also essentially circular (although it does not extend as far posteriorly into the inter-condylar notch nor proximally as does that of the FS prosthesis).

Given that the floor of the natural trochlea is circular as viewed from the side, it is hardly surprising that this circular surface is replaced by some other shape (for example on with a rounded corner half way along its track) there should be unsatisfactory symptomatic results. By analogy, if the natural femoral head (which is circular) were to be replaced by a prosthetic head which had a "corner" on its circumference, one would expect dramatically unsatisfactory symptomatic results when such a prosthesis was articulated with an unreplaced acetabulum. These results might be improved by replacing the acetabular surface (by analogy with the patella surface) but wear might be expected in the long term.

4. Summary

We believe that patellofemoral complications after knee replacement can for practical purposes be eliminated by attention to the design of the trochlea surface on the femoral component. This surface should be circular as viewed from the side over the loaded part of the patella track. It should be deep enough positively to retain the patella and (since the anterior cruciate ligament will be removed) it should extend posteriorly into the inter-condylar notch to provide an articular for the patella well into flexion. Proximally the trochlea extend for about 2 cm above the natural articular surface. The trochlea should be vertical distally and inclined laterally as it extends onto the front of the femoral surface. Overall, such a track can be straight. It is perhaps preferable to displace the trochlea surface slightly to the lateral side of the femoral component thus replicating the normal anatomy and reducing the tension in the lateral retinaculum. This step, however, has the disadvantage of necessitating left and right tibial and femoral components.

Given such a trochlea surface, one further speculative point is worthy of mention. It will be appreciated that in the natural knee articular cartilage is present on the femur anterior to the extremity of the tibial articulation and medial and lateral to the patella articulation. Teleologically the question might be asked: why should this surface be cartilage-covered, implying that it carries a compressive load? Perhaps the answer is that these medial and lateral surfaces do indeed carry a compressive load, i.e., that then compressive forces transmitted from the extensor mechanism to the femur are carried partly in the patella itself and partly in the medial and lateral retinaculae. If this is true, the height of the medial and lateral shoulders on a prosthetic trochlea groove may well be important: if the shoulders are high and, like the floor of the groove, circular, it may well be that much of the compressive load is transmitted to the replaced femur via the retinaculae rather than via the patella itself. This observation would help to explain the satisfactory results of our replaced patellae (with uncemented HDP implants) and would account for the observation that replaced patellae at post-mortem or revision surgery are

frequently covered, sometimes almost entirely, by synovial soft tissue. If the articular surface of the patella was carrying substantial load, this synovial soft tissue would be crushed. The fact that it is there suggests that the load is carried elsewhere than on the patella itself, i.e., in the retinaculae.

Thus the key to satisfactory patellofemoral function after TKR may lie not only with the trochlea but also with the design of its shoulders. The management of the patella may be of secondary importance.

References

1) Rand J.A.: Current concepts review. The patellofemoral joint in total knee arthroplasty. J Bone Joint Surg. 76-A. 4:612-620. 1994.
2) Feinstein W.K., Noble P.C., Kamaric E., Tullos H.S.: Anatomic alignment of the patellar groove. Clin Orthop. 331:64-73. 1996.
3) Poilvache P.L., Insall J.N., Scuderi G.R., Font-Rodriguez D.E.: Rotational landmarks and sizing of the distal femur in total knee arthroplasty. Clin Orthop. 331:34-46. 1996.
4) Freeman M.A.R., Samuelson K.M., Elias S.G., Mariorenzi L.J., Gokcay E.I. and Tuke M.: The Patello-Femoral Joint in Total Knee Prostheses: Design Consideration. Journal of Arthroplasty 4 (suppl); S69-S74. 1989.
5) Elias S.G., Freeman M.A.R., Gokcay E.I.: A correlative study of the geometry and anatomy of the distal femur. Clin Orthop. 260:98. 1990.
6 Hollister A.M., Jatana S., Singh A.K., et al.: The axes of rotation of the knee: Clin Orthop. 290:259. 1993
7) Theiss S.M., Kitziger K.J., Lotke P.S., Lotke P.A.: Component design affecting patellofemoral complications after total knee arthroplasty. Clin Orthop. 326:183-187. 1996.
8) Sum J., Andriacchi T.P., Rosenberg A., Galante J.O.: Effect of a nonanatomical femoral trochlea on patella loading and function following total knee replacement. 43rd Annual Meeting, Orthopaedic Research Society. Feb 9-13, 1997. San Francisco, California.
9) Petersilge W.J., Oishi C.S., Kaufman K.R., Irby S.E., Colwell C.W: The effect of trochlear design on patellofemoral sheer and compressive forces in total knee arthroplasty. Clin Orthop. 309:124-130. 1994.
10) Andriacchi T.P., Yoder D., Couley A., Rosenberg A., Sum J., Galante J.O.: Patellofemoral design influences function

following total knee arthroplasty. J. Arthroplasty. 12:243-249. 1997.
11) Yoshioka Y., Siu D., Cooke D.V.: The anatomy and functional axis of the femur: J. Bone Joint Surg. 69A:873-880. 1987
12) Sakai N., Luo Z-P., Rand J.A., An K-N.: In vitro study of patellar position during sitting, standing from squatting and the stance phase of walking. Am J Knee Surg. 9(4):161-166. 1996.
13) Siu D., Rudan J., Wevers H.W., Griffiths P.: Femoral articular shape and geometry. J Arthroplasty 11(2):166-173. 1996.
14) Eckhoff D.G., Burke B.J., Dwyer T.F., Pring M.E., Spitzer V.M., VanGerwen D.P.: Sulcus morphology of the Distal Femur. Clin Orthop. 331:23-28. 1996.
15) Kujala V.M., Osterman K., Kormano M., Nelimarkka O., Hutme M., Taimeta S.: Patellofemoral relationships in recurrent patellar dislocation. J. Bone Joint Surg. 71B:788-792. 1989
16) Levai J.P., McLeod H.C., Freeman M.A.R.: Why not resurface the patella? J. Bone Joint Surg. 65B:448-451. 1983
17) Keblish P.A., Varma A.K., Greenwald A.S.: Patellar resurfacing or retention in total knee arthroplasty. J. Bone Joint Surg. 76B:930-937. 1994.
18) Takeuchi T., Lathi V.K., Khan A.M., Hayes W.C.: Patellofemoral contact pressures exceed the compression yield strength of UHMWPE in total knee arthroplasties. J Arthroplasty. 10:363-368. 1995.
19) Barrack R.L., Wolfe M.W., Waldman D.A., Miciliz M., Bartof A.J., Myers L.: Resurfacing of the patella in total knee arthroplasty: A prospective randomized double-blind study. J. Bone Joint Surg. 79A: 1121-1131. 1997.

Chapter 7
Bone Grafting in Primary and Revision Total Knee Arthroplasty

Thomas P. Sculco
The Hospital for Special Surgery - New York

Bone Grafting for Tibial Deficiency

When severe malalignment occurs in destructive knee joint disease, the articular surface is devastated and associated changes result in underlying bone and soft tissues. Bone loss takes place on both the tibial and femoral surfaces of the knee joint in association with severe angular deformity. In the varus knee bone loss tends to be greater on the tibial surface and in valgus deformities the bone loss tends to be more symmetrical on the tibial and femoral surfaces. The extent of bone deficiency is usually more marked on the posterior aspect of the tibial plateau as often flexion contractures are concomitant with these marked deformities. There is associated asymmetry of soft tissues about the joint complicating the management of these deformities and most commonly soft tissue releases will be necessary on the concave side of the deformity to balance lax soft tissues on the convex side of the deformity.

The management of bone deficits on the tibial surface are varied depending upon the extent and location of the loss of bone. Methylmethacrylate can be used as a filler in smaller defects with or without screw reinforcement. It is not recommended for larger defects as fracture and fragmentation of large unsupported methylmethacrylate columns may lead to implant failure. In the most severe bone deficits augmentation can be effected by using additions to the implant itself or autogenous bone grafting.

The area of bone loss on the tibial surface has a significantly sclerotic bed. The tibial rim is usually destroyed as the deficiency occurs and the femur subluxes (Fig. 1). This produces a deficiency which is concave at its floor and often has a wedge configuration. Defects may be seen with an intact tibial rim but these are much less common. In deficiencies which are 6-12 millimeter in depth, resection of 10 millimeters of upper tibia will generally remove most of the sclerotic bed. If deficits remain after resection of the tibia which are less than five millimeters these can be fenestrated with a drill and filled with methylmethacrylate to support the tibial component.

Bone grafting is the preferred technique in defects which are greater than 12-15 millimeters in depth. Wedge augments (Fig. 2) may be added to the undersurface of the tibial component to fill these areas but there are a number of disadvantages to this technique. Wedge augments tend to add expense to the cost of the implant and the locking mechanism of the wedge augment to the undersurface of the tibial plate usually requires screws which may produce fretting and abrasive metallic debris. These metallic particles may produce an inflammatory reaction similar to polyethylene debris and potentially lead to osteolysis. Additionally limited sizes and configurations of wedges are available and these may not fit the deficit. Most importantly, however, wedges do not restore bone which has been lost by the arthritic destructive process.

Attempts should be made to restore bone which has been lost and reconstruction with a biologic augmentation, autogenous bone, is readily available from the distal femur and can be shaped to fit the area of bone deficiency. Additionally incorporation occurs, and this restores bone stock to the upper femur should revision surgery be necessary.

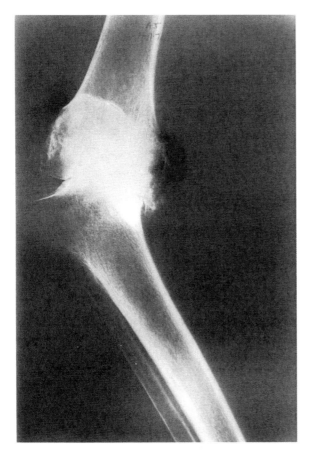

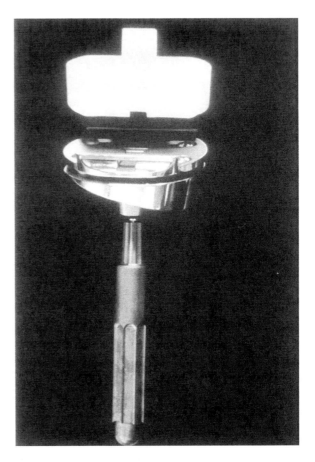

FIG. 1 - Medial tibial deficiency with destruction of peripheral rim and joint subluxation.

FIG. 2 - Tibial wedge augment fixed to tibial baseplate with screws.

Technique of Autogenous Bone Grafting for Tibial Deficiency

The initial tibial proximal bone cut is made utilizing a standard tibial cutting guide in the usual fashion. This tibial cut is conservative and about 8 millimeters of bone is resected from the more preserved tibial plateau. An oscillating saw is then used to create an oblique osteotomy on the side of the tibial defect (Fig. 3a, b). Angled tibial wedge instruments may be used to make this osteotomy. The bony bed of the concave side of the defect is usually very sclerotic and this surface should be resected. The deep surface of the tibial bed should be 80-90% cancellous bone after this oblique osteotomy has been performed. There may be cystic areas in this bed once the sclerotic surface has been removed, and these may be curetted and filled with cancellous bone that is available from bone resection. It is important to remove this sclerotic bone and expose cancellous bone, otherwise consolidation of the graft will be impeded and failure of the

graft may occur (7). The osteotomy should be planar and flat so that a femoral condylar graft will fit intimately with the cancellous bed.

If the implant to be used has a stem for fixation then the peg hole should be made after preparation of the defect bed. This will insure that when the fixation screws are inserted into the graft the stem hole will not be entered. For implants with peripheral fixation peg holes this step is of less importance.

The next step is to remove the distal femoral bone. Generally, the resected distal medial femoral condyle is larger than the lateral condyle and therefore tends to be the better graft material. Having resected the distal femoral condyle, this segment of bone is rotated so that its cancellous surface is coapted against the cancellous surface of the recipient bed (Fig. 4a). The defect should be completely filled with bone graft. There will be an overhanging segment of bone which protrudes above the cut surface of the tibia when the femoral condyle is placed on the upper tibial surface to fill the de-

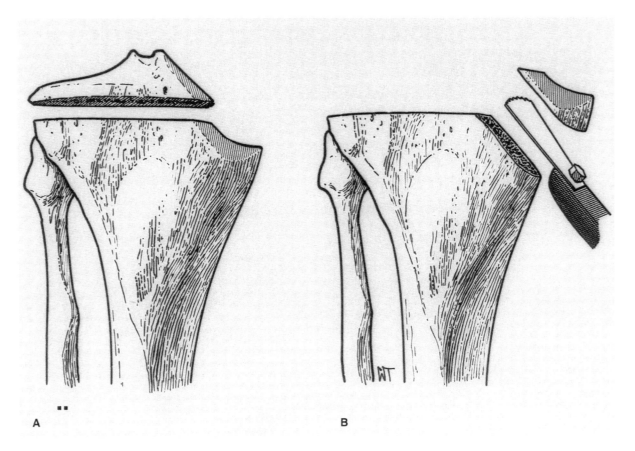

FIG. 3 A - Proximal tibial osteotomy. - B Oblique osteotomy of upper tibial surface to remove sclerotic tibial bed.

fect and this will be resected. If there is any gapping between the bone graft and the recipient bed, the bed must be further resected to create a flat cancellous surface. Once coaptation is precise, two screws are inserted to stabilize the graft to the proximal tibia. They should be inserted from the periphery and not make contact with the metal tibial baseplate. Care must be taken not to crack the graft as the screws are inserted. After the graft has been fixed in position, the overhanging bone should be removed using the resected tibial plateau surface as a guide. At this point the proximal tibia has been reconstituted. On observing the tibia from its upper surface the subchondral bone of the femoral condylar bone graft will act as the peripheral tibial bone of the upper tibia (Fig. 4b).

Cortical screws are generally used to fix the graft and these can be overdrilled proximally to allow a lag effect when inserted (Fig. 5). It is of utmost importance that cement not be allowed to enter the interval between the graft and recipient bed. An excellent method of preventing this from occurring is to cement the femoral component first and use a small portion of doughy cement to caulk the upper surface of the tibia along the line of the graft and host bone. This will harden so that when the tibial cement is inserted it will not penetrate into the graft-tibial bed interface. In the first patient in whom this technique was used, this caulking technique was not used and cement spread into a segment of the interface between graft and tibia. The graft became sclerotic but there was some consolidation in the depth of the graft so that neither collapse nor prosthetic settling occurred (Fig. 6a, b, c).

Postoperative rehabilitation for these patients is the same as for those patients without bone grafting. The tibial implant support is maintained on the more normal side of the tibia and since the graft is securely fixed to the tibia, weight-bearing has not been limited in these patients. Continuous passive motion is employed on the first postoperative day in a manner analogous to that in patients without bone grafting.

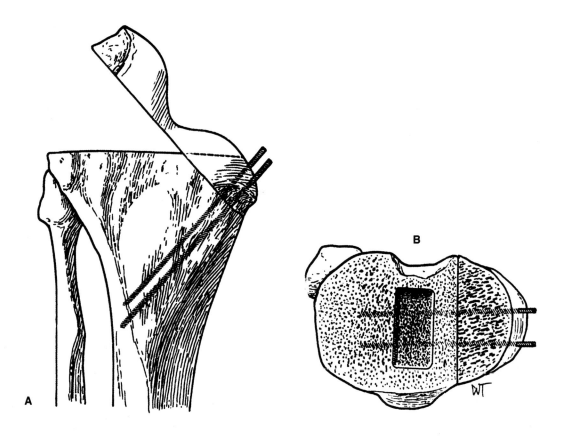

FIG. 4 A - Resected femoral condyle (only one condyle used) being apposed to tibial bed. - B Reconstitution of upper tibial surface after resection of redundant graft.

Results

Forty autogenous bone grafts to the upper tibia have been performed using the technique outlined above over the past fifteen years. The results to date have been excellent with no patient experiencing collapse of the graft and/or loss of implant position. Peripheral resorption of the graft has occurred in 15 % of patients but structural support to the tibial component has not been lost in any patient to date. Because of the complex nature of these knee deformities, a more constrained prosthesis was used in 15 of these knees. The greatest deformities treated included patients with 25 degrees of varus and 30 degrees of valgus. Revision surgery was necessary in one patient because of an incompetent medial collateral ligament after trauma to the knee five years after the primary arthroplasty. This patient was reoperated for severe recurrent valgus deformity and the graft was examined at the time of the procedure and was noted to be

completely consolidated at the interface. Early results with this series were reported by Altchek et al. (2)

Dorr et al. (3) described 24 total knee arthroplasties with proximal tibial defects treated with autogenous bone grafting. In a follow-up period of 3 to 6 years, union and revascularization was demonstrated in 22 of 24 cases by tomogram, bone scan, and bone biopsy. In the two instances in which non-union occurred, the first was attributed to insufficient preparation of the bony bed and the second failure and eventual collapse of the graft was caused by postoperative varus alignment. Clinically, 20 of the 24 postoperative knees had good or excellent results on the Hospital for Special Surgery knee score.

Windsor et al. (18) used the femoral condylar grafting method described here and in addition described a technique developed by Insall that utilizes a self-locking principle in which the bone graft is shaped into a trapezoid. The

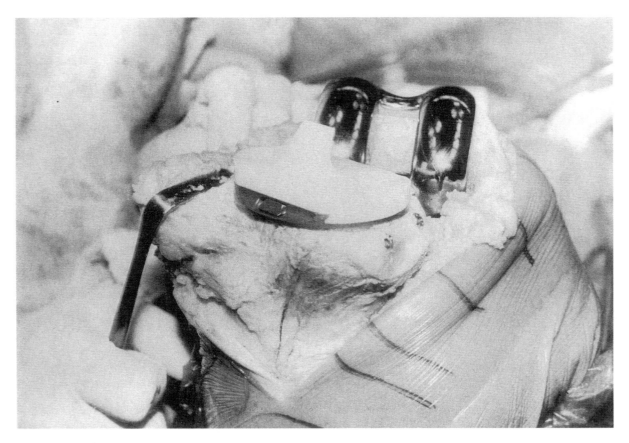

FIG. 5 - Tibial graft in place and fixed with two screws.

graft is then keyed into a created trapezoid defect on the upper tibial surface. K-wires are used to hold the bone block in place during cementing, but are subsequently removed. Over a 5 to 7 year follow-up period, clinical and radiographic results have proved excellent with no radiolucency or collapse in any cases.

Scuderi et al. (12) examined autogenous inlay bone grafting of tibial defects using the Insall technique in 26 total knee arthroplasties. The average Hospital for Special Surgery knee score postoperatively was 89 points with 25 of 26 knees demonstrating a good or excellent result and only one patient had a fair result. All grafts were incorporated within the first year with cross trabeculation between the proximal tibial bone and graft, based on serial roentgenograms. Two knees showed radiolucent lines underneath the tibial component, one of which was due to collapse of the graft, but both were less than 2 millimeters and non-progressive.

Similar results were obtained by Aglietti et al. (1) who described 17 patients with large medial tibial bony defects who underwent autologous bone grafting during total knee arthoplasty. Bone resected from the distal condyles was used to fill the defect and later permanently fixed using one or two cancellous screws. The knees were reviewed over an average of 4 years. The radiographs showed complete union in 14 knees and a partially fibrous union in 3 cases with no evidence of necrosis or collapse, confirmed by bone scans and tomograms. The knee scores demonstrated good or excellent results on 16 of 17 knees, with 1 poor result due to aseptic loosening of the femoral component attributed to excessive postoperative valgus alignment.

Laskin (7) had inferior results in comparison to those reported previously in a technique which employed the posterior femoral condyles rather than the distal femoral bone as the graft material. Twenty-six patients with tibial defects

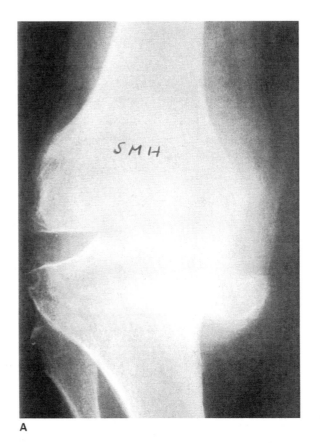

A

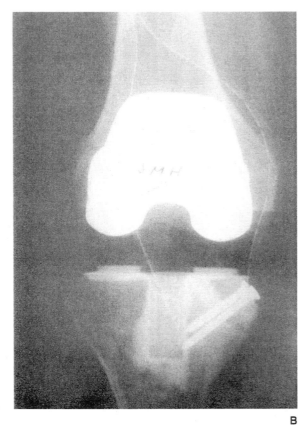

B

C

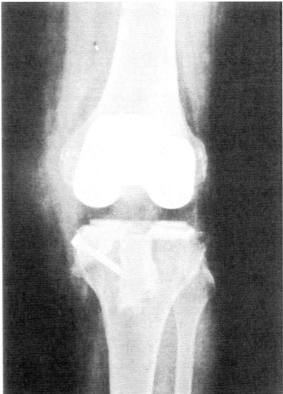

FIG. 6 A - Preoperative radiograph with severe varus deformity and bone loss. - B Immediate postoperative radiograph demonstrating methylmethacrylate in interface between graft and tibial bed. - C 12 years after tibial grafting, graft is sclerotic but has not collapsed and implant is stable.

were reported with a 67% success rate after 5 years follow-up utilizing tomograms and bone biopsy, with 4 knees demonstrating complete collapse and 4 showing radiolucency between the proximal tibia and the graft. However, the sclerotic bed was not removed when the bone graft was inserted and this may explain the inferior results. Also, the author stated that the high failure rate may have been due to excessive use of subchondral and cortical bone rather than cancellous bone. The posterior condyles of the femur consist of a predominant amount of this type of bone rather than cancellous bone seen in distal femoral condylar bone.

Tibial deficiency is almost always seen with severe deformity and particularly if it is biplane or triplane. The area of bone deficiency may be managed in a number of ways depending upon the extent and depth of the defect. Bone grafting is the preferred choice for deficiency which is greater than 12 millimeters. The distal femoral condyle offers signficant cancellous bone for grafting and because of its subchondral surface the upper tibial rim may be reconstituted as part of the grafting process. Bone augmentation by grafting allows an improved bony substrate should revision surgery be necessary. The autogenous bone can be shaped to fill the defect but it is important to the success of the technique that cancellous bone be exposed by excision of sclerotic bone at the tibial bed. Coaptation must be precise between graft and underlying bed. If the surgical technique is accurately performed bone grafting techiques for tibial deficiency have demonstrated excellent long term results in a large number of patients.

Tibial Bone Loss in Plateau Fracture

Tibial bone loss may be significant when plateau fracture occurs and despite internal fixation techniques subsequent tibial surface collapse occurs. Arthritic changes complicate the deformity present on the upper tibial surface. The areas of tibial loss in these patients may be complex and involve both the plateau itself and the tibial rim. Significant areas of depression may persist in these fractures and the tibial surface may be split. Internal fixation plates further complicate the management of these patients.

Management of Tibial Deficiency after Plateau Fracture

If the previous incision is not excessively posterior it is incorporated in the knee arthroplasty incision. Depending upon whether a medial or lateral plateau fracture is present a medial or lateral parapatellar incision is used proximally. The plate is removed after exposure of the proximal tibia. There is usually significant scar in the involved compartment and this must be resected as part of the exposure of the knee joint.

The proximal tibial osteotomy is made in the usual fashion and areas of irregular bone loss will be corrected as part of this procedure. If the remaining deficiency is primarily in the plateau surface and the rim is intact, cancellous bone can be taken from the intercondylar area or the

femoral condyles and morsellized and impacted into the depressed plateau deficit areas. If the peripheral cortical rim of the tibia has also been damaged then distal femoral bone grafting may be used as outlined in the previous section. If autogenous bone is not available to fill both the central plateau and rim defect a wedge may be used in addition to the impaction grafting of the central plateau deficiency (Fig. 7a, b).

An intramedullary press-fit stem is recommended to bypass the screw holes of the internal fixation plate if one is removed. The upper surface of the tibia should be caulked with methylmethacrylate and allowed to harden before inserting the tibial component to prevent cement interdigitating with the bone graft.

The major difficulty with these reconstructions has been wound healing especially if narrow skin flaps are created as part of the exposure. If at all possible a single incision should be used in these patients (Fig. 8). Reconstitution of the upper tibial surface with bone grafting in post-traumatic knees has been successful in most patients. Incorporation of the graft has occurred without exception in my experience.

Femoral Bone Deficiency and Bone Grafting

Angular deformity results in loss of bone both on the femoral and tibial surfaces and this must be addressed during total knee arthroplasty. The most common type of bone loss encountered is tibial plateau deficiency on the medial and posterior tibia as the result of severe varus and flexion deformity. There is associated femoral bone loss in the varus knee but it tends to be less in the distal medial femur and greater in the posterior condylar aspect of the femur. Therefore, in my experience, bone grafting is rarely necessary on the femoral side of the knee joint even in the most severe varus deformities. However, tibial grafting, presented previously, is commonly necessary in these patients.

In the severe valgus deformity the pathologic findings are somewhat different than in the varus knee. The distal lateral femoral condyle tends to be deficient to a greater extent as well as the posterior lateral condylar bone. Bone loss on the femoral side tends to be proportionally similar to what is found on the tibial side in the valgus knee. These distal and posterior surfaces of the femur tend to be extremely sclerotic and frank depression centrally may be present. Soft tissue contracture tends to be more complex on

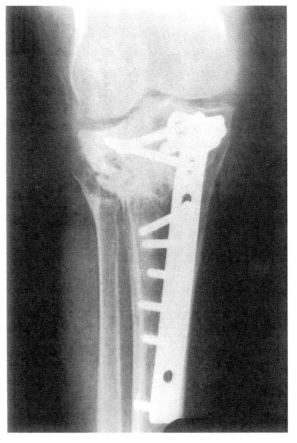 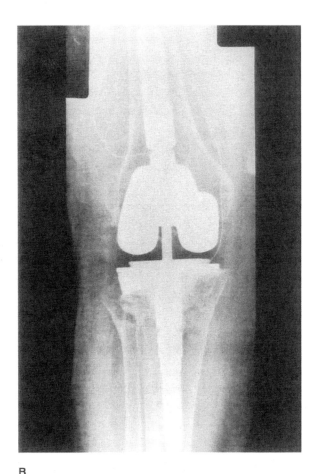

A   B

FIG. 7 A - Tibial plateau fracture treated with plate fixation with severe bone loss. B - Postoperative radiograph demonstrating bone grafting and stem fixation to bypass the screw holes of the plate.

the lateral side of the joint and both tibial and femoral releases may be necessary.

Management of distal femoral bone loss in angular deformity varies depending on extent of bone deficiency. If the deficiency is less than 10 millimeters additional bone may be removed on the opposite femoral condyle, and this will often allow insertion of the femoral component without augmentation of the deficient condyle. As in tibial defects methylmethacrylate can be used to fill small areas of bone deficiency. However, whenever possible it is preferable to achieve coaptation of the implant to the bony surface of the femur. When resecting additional bone from the femur it is important to remember the location of the joint line. In a review that I performed of fifty osteoarthritic knees the distal articular face of the femur was 18-20 millimeters distal to the lower border of the collateral

ligament origin. If this distance is maintained when the implant is inserted, then the joint line will be at approximately its correct level and the surgeon can feel confident that he has restored the joint line.

Increased amounts of distal femoral deficiency (greater than 12-15 millimeters) should be reconstructed by augmentation techniques. Autogenous bone grafting may be performed by utilizing bone from the opposite femoral condyle. The femoral condylar bone is resected from the less affected femoral condyle as it would be normally and this bone is transferred to the deficient side. This grafted bone can be held in place by two screws directly into the condylar graft. Since contact may occur between the femoral component and screws, compatible metals must be used. Care must be taken to insure that the recipient bed is primarily cancellous and that close apposition is present at the graft site. For small grafts in this area K-wire fixation alone may be sufficient. By employing this technique cancellous bone is apposed to a cancellous surface and this ensures high probability of consolidation to the underlying femur. The implant can then be placed directly on the condylar surface of the resected femoral condylar graft.

Modular implants can be used as an alternative method to deal with distal and posterior femoral bone loss. Augments are currently available which can be added to the femoral component in thicknesses to 10 millimeters. When deficiency is greater, I have cemented augments together to increase their thickness to twenty millimeters. When deficiency is of a greater magnitude combinations of distal femoral grafting and augments may be used. Augments also allow for posterior augmentation when deficiency exists. Rehabilitation has not been altered when bone grafting or modular augmentation have been used.

Aside from arthritic angular deformity, bone loss occurs on the femoral side in other clinical circumstances which are amenable to bone grafting techniques. Osteonecrosis of the femoral condyle may produce significant areas of bone destruction. Usually most of the necrotic area is resected with the distal femoral osteotomy but significant bony defects may persist. These are usually managed with morsellized cancellous bone which can be impacted into these defective areas. When the defect is significant, larger segments of cancellous bone can be harvested from the intercondylar area of the femur particularly if a cruciate substituting prosthesis is being used (Fig. 9a, b,c). This cancellous graft can be fashioned to fill these large cavities and impacted into place. The distal femoral surface can then be recreated by using a saw to smooth out the irregular surface. In employing this technique the distal femur can be restored and its face can be prepared for the femoral component.

In patients undergoing total knee replacement after prior supracondylar osteotomy or fracture, bone grafting is usually necessary to the femur if a blade or screw plate composite has been used for fixation. When these are removed from the supracondylar area large defects may be present extending to just above the area where the implant is fixed to bone. If the internal fixation is quite cephalad in the bone it may be left in place and the implant resurfacing may occur below it. However, if the placement

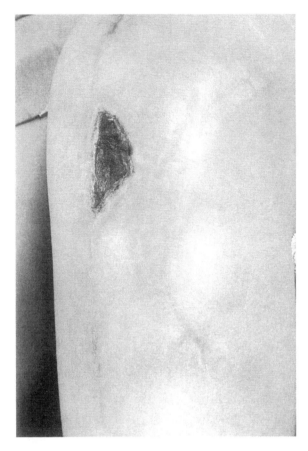

FIG. 8 - Wound slough in area between previous incision for plateau fixation and arthroplasty incision.

of the screw or blade has been lower, then a stress riser is created when the device is removed, and dealing with bone deficiency must be performed. The area where the device is removed can be filled with cancellous bone taken from the intercondylar area or from bone resected from the tibia. The cancellous graft is impacted into these defective supracondylar areas. An intramedullary stem should be used to bypass the weakened area of bone in the supracondylar zone and also to traverse the bone which has been fixed with screws. Bone graft tends to incorporate readily in these patients in my experience (Fig. 10a, b).

Bone loss on the femoral side in the primary knee tends to be less common than tibial deficiency. The principles are similar for both tibial and femoral bone loss. If defects are small and cystic, cancellous impaction techniques can be performed. If defects are larger and more exten-

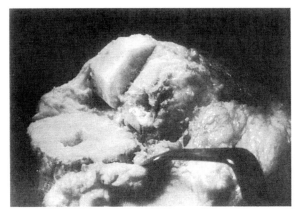

A

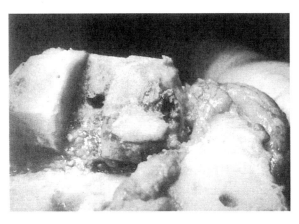

B

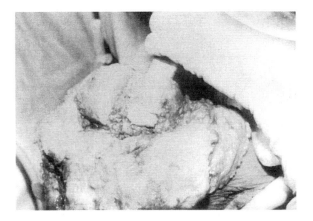

C

FIG. 9 A - Large area of osteonecrosis in femoral condyle. - B Autogenous bone graft apposed to femoral defect. - C Resection of excess autogenous femoral graft.

sive, structural autogenous grafting is necessary to provide support to the implant and effect restoration of bone stock. These structural grafts may be used alone or in combination with modular augmentation to the femoral component. Success in consolidation of these grafts requires careful technique to ensure excellent fixation of the graft and a viable bed onto which the graft is apposed. Autogenous bone is available in the primary knee which is not the case in the revision setting where allografting is an inferior technique to prosthetic augmentation.

Bone Loss in Revision Total Knee Replacement

Failure in total knee replacement requiring revision surgery is often accompanied by significant bone loss and soft tissue asymmetry. When embarking on these complex reconstructions careful preoperative planning is necessary to ensure that these deficiencies will be corrected both by surgical technique and implant selection. The type of bone defect which is present in the revision setting is dictated often by the failure mechanism of the device. A common type of bone failure leading to deficiency can be encountered as the result of excessive asymmetric load particularly in a knee in which malalignment persists after total knee replacement. This is seen in tibial component failure with collapse of the tibial plateau on the compression side of the load and lift off of the implant on the tension side of the tibia. This type of failure is common when the implant is inserted on a sloped tibial cut usually placing the component in excess varus position and the knee is in resultant malalignment.

Although less common in total knee replacement than in hip arthroplasty, osteolysis does occur and lead to bone destruction. Polyethylene debris tends to be a larger particulate size in knee replacement and the inflammatory reaction promoting osteolysis is therefore more muted in the knee. Polyethylene debris may be more catastrophic in the knee due to poor implant design and high polyethylene contact stresses. Bone destruction can be seen as a concomitant component in these knee failures.

A further cause of bone destruction and ultimate deficiency during revision surgery occurs during the surgical reconstruction itself. Poor technique can lead to major bone defects along the distal femoral and proximal tibial face. These defects are created when levering at-

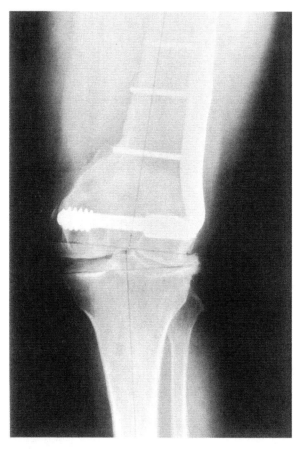

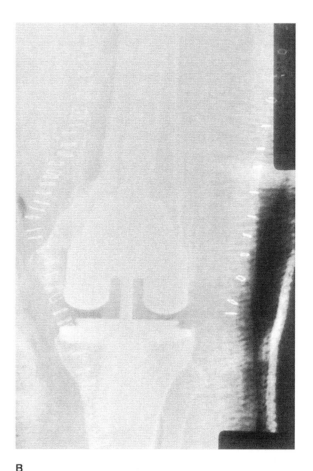

A   B

FIG. 10 A, B - Supracondylar screw plate device removed and treated with femoral grafting and stemmed implant.

tempts to remove implants are made with osteotomes against the underlying bone. It is important that all techniques to remove a cemented or non-cemented implant must be directed at
the cement-implant interface and not the bone-
cement interface. Care must also be exercised
when using slaphammer type devices to remove
implants from the femur and tibia. Fractures of
the femur and tibia may occur with considerable
bone loss as part of these procedures.

An additional mechanism for bone loss in
failed total knee replacement is the pistoning effect of the implant as subsidence is occurring.
This leads to further bone destruction and resorption with progressive bone loss.

Resultant bone loss from any of these mechanisms in revision knee replacement may be
classified into five major categories: (1) cystic,
(2) plateau or condylar defects of femur and tibia, (3) central cavitary defects, (4) fracture/per-
forations, (5) large segmental areas of tibial or
femoral bone loss. The management of these
patterns of bone loss requires knowledge and
implementation of both bone grafting and prosthetic augmentation techniques. Each of these
specific types of bone deficiency will be discussed and their management presented.

Cystic Bone Loss

Cystic bone loss occurs most frequently during removal of a cemented total knee replacement. Methylmethacrylate penetrates into subchondral bone when cementing takes place and
if arthritic cysts are present interdigitation will
take place. When cement is removed from these
areas cystic deficiencies are left on the femur
and tibia which tend to punctate and are less
than one centimenter in diameter. Additionally,

drill holes are often made into sclerotic areas of bone on the tibial and femoral surfaces to improve cement penetration and these areas will also leave cystic bone loss when cement is removed from these holes. Cystic bone deficiency is also seen when osteolysis is present and associated granulomatous inflammatory tissue penetrates into bone leaving focal areas of bone loss. These may coalesce and become quite large cavities. Osteopenic bone promotes cement penetration, and these cystic areas are more common in patients with poor bony substrate.

These cystic defects are easily handled by packing them with bone which is removed as part of the revision. Usually bone is available as the bony surfaces are recut for the revision components and this bone can be fashioned to fit these cystic areas and impacted into place. An impactor is used to compress the cancellous autogeneous bone into these defects (Fig. 11). When the cystic areas are larger autogenous bone can be mixed with allograft and inserted into these deficient areas. Consolidation occurs readily from this type of grafting and bone support for the revision components is maintained. Simple cementing into these defects can be used

to fill these areas, however, bone graft reconstitutes the bony surface and is the preferred technique. The premise of bone preservation and reconstitution is central to this philosophy of grafting rather than using methylmethacrylate as a filler.

Plateau and Condylar Bone Deficiency

Bone loss is commonly seen on the tibial surface in the failed total knee replacement. This is usually the result of prosthetic malalignment with asymmetric loading across the tibial surface. When this failure mechanism occurs a wedge shaped defect develops beneath the tibial component (Fig. 12a, b). As collapse ensues, often the implant is countersunk within the cortical rim of the tibia and a peripheral edge of bone therefore persists. These areas of tibial deficiency may be quite large depending upon the degree of plateau and collapse and defects as large as two centimeters may be seen.

In the revision setting where autogenous bone is not available to fill these defects, appropriately sized wedge augmentation to the under-

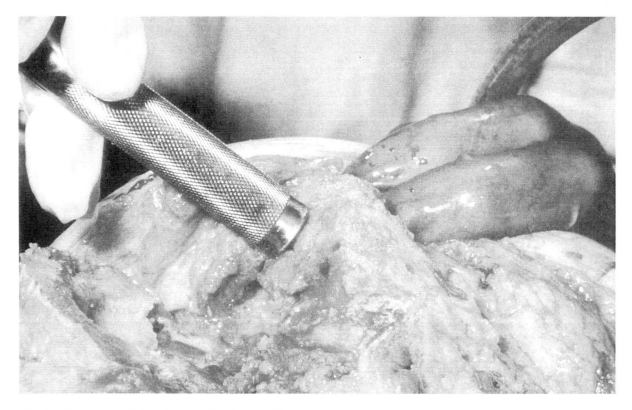

FIG. 11 - Impaction technique for cancellous bone grafting.

side of the tibial component can be used. These augments are available in various configurations and thicknesses and generally fit the wedge shaped tibial deficiency completely. This is particularly true if there is no cortical rim. The proximal tibia is cut utilizing a modified wedge tibial cutting jig to the appropriate angle of the deficiency. If the bone at the base of the defect is sclerotic after refashioning the tibial cut then drill holes can be made into this area to allow penetratioin of methylmethacrylate into bone beneath the defect. If a cortical rim of tibial bone is present, morsellized autogenous bone from the iliac crest with or without allograft may be used to fill the defect with the rim preserved. A stemmed revision component is used to bypass these areas and transfer the load into the medullary canal.

Femoral deficiency generally occurs with collapse of the underlying supporting bone to the femoral component with change of implant position and malalignment. This may evolve when there is poor quality osteoporotic bone beneath the femoral component and collapse ensues. Osteonecrosis involving a large portion of the femoral condyle can also predispose to this pattern of bone loss. Loosening of the femoral component is uncommon after total knee replacement but when it does take place with subsidence of the implant this may also lead to condylar deficiency and implant shift. Most commonly when this type of failure occurs one condyle is involved and this may be secondary to malalignment of the components and limb position (Fig. 13a, b, c).

At the time of revision for this type of failure the bone tends to be of very poor quality and these defects may be quite large. The treatment options are limited to structural allografting or femoral component augmentation and at times a combination of both techniques. Because the defects in the distal femur tend to be so local-

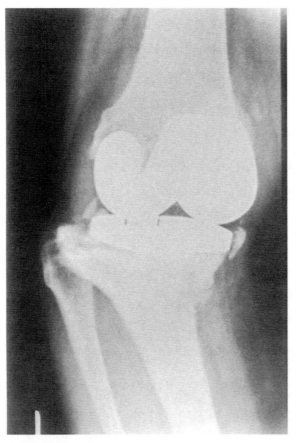

A

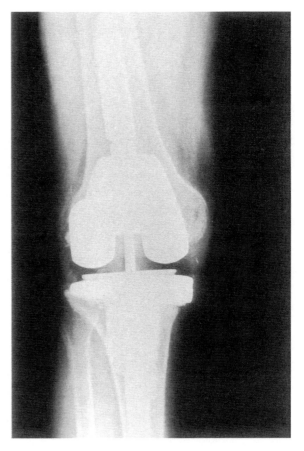

B

FIG. 12 A - Wedge-shaped bone defect with tibial component loosening. - B Wedge tibial augment to fill defect.

ized to one condyle augmentation of the distal femoral component on the defective side resolves this dilemma. A stemmed component is recommended to transfer the load into the medullary bone and away from the deficient distal femur. Currently augmentation is limited in most revision systems to a maximum of 10-12 millimeters. Augments may be cemented together to increase the amount of distal augmentation. Design of newer revision components which will have augmentation added to the distal and posterior femoral components to allow increased augmentation for larger bone defects. At this time posterior augmentation can be made inside the femoral component to fill voids in the posterior femoral condyles but augmentation cannot be added to the posterior condyles to reduce the flexion gap.

Allografting can also be performed to supplement the use of augmentations for femoral and tibial deficiency of the wedge or collapse configuration. Because of the ease at which these deficiencies can be handled with augmentation of the components, full structural allografts are generally not used in these situations.

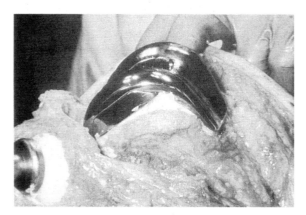

A

B

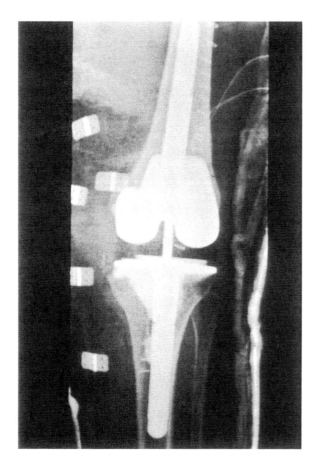

C

FIG. 13 A - Femoral condylar bone loss with marked valgus deformity. - B Lateral femoral augmentation to fill femoral defect. - C Postoperative radiograph demonstrating correction of valgus deformity.

Central Cavitary Bone Deficiency

Central cavitary bone deficiency may occur in both the distal femur or upper tibia. These deficiencies are usually present when stemmed components are removed particularly in osteoporotic bone. The pattern of deficiency tends to be of a funnel type with absence of intramedullary bone and a cortical rim which is usually present. The goal in the management of these deficiencies is to provide structural support to the cavity and attempt to reconstitute biologically the major loss of bone present in these cases. Allografting is necessary in these patients and morsellized bone graft may be used or composites with structural allograft and morsellized bone as a supplement to improve graft to host bone contact.

Femoral head allografts can be shaped to fit these defects and will fill large cavitary defects in most cases. The femoral head is shaped to fit the defect and impacted in place in the distal femur or proximal tibia. Load must be transferred to medullary canal in these patients in that implant support may be poor at the face of the distal femur and proximal tibia. Press fit stems are used which are fluted to improve the stability of the revision component within the deficient bone. In order to accomodate these stems the femoral head is cored with graduated drills until the desired stem diameter has been reached. The allograft is then impacted into the deficiency and the stemmed implant seated through the allograft. Morsellized bone is used to fill smaller deficiencies around the allograft and improve the fit of the stem itself. Often associated wedge defects may be present in the upper tibia or distal femur and these can be managed with augmentation of the implant as described for plateau and condylar defects (Fig. 14a, b, c).

Perforations and Fracture

In patients with multiple knee replacement revisions or poor quality bone perforations or fracture of the upper tibia or distal femur may occur. This most commonly develops during the process of implant and cement removal. In noncemented porous implants which are well-fixed bone loss may also occur during the removal process. If perforation occurs it is important that it is noted at the time of the revision and a stemmed component should be used which bypasses this perforation by at least three centimeters must be used. If tibial or femoral bone is fractured more severely internal fixation should be performed to reconstitute a tubular configuration of the femur or tibia and then stemmed components used to transfer load distal to the fractured area. Allografting and autografting should be performed to reinforce these areas of fracture and perforation.

Segmental Bone Loss

Segmental bone loss of distal femur and proximal femur may occur in patients with multiple revision procedures. Additional injury to bone in patients with deficient bony substrate will lead to devascularized and necrotic bone with large areas of bone deficiency. The attempt at fracture repair in the supracondylar fracture after total knee replacement will often further devascularize bone and lead to large areas of collapse and malalignment. These are catastrophic events and require considerable preoperative planning and skill to effect a stable construct and restore knee joint function.

The management of these segmental defects can be by replacement of bone with an allograft or by a custom or modular implant. If the deficiency is extensive the ligamentous support to the knee is often absent and a constrained implant or hinge device may be necessary to restore knee joint stability. If allografting is used a step cut may be made in the remaining distal femur or proximal tibia and locked into a step cut made in the allograft. The implant is cemented into the allograft and the stems may be cemented or press fit into the host bone. Supplemental strut allografting is used to reinforce the zone of contact between the host and graft bone. If allografting is utililized to deal with these defects several potential problems may arise. Infection is greater in these patients as reported by both Lord (8) and Ghazavi (4). Lord and co-workers (8) reported a 12 per cent infection rate in a series of 283 cases in which massive allografts were used. Ghazavi and co-workers (4) reported three infections in massive allografts in revision knee replacement in a group of 30 patients. Non-union at the allograft-host junction and fracture of the allograft may also occur in these patients. Rehabilitation and weight-bearing is advanced slowly in patients with large allografts. Allografting is the preferred method of treatment in younger patients where all attempts must be made to restore bone stock should further revision surgery be necessary at a later date.

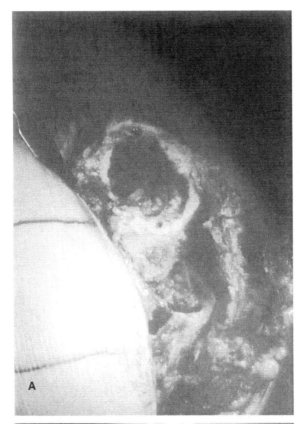

A

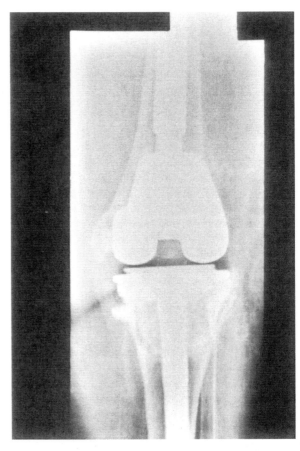

B

C

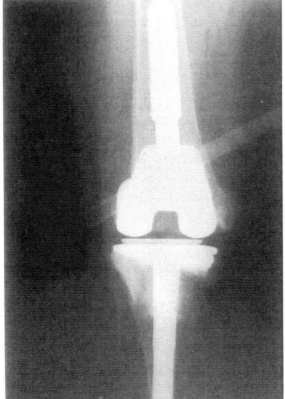

Fig. 14 A - Central cavitary tibial after implant removal. - B Postoperative radiograph of femoral allograft to fill tibial defect. - C 4 year postoperative radiograph demonstrating graft incorporation.

Allografts are non-viable bone and incorporation can occur at the host-graft interface but the bulk of the graft remains dead. Despite this the structural qualities of allografts remain and provide the support necessary for knee function in these complex cases. Revascularization and excessive loading of the graft should be avoided as this promotes resorption of the graft and increases potential for graft collapse. Stemmed components aid in unloading these grafts and transferring the loads away from the graft itself.

Commonly these large segmental areas of bone loss occur in the elderly or low demand patient. Underlying bone is osteoporotic and this contributes to the major loss of bone. Rapid return of ambulatory function is crucial to these patients if the complication of immobility in the elderly patient is to be avoided. Modular implants which substitute for large segmental areas of bone loss is the preferred method in these patients. These can be modified to fill the voids of bone which are present. A hinge type articulation is usually present in these modular segmental devices and this provides immediate stability to the construct. The bone is replaced and ligamentous stability is provided with these devices and the patient can be mobilized and allowed to bear weight on the limb immediately. The need for graft consolidation is obviated with these devices and in the geriatric patient rapid recovery of ambulation is achieved (Fig. 4a, b)

Results with Bone Grafting In Revision Total Knee Replacement

The results with bone grafting in the revision setting must be considered differently depending upon the nature of the underlying deficiency and the type of grafting performed. For localized areas of bone deficiency where morsellized allograft is adequate results have been excellent. Whitesides (16) has reported on the results of 56 cementless revisions. The morsellized bone was taken from a femoral head and all 56 knees demonstrated increased density in the grafted zone. New bony trabeculation was seen in 15 knees with femoral grafting and 21 knees with tibial grafting. Thirty (54%) of the patients had no pain, 17 (30%) had mild pain, 5 (9%) had mild pain and 4 (7%) had severe pain. A stemmed non-cemented component was used in all cases and engagement of the stem against the cortical bone of the isthmus was achieved in all patients. Supplemental screws were used into the tibial baseplate to improve fixation of the implant to bone.

Samuelson (11) reported on a series of contained defects at revision knee replacement utilizing finely milled bone, larger (5-8mm) fragments of bone or larger allograft segments. Of the larger allografts, one on the tibial side and two on the femur did not incorporate. As a rule patients were pleased with the result and 21 patients had mild or no pain.

Ullmark and Hovelius (15) reviewed a small series of three patients treated with impacted intramedullary morsellized allograft similar to the Ling technique for bone grafting of the femoral canal during total hip revision. These patients were followed for 18-28 months and radiographs reviewed. New cortical bone formation was noted in one patient, one patient demonstrated renewed trabecular bone and the third patient showed no bony incorporation. All patients were pain free, however, without absence of implant failure.

Dorr and co-workers (3) reported on 14 revision total knee arthroplasties in which bone grafting was employed. Follow-up evaluation in this series was minimum three years with a range of 3-6 years. The site of the graft varied considerably with local bone being used in 9 procedures, 4 iliac crest grafts and 1 femoral head allograft. The graft failed in 2 cases with only 5 patients achieving an excellent result. There were three patients who required a second revision procedure, one patient with a dislocated implant, one patient with a loose femoral component and one patient who became infected.

Larger allografts in revision knee arthroplasty have tended to incorporate in a diverse group of reports. Harris and co-workers (5) utilized massive allografts in 14 patients with conventional knee implants. Twelve of these patients underwent grafting during revision knee arthroplasty. All revision patients showed evidence of bony incorporation with remodelling at the junction between the allograft and host bone. An excellent result was obtained in six patients, the remaining six patients were considered good results. There were two major complications in this series: a dislocation of the implant and an injury to the anterior tibial artery. The authors proposed five principles with massive allografting techniques in total knee arthroplasty revision: (1) the allograft should be completely fixed with internal fixation, (2) the prosthesis should be cemented to the allograft, (3) there should be respect for the investing soft tissue envelope, (4) the graft should not be trimmed, (5) these grafts may transmit infection and this is a potential danger with the technique.

Tsahakis and co-workers (14) in a series of 19 allografts in 15 revision total knee replacements reported incorporation in all cases. Distal femoral allografts were used in six patients, proximal tibial allografts in 4 patients, and femoral head allografts in 9 patients. Full incorporation of graft to host bone interface occurred by one year. The knee score improved from 29 points to 87 points and the function score increased from 33 points to 85 points. There was no allograft collapse, and there were no infections.

Results with twelve revision total knee arthroplasties utilizing large tibial allografts were documented by Wilde and co-workers (17). Five cases had a contained defect which was treated with appropriately fashioned block allograft of cancellous bone and 7 cases had uncontained defects treated with large structural corticocancellous allografts. On standard radiographs normal trabecular patterns were seen between the graft and the host bone at an average of twenty three months after surgery in 11 of 12 knees. Single photon-emission computed tomography scans were done in 5 patients and 4 showed uniform uptake to demonstrate ongoing incorporation. The one patient who did not have activity on scanning did have trabeculation on routine radiographs. A Total Condylar III prosthesis was necessary in 11 of the 12 patients in this series. There was no evidence of graft collapse and no infections. Seven cases were excellent, 2 good and 2 fair.

Mow and Wiedel (10) reported on 13 patients undergoing revision total knee replacement in which 15 structural allografts were used. Follow-up averaged 47 months and all grafts showed healing at the host-graft junction. There were no infections and no allograft collapse in this series. Overall HSS scores in these patients improved from 47 preoperatively to 86 postoperatively.

Mnaymneh and co-workers (9) reviewed the results of 14 allografts in 10 patients undergoing revision total knee arthroplasty. There were 3 distal femoral allografts, 3 proximal tibial grafts and 4 patients with both femoral and tibial grafts. The grafts were quite large and ranged from 6-16 centimeters on the femoral side and 3-11 centimeters on the tibial side. Constrained implants were used in 7 cases with a hinge being used in 2 patients. The allografts were secured to underlying host bone with both intramedullary stem and extramedullary plate and screw fixation. All seven tibial allografts united and five of seven femoral grafts incorporated. Two patients demonstrated inadequate healing at the ligament-allograft junction and one patient had a late infection. There was one dislocation in this series. Follow-up was from 26-69 months and averaged 40 months. The patients had severe bone loss and HSS scores improved but to only 67 in this complex series of patients.

Infection was noted to be more of a problem in allografts for revision total knee replacement in a series by Stockley and co-workers (13). There were 32 allografts used in 18 revision and 2 complex primary arthroplasties in this group of patients with large bone defects. Average follow-up in this series was 4.2 years. All grafts went on to incorporate but two grafts fractured and there were three deep infections in the group. These infections were attributed to persistent infection from previous implant surgery.

Management of supracondylar fracture after total knee replacement can be particularly difficult if bone is severely osteoporotic. Marked comminution may occur and obviate the ability to internally fix these fractures. Kraay and co-workers (6) reported on the results of four patients undergoing distal femoral replacement with allograft/prosthetic reconstruction for treatment of these complex supracondylar fractures in patients with total knee arthroplasties. All patients were followed for at least two years and the average knee score was 83. One patient went on to full union and one to a partial union at the graft site. There was no evidence of allograft resorption or mechanical failure of the allograft in these patients.

Technique of bone grafting in revision total knee arthroplasty has to be individualized to the bone deficiency present at the time of the revision. Careful preoperative planning is mandatory to determine the exact degree of bone loss. Three dimensional scanning procedures can be of help in these more complex cases. A full array of modular implants with varying degrees of constraint are often necessary to supplement the bone grafting procedures performed, and thorough preoperative planning facilitates this. Grafting techniques may be as simple as using available bone to fill small craters and defects. More substantial loss requires the use of bulk allografts from femoral head or distal femur and proximal tibia. These must be well-fixed and as a rule cementing the allograft to a stemmed revision knee component is the best technique. Overall results reported have been encouraging but these cases are among the most challenging and should be approached with considerable experience in total knee arthroplasty. Underlying bone and soft tissue substrate is poor in these cases and if technical difficulties are encountered because of inadequate experience of planning results may be severely compromised.

References

1) Aglietti P, Buzzi R, Scrobe F.: Autologous bone grafting for medial tibial defects in total knee arthroplasty. J. Arthroplasty 1991, 6 (4): 287-294.

2) Altchek D, Sculco TP, Rawlins B.: Autogenous bone grafting for severe angular deformity in total knee arthroplasty. J. Arthroplasty 1989, 4 (2): 151-155.

3) Dorr LD, Ranawat CS, Sculco TP, McKaskill B, Oriesek BS.: Bone grafting for tibial defects in total knee arthroplasty. Clin Orthop. 1986, 205:153-165.

4) Ghazavi MT, StockleyI, Yee G, et al.: Reconstruction of massive bone defects with allograft in revision total knee arthroplasty. J. Bone Joint Surg. 79: 17-27, 1997.

5) Harris AI, Poddar S, Gitelis S. et al.: Arthroplasty with composite of an allograft and a prosthesis for knees with severe deficiency of bone. J. Bone Joint Surg. 77A: 373-80, 1995.

6) Kraay Mj, Goldberg VM, Figgie MP. et al.: Distal femoral replacement with allograft/prosthetic reconstruction for treatment of supracondylar fractures in patients with total knee arthroplasty. J. Arthroplasty, 7:7-16, 1992.

7) Laskin RS: Total knee arthroplasty in the presence of large bony defects of the tibia and marked knee instability. Clin Orthop. 1989; 248:66-70.

8) Lord CF, Gebhardt MC, Tomford, WW, et al.: Infection in bone grafts: incidence, nature, and treatment. J. Bone Joint Surg. 70A: 369-74, 1988.

9) Mnaymneh,W, Emerson RH, Borja F et al.: Massive allograft in salvage revision of failed total knee arthroplasty. Clin Orthop. 260:144-152, 1990.

10) Mow CS, Wiedel JD.: Structural allografting in revision total knee arthroplasty. J Arthroplasty. 11:235-243, 1996.

11) Samuelson KM.: Bone grafting and noncemented revision arthroplasty of the knee. Clin Orthop. 226:93-101, 1988.

12) Scuderi GR, Insall JN, Haas SB, Becker-Fluegel MW, Windsor RE: Inlay autogenic bone grafting of tibial defects in primary total knee arthroplasty. Clin Orthop. 1989, 248:93-97.

13) Stockley I, McAuley JP, Gross AE: Allograft reconstruction in total knee arthroplasty. J. Bone Joint Surg. 74B:393-402, 1992.

14) Tsahakis PJ, Beaver WB, Brick GW: Technique and results of allograft reconstruction in revision total knee replacement. Clin Orthop. 303: 86-93, 1994.

15) Ullmark G, Hovelius L.: Impacted morsellized allograft and cement for revision total knee arthroplasty: A preliminary report of 3 cases. Acta Orthop Scand. 67 (1): 10-18, 1996.

16) Whiteside LA.: Cementless revision total knee arthroplasty. Clin Orthop. 286:160-170, 1993.

17) Wilde AH, Schickendabtz MS, Stulberg BN, et al. The incorporation of tibial allograft in total knee arthroplasty. J Bone Joint Surg. 72A: 815-822, 1990.

18) Windsor RE, Insall JN, Sculco TP. Bone grafting of tibial defect in primary and revision total knee arthroplasty. Clin Orthop. 1986, 205:132-137.

Chapter 8
Total Knee Arthroplasty Following High Tibial Osteotomy

Charles L. Nelson, Steven B. Haas
The Hospital For Special Surgery - New York

Valgus high tibial osteotomy has been advocated for the treatment of isolated medial compartment osteoarthritis. Successful results have been obtained in eighty to ninety percent of patients in the short term (1). However, with longer follow-up progressive arthritic deterioration has developed in more patients requiring conversion to total knee arthroplasty (1). Conversion of a high tibial osteotomy to a total knee arthroplasty introduces unique challenges not typically encountered during primary total knee arthroplasty.

The results of total knee arthroplasty following high tibial osteotomy have varied in the literature with some reports describing results comparable to primary total knee arthroplasty (2-4), and others describing results approaching those of revision total knee arthroplasty (5-7). The discrepancy between these series may be secondary to the fact that knees requiring knee replacement following high tibial osteotomy represent a heterogeneous group, with varying degrees of coronal and sagittal plane deformity, bone loss ligament imbalance, patella infera and soft tissue compromise. Conversion of a high tibial osteotomy without significant preoperative deformity, without patella infera, and without a compromised soft tissue envelope is probably similar to a primary total knee arthroplasty both in terms of technical difficulty and results. On the other hand, converting a severely overcorrected high tibial osteotomy with marked lateral soft tissue scarring, medial and posteromedial ligamentous laxity and significant patella infera, probably approaches a revision total knee arthroplasty in terms of technical difficulty, need for more constrained prostheses, and anticipated results.

Indications

Conversion of a high tibial osteotomy to a total knee arthroplasty is recommended when a patient having undergone a previous high tibial osteotomy develops knee pain unresponsive to conservative or minimally invasive measures. The history, physical examination and radiologic studies should demonstrate that the patient's knee pain is secondary to a degenerative or arthritic condition involving the knee. Extra-articular sources of knee pain such as referred or radicular pain from the hip or lower back should be ruled out. The surgeon should attempt to exclude poorly understood pain syndromes such as reflex sympathetic dystrophy. Inflammatory conditions of the soft tissue about the knee must be excluded as well, as these are not likely to benefit from total knee arthroplasty. Total knee arthroplasty may not be indicated for patients with intra-articular loose bodies or meniscal pathology. These conditions may benefit from arthroscopic procedures depending on the degree of arthritic involvement.

Total knee arthroplasty is obviously inappropriate when the patient in unlikely to benefit from procedure, or is likely to be made worse. Once infection, reflex sympathetic dystrophy, and additional sources of pain unlikely to respond to total knee arthroplasty have been effectively screened, additional relative contraindications for total knee arthroplasty following high tibial ostetomy include Charcot arthropathy, medical comorbidities which predispose to unacceptable risk, and soft tissue coverage problems that either are not reconstructable or where reconstruction is inappropriate. The patient needs to understand the occupational and recreational restrictions imposed by a total knee arthroplasty prior to the surgical procedure.

Preoperative Planning

Preoperative planning is critical once a decision to proceed with total knee arthroplasty in a patient with a previous high tibial osteotomy has been finalized. The history, physical examination, and radiographic studies should be reviewed for evidence of severely overcorrected high osteotomies, or excessively unstable knee. Both of these situation may be associated with a poorer prognosis, and may require special surgical techniques or more constrained implants. The type of hardware utilized to stabilize the previously performed high tibial osteotomy may also dictate the type of prosthesis required. For example, following removal of a plate, utilization of a tibial tray with a stem augment may be necessary to bypass old screw tracts and avoid creation of stress risers.

The condition of the soft tissue is critical to preoperative planning in these cases. The configuration and number of previous incisions should be noted. When there is significant concern that wound healing may be compromised, the surgeon may wish to remove the hardware, allow wound healing, and perform the total knee arthroplasty several weeks later as a second stage. In one se-

ries which reported a higher complication rate for total knee arthroplasty following high tibial osteotomy than for total knee arthroplasty following failed unicompartmental arthroplasty, the higher complication rate was secondary exclusively to wound problems, or infections directly related to wound problem (8).

Evaluation of radiographs must be performed with an understanding that the previous osteotomy procedure alters the anatomy of proximal tibia. Because of the flare of the proximal tibia, the width at the proximal site of the osteotomy is greater than at the distal site of the osteotomy. Maintenance of the medial periosteal hinge with removal of the laterally based wedge and closure of the wedge shaped defect changes the shape of the proximal tibia. Following high tibial osteotomy, there is a step-off at the lateral proximal metaphysis resulting in a more pronounced tibial flare at the lateral proximal tibial metaphysis. The tibial medullary canal becomes more offset medially relative to the tibial articular surface. In addition, because there was a greater quantity of bone removed from the lateral side than the medial side at the time of the prior osteotomy procedure, the proximal tibial articular surface usually has a valgus configuration rather than the normal three degrees of varus configuration. Consequently, preoperative planning will usually indicate resection of a greater amount of bone from the medial tibial plateau than from the lateral tibial plateau (6).

The anatomy of the proximal tibia is altered in the sagittal plane as well. Because the osteotomy is performed in the metaphyseal region where the posterior slope of the tibia changes from seven degrees at the articular surface to neutral at the tibial diaphysis, there is a tendency toward decrease of the normal posterior slope of the articular surface with removal of the wedge. Moreover, the technical difficulty in making the osteotomy cuts perpendicular to the long axis of the tibia in the sagittal plane has resulted in more significant decreases in the normal posterior slope of the tibia in many cases than would be anticipated. A previous study has documented the decrease in the normal posterior slope of the tibial articular surface following high tibial osteotomy (6). In some cases the slope is even reversed to an anterior slope. These patients also have a higher incidence of patella infera (Fig. 1) (6, 9). This is believed to be secondary to scarring of the patellar tendon following the osteotomy procedure, or contracture of the patellar tendon during immobilization. A recent study suggested the incidence of patella infera following high tibial osteotomy

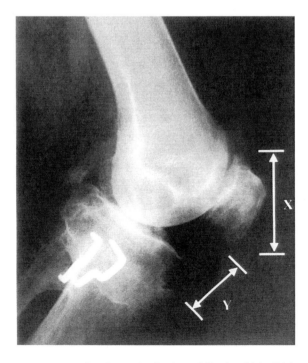

FIG. 1 - Lateral radiograph of a knee following high tibial osteotomy demonstrating patella infera. Note that the Insall-Salvati ratio (X/Y) of length of the patella to the distance from the inferior pole of the patella to the tibial tubercle is greater than 1:20.

was less in patients in whom early range of motion of the knee was begun following the osteotiomy procedure (Fig. 2) (10).

We routinely obtain a standing anteroposterior, lateral and Merchant view of the involved knee. We strongly recommend templating the radiographs preoperatively, as in some cases where the medullary canal is excessively offset medially, a custom or noninventory component with an offset stem may be required (Fig. 3). Preoperative templating in some cases allows determination of the necessity of removal of hardware. This may be more safely performed as a separate procedure prior to total knee arthroplasty to decrease risks of wound problems at the time of total knee arthroplasty. The presence of patella infera can be determined from the lateral radiograph as described by Insall and Salvati (11). Patella infera results in more difficult exposure and increases the risk of avulsion of the patellar tendon insertion during surgery (5, 6). The inclination of the tibial plateau can also be determined from the lateral radiograph. Anterior slope of the tibia may

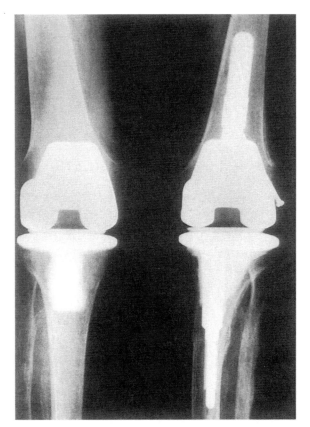

FIG. 3 - Anteroposterior radiograph demonstrating the use of a prosthesis with a custom medially offset stem for a total knee arthroplasty following high tibial osteotomy on the left side.

result in excessive posterior bone removal during tibial resection (6). The medial and lateral thickness of the resected specimen can be templated and compared to the resected specimen at the time of surgery, providing an additional clue to alignment. In some cases, bone grafting or augments may be required to replace bone loss secondary to overcorrected tibial osteotomies.

Surgical Techniques

Antibiotics are administered prior to induction of anesthesia. Following induction of anesthesia, prep and drape of the lower extremity are performed in standard fashion. The total knee arthroplasty procedure can be performed with or without tourniquet control, although we typically utilize a tourniquet. The incision is determined based upon prior knee incisions and the need for hardware removal as outlined below.

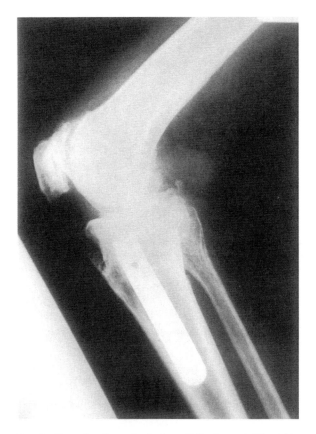

FIG. 2 - Lateral radiograph of a knee following a rigidly stabilized high tibial osteotomy in which early postoperative motion was instituted demonstrating the absence of patella infera.

Previous transverse incisions can be ignored, and a standard anterior midline incision can be made (6). If staples were utilized for fixation, these can be left in place so long as they do not preclude resection of the tibia at a suitable level to create a stable platform. If necessary, staples can be bent to allow passage of the tibial stem or keel (Fig. 4). When removal of staples is necessary, this can generally be performed through the anterior midline incision by raising a full thickness flap laterally without major risk of wound compromise (Fig. 5). It is critical that skin flaps be developed below the deep fascia to maximize perfusion to the overlying skin and minimize the risk of wound complication in these patients.

Following prior lateral longitudinal incisions, several options exist. The best option for a particular patient depends on the following factors: the wound healing status of the particular host; the exact location of the prior lateral longitudinal in-

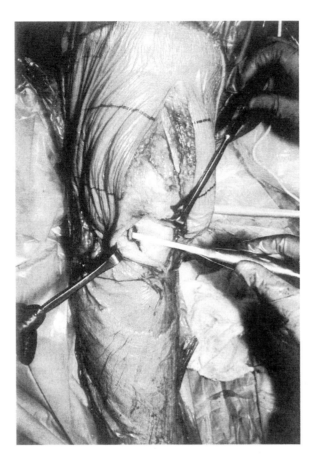

FIG. 5 - Intraoperative photograph demonstrating staple removal through a midline anterior incision. Care must be taken to maintain dissection bellow the deep fascia during development of the lateral flap. A narrow osteotome is useful to initially disengage the staple from the tibia. Needle nosed pliers can then be utilized to extract the staple.

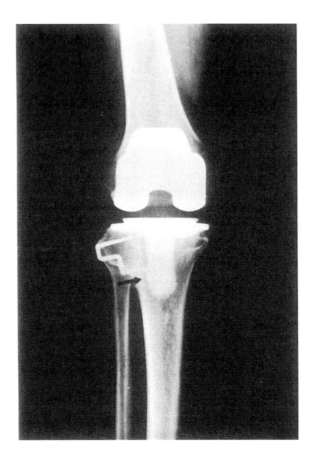

FIG. 4 - Anteroposterior radiograph of the right knee following conversion of a high tibial osteotomy to a total knee arthroplasty demonstrating fracture of the staple (arrow) in order to allow placement of a tibial component without hardware removal.

cision; and the surgeon's experience and technical expertise, A more medial than normal anterior midline longitudinal incision can be utilized, leaving as large a skin bridge as possible. Previous experience with tibial pilon fractures and skin flaps suggests maintaining a skin bridge of at least a 7 cm (Fig. 6) (12,13). This option may not provide sufficient exposure for removal of lateral hardware, particularly in cases involving internal fixation with blade plates or L-plates. In this case, we recommend removing the hardware prior to the total knee arthroplasty, allowing wound healing, and subsequently performing the arthroplasty procedure as a second stage several weeks latter. Alternatively, the lateral longitudinal incision can be utilized, allowing removal of the implant and exposure of the knee through a lateral parapatellar arthrotomy (14, 15). This approach often

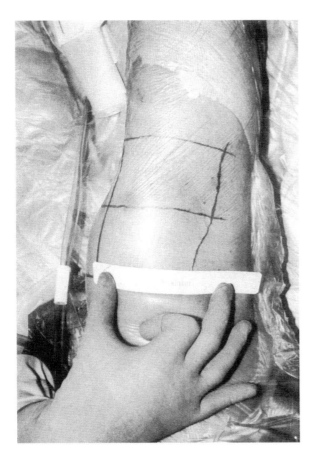

FIG. 6 - Photograph demonstrating proper planning of a midline longitudinal incision in a patient who underwent a previous high tibial osteotomy through a lateral longitudinal incision. The midline longitudinal incision has been positioned in order to maintain a wide skin bridge (8.5 cm). In most cases a skin bridge of at least 7 cm is possible without compromising exposure of the knee.

lateral longitudinal incision and the oblique incision should be between forty-five and sixty degrees to minimize the risk of wound healing problems (16). This approach has been successfully utilized at our institution to remove lateral L-shaped plates and blade plates and to perform medial arthrotomies as a single stage following prior lateral longitudinal incisions without subsequent wound healing problems. A more conservative option involves exposure of the knee through an anterior midline incision, maintaining at least a 7 cm skin bridge. The distal screws can generally be removed without difficulty through the anterior midline incision by raising a small full thickness flap laterally deep to the deep fascia, and

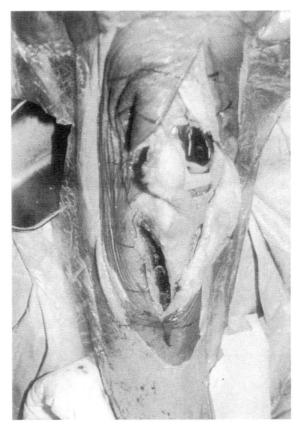

FIG. 7 - Intraoperative photograph of the right knee following removal of a lateral blade plate and implantation of total knee components as a single procedure. Note that the distal aspect of the lateral longitudinal incision was utilized for removal of the blade plate. The incision was then carried obliquely at the level of the tibial tubercle across the patella to the mid thigh. A sixty degree angle was maintained between the unutilized proximal aspect of the previous lateral longitudinal incision and the oblique medial extension. This patient had had the same technique utilized on left knee at the time of conversion to total knee arthroplasty. The wounds of both knees healed uneventfully.

requires a tibial tubercle osteotomy in order to evert the patella and expose the knee adequately. A third option involves utilizing the distal aspect of the lateral longitudinal incision, and extending the incision obliquely in a medial direction at the patella. Plate removal can be performed from the distal aspect of the incision (Fig. 7). The fascia over the tibialis anterior is incised along the tibial flare just distal to Gerdy's tubercle leaving a small cuff for repair. The muscle is then stripped in a subperiosteal fashion being careful not to injure the anterior tibial artery as it enters the anterior compartment. Following plate removal, a flap developed deep to the deep fascia and superficial to the patellar tendon and tibial tubercle allowing a standard medial parapatellar arthrotomy to be performed through this incision. We recommend that the angle between the proximal aspect of the

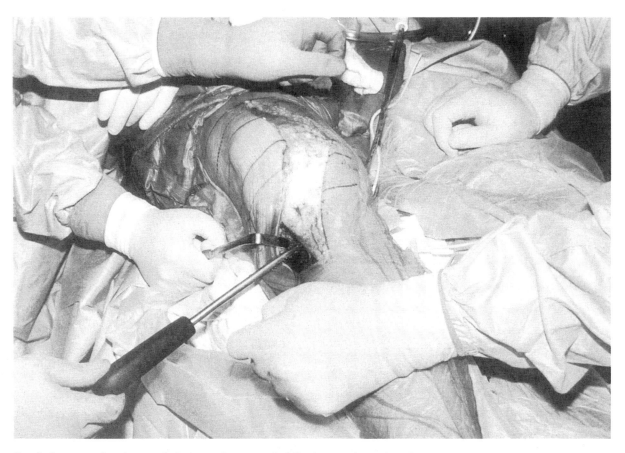

FIG. 8 - Intraoperative photograph demonstrating removal of distal screws from a lateral L-plate through a midline longitudinal incision following development of a short full thickness skin flap.

stripping the tibialis anterior in a subperiosteal fashion, and exposing the screws (Fig. 8). Removal of the proximal posterior screws of an L-plate is completed through a 1-2 cm incision in line with the prior lateral incision (Fig. 9). The plate is extracapsular, typically it is firmly adherent to the underlying bone, and can be left in place as it does not preclude placement of the tibial component (Fig. 10). This technique minimizes trauma to the lateral soft tissues, thereby minimizing the risk of wound complications. Utilization of a small portion of a prior lateral longitudinal incision is also applicable following extreme posterior placement of staples through such an incision (Fig. 11), where removal through an anterior midline incision is not possible.

Inverted L-shaped incisions allow anterior midline incisions by utilizing the longitudinal limb of the prior incision as the inferior aspect of the longitudinal incision and extending the incision in a proximal direction (6). The result is an incision similar to the anterior midline incision utilized with a prior transverse incision, with the

exception that in some cases the incision may end more laterally secondary to placement of the longitudinal limb of the prior inverted L-shaped incision. In this case a small full thickness medial flap may need to be raised to allow medial parapatellar arthrotomy.

We prefer to expose the knee through a medial parapatellar arthrotomy. Surgeons interested in performing lateral parapatellar arthrotomies with concurrent tibial tubercle osteotomies are referred to approach as described by Buechell (14). We prefer to make the distal aspect of our arthrotomy 1 cm medial to the patellar tendon. The resulting cuff of tissue adds support to the patellar tendon, decreasing the chance of avulsion, and facilitates closure of the arthrotomy at the completion of the case (6). A medial subperiosteal sleeve is developed with a scalpel, being careful to protect the medial collateral ligament. Elevation of the scarred patellar tendon from the proximal tibia may be necessary to allow eversion, however, care must be exercised to not disrupt the patellar tendon insertion into the tibial tubercle.

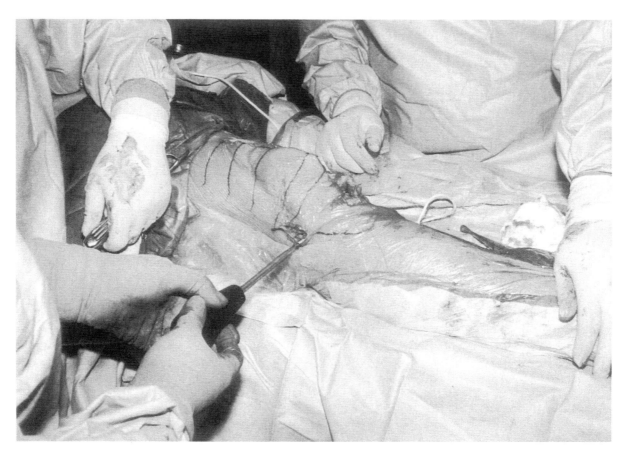

FIG. 9 - Intraoperative photograph demonstrating removal of a proximal L-plate screw through a short lateral incision incorporated within the patients prior to lateral longitudinal incision.

The fat pad is released from the lateral meniscus. In many cases, particularly cases with patella infera, there may be difficulty with patellar eversion. Tight lateral structures need to be released. In some cases, a formal lateral retinacular release may be necessary prior to patellar eversion to prevent excessive tension on the patellar tendon insertion. A pin through the patellar tendon and tibial tubercle helps protect against avulsion of the patellar tendon insertion. If patellar eversion cannot be performed safely at this stage, a rectus snip may be required. Rarely is a quadriceps V-Y plasty or tibial tubercle osteotomy necessary. Following eversion of the patella, the knee is flexed with the foot externally rotated to protect the patellar tendon insertion. Generous release of the patellofemoral ligaments facilitates exposure of the lateral tibial plateau without undue tension on the patellar tendon insertion.

Exposure of the knee is completed with incision of the anterior cruciate ligament, and anterior subluxation of the tibia. We recommend use of an extramedullary guide during the tibial resec-

tion. The medullary canal may be displaced medially secondary to the previous osteotomy procedure potentially making intramedullary assessment less accurate. The tibial resection should remove minimal bone from the more deficient side allowing for the creation of a stable platform perpendicular to the long axis of the tibia. Usually this results in a greater thickness of resected bone medially (Fig. 12). When resection of more than five to ten millimeters of bone from the medial side is necessary in order to create a stable platform, we recommend utilization of metal augments or allografts to substitute for the deficient bone and utilization of a stemmed tibial component rather than excessive bony resection. If an anterior slope of the tibial articular surface was noted on the preoperative lateral radiograph, we recommend resection of the tibia be done with a minimal posterior slope to avoid creating an excessively large flexion gap in comparison to the extension gap. If the knee is subsequently noted to be tight in flexion, a second tibial resection creating a normal posterior slope can be per-

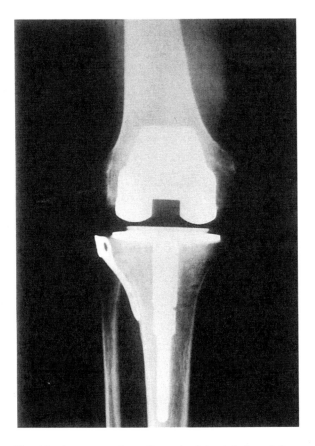

FIG. 10 - Anteroposterior radiograph of the right knee following conversion of a high tibial osteotomy to a total knee arthroplasty demonstrating removal of screws allowing placement of the tibial component without plate removal. Note the stem extension on the tibial component bypassing potential stress risers following screw removal.

formed. The resected specimen should be compared to the anticipated resection from the preoperative template. The tibial alignment is checked using an alignment block and rod. In cases of marked bone loss or severely overcorrected high tibial osteotomies, bone grafting or augments may be required for deficiencies of the lateral tibial plateau.

Following tibial resection, the femur is prepared at the discretion of the operating surgeon using standard cutting guides. The menisci are resected with a laminar spreader in the opposite compartment. We leave a small rim adjacent to the medial meniscus to avoid injury to the medial collateral ligament. Posterior osteophytes are osteotomized with curved osteotomes, and removed using angled curettes.

Our preference is to resect the posterior cruciate ligament and use a posterior-stabilized prosthesis. We believe the results are more re-

producible using a posterior cruciate-substituting prosthesis in these patients as the posterior cruciate ligament and posterior medial capsule may be lax in this setting. If use of a posterior cruciate-preserving prosthesis is entertained, advancement of the posterior cruciate ligament may be necessary for appropriate balance (7).

Flexion and extension gaps are checked using spacer blocks and laminar spreaders. There may be a larger flexion than extension gap noted, particularly following conversion high tibial osteotomies associated with anterior tibial slopes on the lateral radiographs secondary to resection of a significant amount of bone posteriorly. This is best minimized by resecting the tibia with minimal posterior slope. Increased distal femoral resection and utilization of a thicker polyethylene equalizes flexion and extension gaps in this setting at the expense of joint line elevation and increased relative patella infera. Another option is to upsize the femoral component, if necessary utilizing posterior augments.

Flexion and extension gaps are also checked for medial and lateral balance. We prefer to remove all osteophytes prior to ligament releases as ligament balance may be improved following removal of osteophytes. Appropriate ligament releases are performed as necessary. When necessary, we perform a medial subperiosteal release from the tibia as a continuous sleeve as described by Insall (18). When the lateral side is tight in extension, we perform our lateral release in extension with a laminar spreader in place. We palpate the posterolateral capsule and iliotibial band, releasing structures in an incremental fashion based on how tight individual structures feel, and repeatedly reassessing stability. Usually this initially involves releasing the posterolateral capsule. We release the posterolateral capsule below the popliteus tendon. If necessary, we release the iliotibial band incrementally from anterior to posterior at the resected surface of the tibia also with the knee in extension. In cases where the flexion space is trapezoidal with a tight lateral side, release of the lateral collateral ligament and/or popliteus from the femur is performed with the knee in flexion. We attempt to avoid complete subperiosteal stripping of the lateral collateral ligament and popliteus from the lateral femoral epicondyle as this results in lateral flexion instability and/or osteonecrosis of the lateral femoral condyle (18). In cases of marked ligamentous imbalance, a more constrained implant may be required (18). When an excessive lateral release is necessary, predisposing to peroneal nerve palsy or lateral flexion instability, one option is to perform a more conservative release, accepting some mild imbalance, and using a constrained condylar style prosthesis. This technique is most applicable in the elderly low demand patient. Alternatively, an advancement of the lax medial collateral ligament, medial hamstring tendons and posterior cruciate ligament can be performed as described by Krackow (17), although we have no experience with this technique. This technique is technically demanding, and requires more protected postoperative rehabilitation (17).

must be performed as the posterior cruciate ligament may not be functional in this setting (17). We recommend balancing the posterior cruciate ligament utilizing the techniques described by Ritter (19), and by Swany and Scott (20). The posterior cruciate ligament should be assessed with the patella reduced and tracking appropriately in the trochlear grove (20). Lift off of the anterior portion of the tibial tray with flexion indicates an excessively tight posterior cruciate ligament (19, 20). The knee should be stable to anteroposterior displacement at 90 degrees of flexion, and the

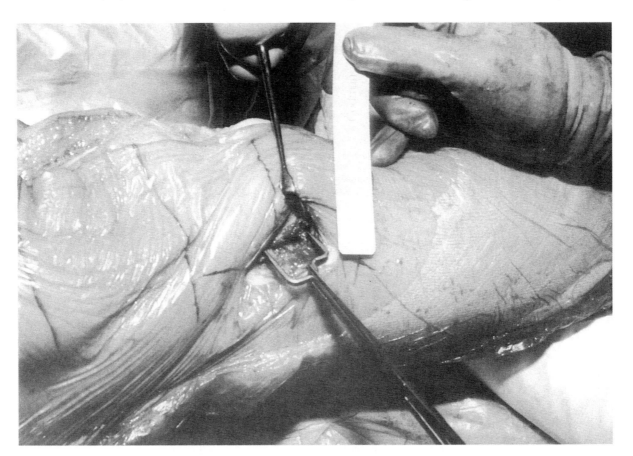

Fig. 11 - Intraoperative photograph demonstrating removal of an extremely posteriorly placed staple through a short lateral incision incorporated into a previous lateral longitudinal incision. Note the ruler demonstrating an 8 cm skin bridge between incisions.

The trial components are inserted. The knee is taken through a range of motion and patellar tracking, ligament balancing and stability are checked. We do not perform posterior cruciate ligament-retaining total knee arthroplasty following high tibial osteotomies because of the issues discussed above. However, if utilization of a posterior cruciate-retaining prosthesis is entertained, a careful assessment of anteriorposterior stability

posterior cruciate ligament should deflect only 1-2 mm with firm digital pressure in this position (20). In cases of patella infera, care must be taken to ensure that the patellar component does not impinge on the tibial tray in extension. If this occurs, our preference is to utilize a smaller patellar polyethylene, and place it more superiorly on the patella. The inferior aspect of the patella which is not supporting the component can then be thinned

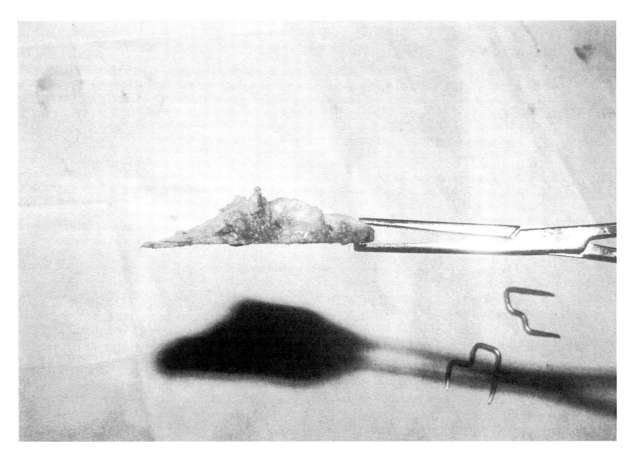

FIG. 12 - Photograph of the resected tibial specimen of a patient who underwent conversion of a high tibial osteotomy to a total knee arthroplasty demonstrating minimal resection of lateral bone. Note the greater thickness of the medial aspect of the resected specimen.

with a burr, being careful not to damage the patellar tendon. We prefer to avoid moving the joint line distally with distal augments in this setting. Once satisfactory patellar tracking, ligamentous balance and stability are demonstrated, the components are implanted in standard fashion.

Postoperative rehabilitation must be individualized based on the particular procedure performed. Most total knee arthroplasties following high tibial osteotomies can be rehabilitated as if they had a primary total knee arthroplasty. In settings at substantial risk for wound complications secondary to the need to raise large flaps or have parallel incisions, we prefer to keep the knee immobilized until the first postoperative day and start continuous passive motion at 0-30 degrees at that time. We increase range of motion more slowly in these patients. In cases of severely overcorrected high tibial osteotomies or significant bone loss requiring either bone grafting or augments, postoperative rehabilitation mimics that following revision total knee arthroplasty.

Complications

The complications following conversion of high tibial osteomies to total knee arthroplasties are the same as for primary or revision total knee arthroplasty. These included extensor mechanism problems, wound healing problems, infection, arthrofibrosis, instability, aseptic loosening, reflex sympathetic fracture, malalignment, blood loss, neurovascular injury, compartment syndrome, deep venous thrombosis, pulmonary embolism, and death as well as complications associated with anesthesia or medical comorbidities. Extensor mechanism problems can be further subdivided into patella infera, patellar ligament avulsion, patella fracture, quadriceps tendon rupture, patellar subluxation or dislocation and patella clunk syndrome.

Several series have noted higher rates of some of these complications for total knee arthroplasty following high tibial osteotomy with primary total knee arthroplasty (3, 5-8). Complications in which studies have noted increased rates of complications in post-osteotomy patients compared with patients not having had previous osteotomies include wound healing problems and infection (6, 8). One series noted greater blood loss in post-osteotomy patients undergoing total knee replacement that in their patients undergoing primary total knee replacement (3).

Surgeons have also made reference to increased risk of patellar tendon avulsion and patellar subluxation in post-osteotomy patients (5, 6). However, these complications have not been reported in their respective series. Nevertheless, extreme caution should be exercised when everting the patellar mechanism in these patients to avoid patellar tendon avulsion. A quadriceps snip or controlled tibial tubercle osteotomy is a much more favorable situation than patellar tendon avulsion.

Instability has been recognized as a complication following conversion of high tibial osteotomies to total knee arthroplasties (4, 17). However, to our knowledge, no series has documented increased rates of instability in these patients compared with primary total knee arthroplasty. This is probably secondary to utilization of more constrained prostheses or ligament advancing techniques in those patients with more severe deformities in these series.

Several series have noted decreased range of knee motion and/or high rates of manipulation in the post-osteotomy patients, but these authors have not addressed whether they noted increased rates of arthrofibrosis (2, 3, 6). In addition, at least three series had poor results in patients subsequently diagnosed with reflex sympathetic dystrophy (5-7).

There is theoretically an increased risk of neurovascular injury or compartment syndrome if removal of a lateral plate is necessary secondary to stripping of the anterior compartment muscles from the tibia. Care should be taken to strip the anterior compartment muscles in the subperiosteal plane. We recommend avoiding tight closure of the anterior compartment fascia, and placement of a hemovac or constavac drain deep to the anterior compartment fascia at the completion of the case.

When the principles of appropriate patient selection, proper preoperative planning, meticulous surgical technique, intelligent prosthetic component selection, and appropriate postoperative rehabilitation are adhered to, these complications can be minimized. We cannot overemphasize respect for the soft tissues in this setting to avoid wound complications and infection.

References

1) Berman, A.T., et al.: Factors Influencing Long-term Results in High Tibial Osteotomy. Clin. Orthop., 1991. 272: p. 192-8.
2) Amendola, A., et al.: Total Knee Arthroplasty Following High Tibial Osteotomy for Osteoarthritis. J. Arthroplasty, 1989. S12: p. S11-7.
3) Bergenudd, H., A. Sahlstrom, and L. Sanzen: Total Knee Arthoplasty After Failed Proximal Tibial Valgus Osteotomy. J. Arthroplasty, 1997. 12(6): p. 635-8.
4) Staeheli, J.W., J.R. Cass, and B.F. Morrey: Condylar Total Knee Arthroplasty After Failed Proximal Tibial Osteotomy. J. Bone Joint Surg., 1987. 69-A: p. 28-31.
5) Katz, M.M., et al.: Results of Total Knee Arthroplasty After Failed Proximal Tibial Osteotomy for Osteoarthritis. J. Bone Joint Surg., 1987. 69-A: p. 225-233.
6) Windsor, R.E., J.N. Insall, and K.G. Vince: Technical Considerations of Total Knee Arthroplasty After Proximal Tibial Osteotomy. J. Bone Joint Surgery, 1988. 70-A: p. 547-55.
7) Mont, M.A., et al.: Total Knee Arthroplasty After High Tibial Osteotomy. Clin. Orthop., 1994. 299: p. 125-30.
8) Jackson, M., P.P. Sarangi, and J.H. Newman: Revision Total Knee Arthroplasty. J. Arthroplasty, 1994. 9(5): p. 539-542.
9) Scuderi, G.R., R.E. Windsor, and J.N. Insall: Observations of Patellar Height After Proximal Tibial Osteotomy. J. Bone Joint Surg., 1989. 71-A: p. 245-8.
10) Westrich, G.H., et al.: New Observations of Patella Height After High Tibial Osteotomy With Intraoperative Fixation and Early Range of Motion. American Academy of Orthopaedic Surgeons, 64th Annual Meeting. 1997. San Francisco, CA.
11) Insall, J.N. and E. Salvati: Patella Position in the Normal Knee Joint. Radiology, 1971. 101: p. 101.
12) Mast, J.: Fractures of the Tibial Pilon. Clin. Orthop., 1988. 230: p. 68-82.
13) Craig, S.M.: Soft Tissue Considerations in the Failed Total Knee Arthroplasty, in The Knee, W.N. Scott, Editor, Mosby: St. Louis. p. 1279-95.
14) Buechel, F.F.: A Sequential Three Step Lateral Release for Correcting Fixed Valgus Knee Deformities During Total Knee Arthroplasty. Clin. Orthop., 1990. 260: p. 170.
15) Keblish, P.A.: Valgus Deformity in Total Knee Replacement. Orthopaedic Transactions, 1985. 9(1): p. 28-9.
16) Wright, P.E.: Basic Surgical Technique and After Care. In: Campbell's Operative Orthopaedics, A.H. Crenshaw, 1992, Mosby: St. Louis. p. 2976.
17) Krackow, K.A. and J.L. Holtgrewe: Experience with a New Technique for Managing Severely Overcorrected Valgus High Tibial Osteotomy at Total Knee Arthroplasty. Clin. Orthop., 1990. 258: p. 213-24.
18) Insall, J.N.: Surgical Techniques and Instrumentation in Total Knee Arthroplasty. In Surgery of the Knee, J.N. Insall, 1993, Churchill Livingston: New York. p. 779-784.
19) Ritter, M.A.: Posterior Cruciate Ligament Balancing During Total Knee Arthroplasty. J. Arthroplasty, 1988. 3: p. 323-6.
20) Swany, M.R. and R.D. Scott: Posterior Polyethylene Wear in Posterior Cruciate Ligament-retaining Total Knee Arthroplasty. J. Arthroplasty, 1993. 8: p. 439-45.

Chapter 9
Total Knee Arthroplasty in the Stiff Knee

Thomas P. Sculco, Ermanno A. Martucci*

The Hospital for Special Surgery - New York
* Rizzoli Orthopaedic Institute - Bologna

Introduction

Total knee arthroplasty in the stiff or anky-losed knee is an extremely demanding technical procedure (Fig. 4). The challenge begins in the work-up and evaluation of these patients by assessing the cause of their stiffness and the degree to which it interferes with activities of daily living. Preoperative planning directs surgical management by deciding which type of surgical exposure is utilized, and whether a custom prosthesis is necessary based upon clinical and radiographic examinations. Surgical performance is centered on the same principles as in less challenging primary cases: adequate exposure, soft tissue balancing of symmetric flexion and extension gaps, maintenance of the joint line, and proper patellofemoral kinematics. Prior studies have detailed the results, as well as the complications of this procedure. These experiences have shown that in the properly indicated patients, successful results can be achieved through careful surgical technique and adherence to an aggressive postoperative physical therapy protocol.

Indications

Although opinions vary, the knee joint is considered stiff if there is less than a 50 degree arc of motion. An ankylosed knee may present in flexion or extension depending on the pathology present. The more complex stiff knees should be approached as if planning revision knee replacement. Before considering an arthroplasty, one must absolutely rule out low-grade sepsis as the cause of the stiffness. Pre-operative knee aspiration should be performed if there is any suspicion of infection. Knee stiffness may result from the arthritic process itself or prior injury to the knee, prior knee surgery, prior infection, reflex sympathetic dystrophy, neuromuscular disorder, such as stroke or Charcot deformity secondary to diabetes. Ankylosis, especially in flexion, may be the result of inflammatory arthridites, such as rheumatiod arthritis or psoriasis.

The underlying cause of the pathology may have a significant effect on the results of the arthroplasty. Mechanical derangement of the internal knee structures caused by injury or prior surgery may be successfully addressed through the proper soft tissue management during surgical exposure. However, patients with reflex sympathetic dystrophy (RSD) or neuro-muscular deformities must be approached with caution. One absolute contraindication to arthroplasty in this patient population is the knee which is stiff or ankylosed secondary to extensor mechanism disruption or incompetence. Allograft reconstructions of the patellar tendon have all reported poor functional results.

Preoperative Evaluation and Surgical Planning

Work-up should start with a thorough history and physical examination. Preoperative range of motion must be documented, along with any contractures, scars, or angular deformity. It is important to clearly define knee motion and whether the knee is stiff in extension or flexion. If the knee is stiff in flexion, the ex-

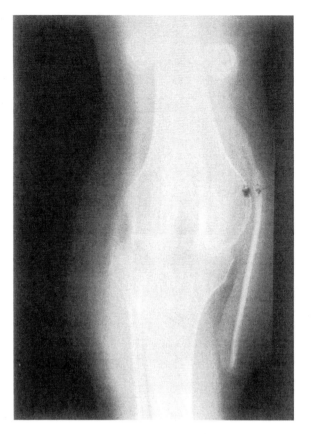

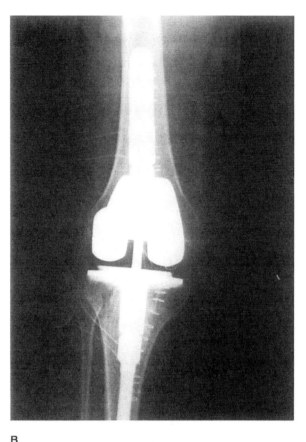

A   B

FIG. 1A-B - Arthroplasty in a knee previously submitted to arthrodesis.

tensor mechanism will generally be more elongated and need for extensor lengthening procedures is less. If the knee is stiff in extension then there is always associated extensor contracture, which will require quadriceps lengthening in some manner. It is important for the surgeon to realize this preoperatively and be prepared to use various techniques based on degree of flexion present in the stiff knee. Complete motor, sensory, and vascular assessment of the extremity should be performed including pulse venous recordings, especially if the patient is a diabetic. Ankle/brachial index of less than 0.4 has been associated with a need for vascular reperfusion. In addition, the patient's overall condition must be evaluated preoperatively to assess whether compliance with a rigorous postoperative physical therapy protocol can be achieved.

Laboratory work-up should include CBC, ESR C-reactive protein. Knee aspiration should be performed and sent for cell count and culture. New polymerase chain reaction techniques have increased the sensitivity of aspiration culture to 98%. The procedure should be performed twice to increase the sensitivity of the test. If the patient has been on antibiotics up to a week prior to the aspiration, he should be brought back in 2 weeks to insure against a false negative result.

Radiographic assessment must include anteroposterior (AP), lateral and patellar views, Long axis AP views can be used to properly align the mechanical axis of the extremity. More sophisticated studies such as CT or bone scans may be used to assess bone stock or further attempt to rule out infection. By combining the clinical and radiographic preoperative data, a thoughtful surgical plan can be constructed to determine the quality and/or deficiency of bone stock and how to properly address this concern; type of surgical exposure; and, finally, choice of prosthesis. Since most if not all of the ligamentous and other soft tissue structures are all contracted, a posterior cruciate-sacrificing design should be employed. One must contemplate that symmetric and balanced flexion and extension gaps will not be achieved.

In knees that have severe limitation of motion, flexion instability after releases may require constrained implants, therefore a constrained polyethylene with long stem tibial and femoral components should be available. Custom prostheses can be employed, especially in the ankylosed knees of rheumatoid patients and patients with psoriasis. These patients typically have very small joints with very narrow intramedullary canals.

Surgical Technique

Wide exposure is necessary for successful outcome. The most technically difficult aspect of this procedure is gaining adequate exposure. The position of the skin incision must respect prior approaches performed. Wide dissection superficial to the deep fascia will compromise the blood supply to the skin, therefore it is not recommended. Parallel incisions should have at least a 6-7 cm skin bridge between them to guarantee the epidermal blood supply to the intervening skin segment. If the patient has had a

fusion with atrophy of the overlying tissues, evaluation by plastic surgery may be necessary to determine whether the patient may require a tissue expander prior to sugery.

If there has been no prior surgery, a standard midline approach is recommended. Once the capsule has been entered, establishment of the lateral and medial gutters may be required for flexion of the knee. Perhaps the most difficult aspect of the procedure will be everting the patella. In cases in which the knee is fused, the patella may actually be ankylosed to the trochlea. In this instance, an osteotome can be used to separate the two. Application of revision type exposure may be necessary in order to obtain satisfactory exposure. In the stiff knee there is severe periarticular fibrosis proximally and distally. This must be released subperiosteally extensively around the distal femur and proximal tibia. Dissection should begin at the surfaces of the distal femur and continue until the femur is devoid of tissue. If there is an associated flexion contracture, extensive posterior subperiosteal release is necessary from the femur and tibia. After release about the femur similar radical subperiosteal dissection should be performed around the tibial circumference. In cases of moderate limitation of motion, soft tissue release can be less radical and this dissection alone may allow mobilization of the knee.

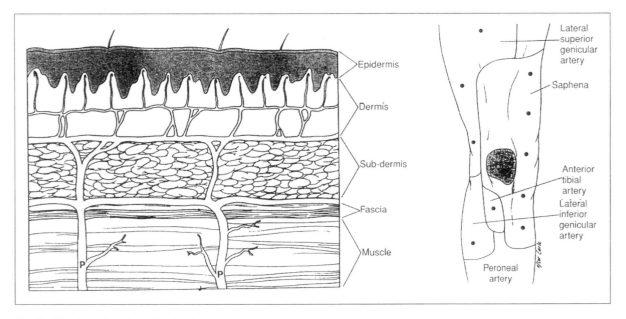

FIG. 2 - Blood supply to the skin of the knee.

After skeletonization of the femur and tibia has been performed, care must be taken in knee flexion not to avulse the insertion of the patellar tendon. A lateral patella release should be performed to assist in patella eversion. Often the skin is adherent to the subcutaneous tissues in these complex stiff knees and subcutaneous dissection may be necessary to mobilize the skin from the adherent deep soft tissues. This also facilitates skin closure.

If the extensor mechanism is still contracted preventing exposure, quadricepsplasty exposures may be utilized at this point. The quadriceps snip (Fig. 1) can provide wide exposure with minimal risk to the extensor mechanism. At the proximal end of the medial parapatellar approach. The rectus tendon is divided in an oblique manner in a superior and lateral direction. The patella is everted and knee flexed, with care taken not to avulse the patellar tendon insertion. An advantage to this approach is that no alteration in postoperative range of motion or weight bearing is required. If this approach is inadequate, it can be extended into a Coones-Adams inverted V-Y quadricepsplasty (Fig. 2). In this approach, the incision into the quadriceps tendon is extended laterally and distally through the tendinous insertion of the vastus lateralis and the lateral retinaculum. The superior lateral geniculate artery, providing blood supply to the patella, can be preserved by curving the incision laterally underneath the edge of the vastus lateralis through its tendinous insertion into the retinaculum. It is important to restrict the lateral extent of the release if possible. In the most severe cases allowing the tongue of quadriceps to slide distally and suturing the tendon end-to-end proximally can perform a formal lengthening of the quadriceps tendon. If lengthening is performed in the fashion the knee should be placed in 30-40 degrees of flexion and the lengthening performed at that level. If the tendon is lengthened greater than this an extensor lag may persist permanently. If the tendon is repaired in less flexion then more stiffness will persist. Postoperatively if a formal V-Y lengthening has been performed rehabilitation must be altered. The knee should not be allowed to flex greater than 45 degrees of flexion for 3-4 weeks. If greater than 45 degrees of flexion is allowed immediately postoperatively there is a risk of disruption of the quadriceps repair. All patients will have an extensor lag after quadricepsplasty, but it generally resolves at 4-6 months.

Tibial tubercle osteotomy (Fig. 3) has been used in difficult knee arthroplasty exposures since 1983. To perform this osteotomy, the incision is extended distally along the proximal tibia until the medial 10 cm of the tibia is exposed. The osteotomy should encompass at least 8 cm of bone to facilitate healing. The bone cut is made with an oscillating saw from medial to lateral and curved at the distal end to protect against fracture. The osteotomy is continued with curved osteotomes to but not through the lateral cortex. The osteotomes are raised to de-

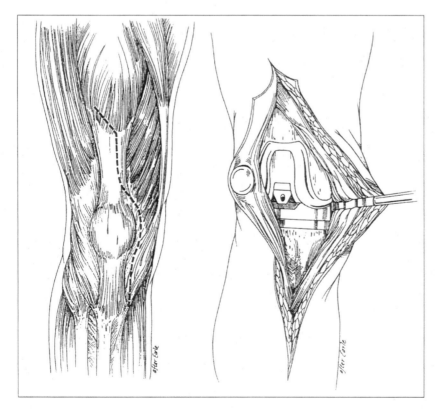

Fig. 3 - Quadriceps "snip."

tach the lateral edge leaving a periosteal soft tissue hinge. Two or three wires are passed to encompass the tubercle during closure. In a review of 136 osteotomies, the mean postoperative range of motion was 93.7 degrees. Nonunion, fracture and infection have been reported in case reports after this procedure. It must be remembered that tibial osteotomy does not deal with the extensor pathology, which is proximal. Quadriceps lengthening is needed, particularly in markedly stiff knees in extension.

Once the knee has properly been exposed, the general rules for balanced and symmetrical flexion and extension gaps apply. Due to the severity of soft tissue contractures in the contracted knees, the posterior cruciate ligament is always sacrificed. When extensive subperiosteal releases have been performed to mobilize stiff knees, there is often increased laxity in flexion. A constrained implant with an elevated polyethylene post must be used in these patients to provide increased stability in flexion. Additionally the femoral component should be moved posteriorly as much as possible to decrease the flexion gap. Custom implants with posterior femoral augmentation may be needed in extremely rigid knees, especially in extension. The prosthesis chosen should have options available for augmenting the femur or tibia to recreate the anatomic joint line. It is often difficult to determine the original joint line of the knee. On a radiograph, the fibular head and inferior pole of the patella

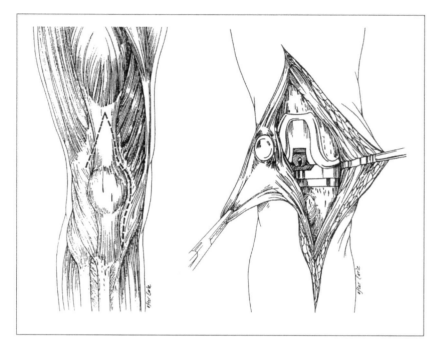

FIG. 4 - Modified V-Y quadricepsplasty: the lateral incision is lateral to the vastus lateralis, and it is posteriorly directed to save the superior lateral geniculate artery.

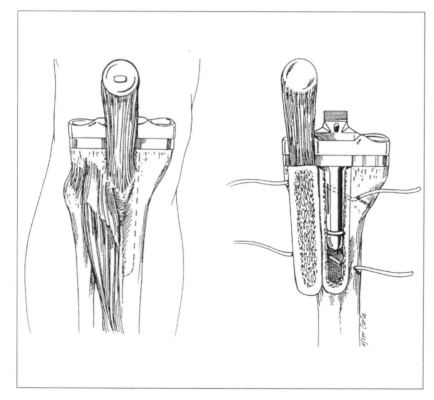

FIG. 5 - Osteotomy of the tibial tubercle.

offer helpful guidelines. The inferior pole of the patella should be above the joint line and the fibular head below it. For operative inspection, the normal joint line is normally 14-16 mm distal to the origin of the posterior cruciate ligament and approximately 25-30 mm distal to the medial epicondylar eminence. Care should be taken to not "overstuff" the patellofemoral articulation, as it will encourage redevelopment of a flexion contracture. This point is crucial: If proper soft tissue balancing of symmetrical flexion and extension gaps cannot be present, a constrained type polyethylene spacer and femoral component must be in the operating, theater otherwise failure will be imminent. Considering the stiffness of the soft tissues, larger prosthetic interface stresses are present so long stem components should be used.

Postoperative Management

Drains and/or splints are removed on the first postoperative day and the patient is placed in a continuous passive motion machine from 0 to 30 degrees of flexion. The flexion is increased 10 degrees a day or as tolerated. If the patient's deformity was in flexion, care should be taken to evaluate the neurovascular status of the lower extremity due to the contracted nature of the tissues in the posterior aspect of the knee. Additionally, the knee should be placed in a knee immobilizer while sleeping to avoid re-accumulation of the flexion deformity.

The next postoperative day, the patient starts weight-bearing with a walker. Physical therapy concentrates on strengthening and stretching the quadriceps mechanism. However, the expectations of the patient must be realistic and should be discussed preoperatively.

The goal is to improve a knee with poor function, not to create a normal one. In-patients with less than 50 degrees of arc flexion pre-op could expect 80-90 degrees of flexion post-operatively. Knee motion in normal gait has found that 65 to 70 degrees of flexion is needed in the swing phase on level ground. Ninety degrees is required to descend stairs and 105 degrees is needed to rise from a low chair.

Results

There have been conflicting reports regarding the outcome of total knee arthroplasty in patients with stiff or ankylosed knees. One difficulty in assessing these reports are the paucity of patients. The largest series of patients was reported from the Hospital For Special Surgery, with an average 6 year follow-up on 86 patients. All of their patients had stiff knees defined as less than 50 degrees of total arc of motion. Three of the patients had auto-fusions, while none of their patients had a previous operative bony fusion. Knee scores improved from an average of 38 to 80 and range of motion increased from 36 degrees to 93 degrees. However, a 7% aseptic loosening rate and an 11% complication rate was reported including two peroneal nerve palsies. Cameron reported on seventeen cases of operative knee fusion takedown with an average 5-year follow-up. Average flexion was reported as 83 degrees. However, a 53% complication rate was reported, with 2 patients requiring re-fusion due to patella tendon loss. One third were rated as excellent, one third as good, and one third poor. One common theme in all of the author's conclusions is that good results are attainable, but considering the possible complications, decisions to go ahead with this kind of sugery should be made with trepidation.

References

1) Aglietti P; Windsor R; Buzzi R; Insall J: Arthroplasty for the stiff or ankylosed knee. J. Arthroplasty; 41(1): 1-5; 1989.

2) Bradley GW; Freeman MAR; Albrektson BJ: Total Prosthetic Management of Ankylosed Knees. J. Arthroplasty. 2; 179-185; 1987.

3) Cameron HU; Hu C: Results of Total Knee Arthroplasty Following Takedown of Formal Knee Fusion. J. Arthroplasty; 11(6); 732-737; 1996.

4) Kim Y; Cho S; Kim J: Total Knee Arthroplasty In Bony Ankylosis In Gross Flexion. J. Bone Joint Surg.; 81(B); 296-300; 1999.

5) Montgomery WH; Insall J; Haas S; Becker M; Windsor R: Primary Total Knee Arthroplasty In Stiff and Ankylosed Knees. Amer J. Knee Surg; 11(1); 20-24; 1998.

6) Naranja RJ; Lotke PA; Pagnano M; Hanssen AD: Total Knee Arthroplasty in a Previously Ankylosed or Arthrodesed Knee. Clin. Orthop. Rel. Res.; 331; 234-237; 1996.

7) Scott RD; Siliski JM: The Use of a Modified V-Y quadriceps-plasty during total knee replacement to gain exposure and improve flexion in the ankylosed knee. Orthopedics; 8(1): 45-48; 1985.

8) Sculco TP; Faris PM: Total Knee Replacement In the Stiff Knee. Tech. Ortho.; 3(2): 5-8; 1988.

9) Whiteside LA; Ohl MD: Tibial Tubercle Osteotomy For Exposure of the Difficult Total Knee Arthroplasty.

10) Windsor RE; Insall JH: Exposure in Revision Total Knee Arthroplasty: The Femoral Peel. Tech. Orthop.; 3(2): 1-4; 1988.

Section 3
PROSTHETIC SELECTION

Chapter 10
Unicompartmental Knee Arthroplasty

Nikolaus M. Boehler
Orthopaedische Abteilung Linz

The idea of unicompartmental knee arthroplasty (UKA) was first conceived by McKeever and Elliot in 1952 while doing work to develop metallic tibial plateau prostheses. In 1958, McIntosh reported (22) the use of a prosthesis with a vitallium tibial plateau.

At the John Charnley Clinic, Gunston developed a plastic and metal prosthesis during the early 70s. This type of prosthesis was modified by the Mayo Clinic and called the "Polycentric Knee."

Marmor carried out most of the early scientific work on UKA. He created his own "Marmor prosthesis," developed the correct indications, and in 1977 began publishing studies (11).

Halfway through the 80s, discussion surrounding the use of UKA was controversial due to the fact that Insall and Aglietti (15) published unsatisfactory results. On the other hand, Cartier, Scott (7, 29) and many others could demonstrate that they had instead obtained satisfactory results.

The controversy continues today, but after learning about the technical principles and careful indications of the method, I am convinced that there will always be a place for UKA.

Indications

Many countries are still discussing whether there is a place for UKA at all, while at the same time the results obtained when the method is used are more and more convincing.

There are two different standpoints:

1. Against use of UKA: it is best to replace the entire knee, as the other compartments will eventually wear out.

2. For use of UKA: it is a basic principle of orthopaedics to save all of the normal tissue, knowing that any device used will always be inferior to the natural joint.

For those who believe in UKA, patient selection is one of the most important factors in achieving good results.

The traditional indication is osteonecrosis of the femoral condyle (Ahlbaeck's disease). In patients with this pathology, the decision whether or not to implant a UKA can easily be made by X-ray assessment or MRT.

In patients with knees with degenerative arthritis, patient selection must be done carefully, monitoring several criteria.

Criteria Related to the General Circumstances of the Patients

Patients below the age of 60 years should only be selected for the use of UKA under special circumstances. The best candidates are not active patients over the age of 70, or those with multiple degenerative joint involvement. Heavy patients, exceeding 80 kg in weight, and patients engaged in demanding sports activities are poor candidates for UKA. In younger, heavy or very active patients, a high tibial osteotomy, over the age of 70, and total knee replacement might be favored.

On the other hand, UKA is more predictable if it is compared to high tibial osteotomy; early results are much more satisfying, and postoperative rehabilitation remains shorter. Therefore, even in patients aged under 60 years, UKA might be used for appropriate candidates.

If we compare it to total knee replacement, UKA offers the advantage of easier and faster postoperative management, better range of movement, and if complications such as infection or loosening occur, further surgery is easier.

Soft Tissue Related Criteria

Both the posterior cruciate and the anterior cruciate ligaments must be intact (9, 10, 27, 35).

Minor degrees of collateral ligamentous laxity in the affected compartment can be corrected by the implant. In cases of severe laxity in the affected compartment, with overcorrectability or combined laxity of the medial and lateral collateral ligament, there is a high chance of destruction of the second femoral compartment and the need for TKA.

Flexion contractions of more than 10 to 15 degrees are also a contraindication to the use of UKA if they cannot be corrected.

Osteocartilaginous Related Criteria

The use of UKA should be limited to monocondylar destruction caused by non-inflammatory joint diseases; UKA is contraindicated when a second compartment is involved.

Osteoarthritis of the patellae is a contraindication only in case of anterior knee pain in the patellar region. In addition, more extensive cartilage deficit has to be considered a contraindication. On the other hand, we do not feel that pain-free osteoarthritis at the patellofemoral joint with some osteophytes contraindicates UKA.

Decision-making with Imaging Techniques

The following imaging techniques should be used:
  a) Radiographs;
  b) MRT to detect a vascular necrosis and loose bodies;
  c) Bone scan, mainly in cases where vascular necrosis is suspected, when MRT is not available.

Recommended Preoperative Radiographic Evaluation

The following are essential:
1. AP view radiographs in extension under single leg weight-bearing conditions; this can demonstrate the state of the cartilage on the affected compartment, a lateral dislocation with a defect on the non-affected compartment (kissing lesion), and the degree of the deformity.
2. AP view radiographs in 20° flexion (Rosenberg) (28); these allow us to demonstrate the definite state of the cartilage eliminating the influence of the residual anterior meniscus.
3. A lateral weight-bearing radiograph in maximum extension to demonstrate whether there is a flexion contracture or a genu recurvatum. The quadriceps muscle should be contracted to show the level of the patella. Furthermore, anteroposterior subluxation can be shown in case of ACL rupture.
4. Patella tangential view radiographs with the leg in 30° of flexion show the state of the patellofemoral compartment.

The following are recommended:
5. Long films including hip, knee and ankle on single leg weight-bearing conditions can determine the overall femoral and tibial axes.
6. Varus and valgus stress films can demonstrate the condition of the collateral ligaments and show the thickness of the unaffected tibiofemoral compartment.
7. Template the knee in order to see the extent of the defects on the femoral and tibial site and to define the area of bone cuts. The position of the tibial implant should follow the femoral joint line.

UKA Design

If we take a general look at the large number of implants on the market, we may discern three general designs.

1. The Resurfacing Type

Implants of this type use femoral fixation in the subchondral bone and typically a flat tibial plateau (Fig. 1). The advantage to using this type of implant is minimal bone loss as a result of surgery. The operation itself is technically simple, but it does require an experienced surgeon for implant positioning.

The rate of implant loosening on the femoral and tibial site is low.

The disadvantage might be more extensive polyethylene wear, especially in implants using an inlay with a 6 mm polyethylene or less. If we use a PE thickness of more than 6 mm and surface hardening with ODH on the femoral implant, wear is substantially reduced (2, 3, 31, 32).

2. Resection type UKA

Femoral fixation lies in the cancellous bone. Resection is guided by instrument, and it is similar to the technique of total knee arthroplasty. Intramedullary positioning is often used.

The advantage of this type resides in the very accurate positioning of the femoral implant using a technique that is well-known to TKA surgeons. Thus, the learning curve is shorter.

One of the drawbacks is that there is greater loss of bone stock as compared to when the resurfacing type is used, and there is also a higher loosening rate due to fixation in softer cancellous bone (14, 18).

3. The mobile bearing type

This was first invented by J. W. Goodfellow. Advantages to using the method reside in the reduction of polyethylene wear combined with reduced stress on implant fixation.

A disadvantage is that a higher rate of implant dislocation can be observed. Ligament tension and implant positioning has to be carried out very carefully to avoid early complications. The learning curve for adequate implantation is longer as compared to when other types are used.

Principles of surgery

Surgical Approach

The surgical approach should include a standard incision for a complete overview of the knee joint. The reason for this is that the surgeon must see the apposite compartment as a reference for the resection level and for the cutting angles.

The extent of the degenerative changes in all three compartments must be monitored.

Another important reason for the incision to be adequate is to provide a second line of defense, meaning the possibility to use the same approach for secondary surgical interventions.

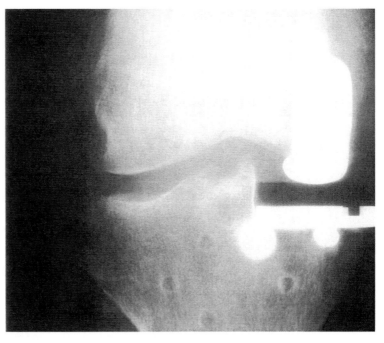

FIG. 1 - Overcorrection or a 6° anatomical axis is the main reason for early problems in UKA. Undercorrection keeping the knee in a slight varus has to be achieved.

A medial parapatellar, midvastus or subvastus approach should be chosen to implant a UKA in the medial compartment. We personally prefer the midvastus, which allows us a good overview together with the preservation of optimal function of the vastus medialis muscle.

The implantation of a UKA in the lateral compartment is done by a lateral or medial parapatellar approach normally without osteotomy of the tibial tuberosity.

Bone Preparation

Bone preparation should follow some typical requirements. The tibial cut should be right at the *eminentia intercondylaris* and immediately beside the cruciate ligament insertion: Care must be taken to avoid rotation failures by making this cut. Accurate instrumentation has to define this position. Complete coverage after bone resection had to be provided by the implant. Therefore, the instrumentation has to allow for an additional sagittal cut in case of mismatch in AP and medial-lateral direction.

In the frontal plane, the horizontal cut should follow the former joint line. This is not necessarily the right angle position to the tibial axis.

Femoral preparation should allow for fixation in the subchondral bone for optimal preservation of bone stock and optimal load transfer. Using this principle, we had no single aseptic implant loosening on the femoral site with our type of Alloflex UKA. It is important to consider that we have to restore the adequate joint line in relation to the apposite compartment. Therefore, an additional femoral resection has to be carried out in case of a minimal bony defect on the femoral condyle to avoid distalization of the implant joint line.

Proper centering of the femoral component in relation to the tibial component has to be established especially with the knee in extension. This has to be monitored in flexion and extension before the definite femoral cuts are made.

Selection of the proper implant

On the femoral site, we use the smallest implant that covers the pre-existing defect. Care must be taken so that there is minimal contact between patellar cartilage and femoral implant.

On the tibia, we use the implant that provides full coverage of the resected area. The implant must not overlie the cortical bone of the tibia, affecting the collateral ligament. Alteration of the collateral ligament or the pes anserinus in this manner is a typical source of postoperative pain (29).

The minimal thickness of the polyethylene component should be 6 mm or better 8 mm in case of a metal backed implant, and 9 mm or better 10 mm in case of an All-Polyethylene Tibial Implant.

Undercorrection

It is very important that postoperative and undercorrection of the physiological mechanical axis be achieved. The mechanical lot must lie on the operated compartment and away from the apposite compartment. Otherwise, rapid deterioration of the non-replaced compartment is to be expected.

Furthermore, overcorrecting frequently causes excessive and painful tension of the medial collateral ligament in case of varus deformity (Fig. 2).

Overcorrecting occurs mainly in medial monocondylar replacement. The reason for this is that the deformation in case of a genu varum mainly affects the proximal tibia. Because of the destruction or bone loss of the femoral condyle, the height of the femoral implant might be greater than the amount of the resected bone leading to a valgus deformity.

Overcorrection can be avoided by a somewhat deeper femoral resection but even in this case the femoral implant has to lie on the subchondral sclerotic bone. Otherwise, an addi-

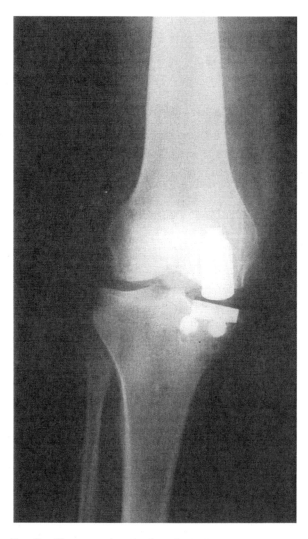

FIG. 2 - The cementless implanted Alloflex UKA with PE thickness exceeding 6 mm permist long-lasting good results.

tional tibial cut or the use of a lower tibial plateau has to be chosen.

Implant stability has to be achieved intraoperatively without any cementing, especially in the flexed knee position. If any lift-off or rotation of the tibial plateau can be seen during knee movement, pressure on the implant has to be reduced.

This can be done by making an additional resection on the tibial site, or by enlarging the posterior slop (i.e., anteroposterior reclination).

Ligamentous tension

In order to create a pain-free knee with almost normal motion, protective laxity of the medial collateral ligament in case of genu varum has to be achieved. This laxity should be tested at 15° of flexion, allowing for a 2 to 4 mm medial opening.

The anterior cruciate ligament has to be preserved. In case of anterior or posterior laxity, progressive posterior subluxation followed by excessive polyethylene wear has to be expected (10, 13).

Results

Early Results

Early results are excellent, as postoperative time of recovery is much faster as compared with high tibial osteotomy and total knee arthroplasty. Ivarsson (16) revealed in his studies that rehabilitation 6 months after UKA is much better in terms of muscle torque, maximal gait velocity, and duration of single leg support, as compared with the status 12 months postoperatively following high tibial osteotomy. Laurencin (21) demonstrated in a comparative study a better return of proprioception and a somewhat better mobility, in a patient group with UKA on one knee, and TKA on the other.

According to the literature, the postoperative range of motion is excellent, and the average flexion lies between 105° (6, 17) and 120° or more (4, 5, 26, 30, 37).

Long-term results

These results depend very much on the type of design.

The resurfacing type

The best results could be found with the resurfacing type of UKA. Marmor himself re-

ported 70% satisfactory results following 60 UKA with a minimum 10 year follow-up: 38 of these were excellent or good, but there were 21 failures due to poor patient selection adn the use of 6 mm tibial components (26): Heck reported a 91.4% survival rate after 10 years in a study conducted on 294 knees (12).

Cartier (7, 8) also published very satisfying results after 10 year follow-up using the Marmor implant. He published a survival rate of 93% and 95% excellent and good results in a study of 149 Marmor UKAs. Koshino (20) using the YMCK and the Marmor implant published an 80% survival rate with an HSS score of 83, in a study of 67 UKAs over 10 to 25 years. Scott (30) published 100 ERA 1 UKAs with a 10 year follow-up showing an 85% survival rate in 1991.

The resecting type

The published results when the resecting type of UKA was used were inferior to the results of the resurfacing type. In 1990, Wanivenhaus (36) observed 14 loose PCA implants out of a total of 19.

Rosenberg studied 62 Miller Galante UKA implants and found a 14% incidence of progressive radiolucent lines after just 2 to 5 years postsurgery. In 1993, Swank (34) published a total failure rate between 4 and 8 year follow-up of 12% and an additional 17% of radiological evidence of impeding failure. Knight found a 33% failure rate and 41% unsatisfactory results when he studied 43 PCA implants (18).

The mobile bearing type

Results obtained with the mobile bearing type are not homogeneous. The reason for this might be the somewhat higher learning curve with this type of prosthesis. Goodfellow himself published with the Oxford UKA after 10 years a 95% survival rate while studying 53 lateral implants and a 76% survival rate while studying 53 lateral implants for 8 years. Argenson published the results of a study that included 472 Oxford implants in a multicentric study that after 5 years revealed a 93% medial and 80% lateral survival rate. Carr followed 121 Oxford knees and after 4 years found a survival rate of 99% (6).

In 1997, Stenstrom (33) published the results of the Swedish knee arthroplasty project showing a 5 year survival rate of the Oxford knee of 90%, the PCA of 85%, and the St. George and Marmor of 95%. In the same project, Knutson (19) revealed that there was significant deterioration after 6 to 8 years with the PCA, but also with the medial Oxford UKA.

In short, one may say that the resurfacing type of UKA still provides the best results in the follow-up period up to 10 years. The survival rate of the resecting type is much lower because of a higher rate of implant loosening. The mobile bearing type shows a higher rate of early problems occurring, in the long run after 10 years or more, and there might be some advantage with regard to reduced polyethylene wear.

Revision

Revisions are carried out when there is implant loosening, polyethylene wear, destruction of primarily uninvolved compartments, infection and implant failures like dislocation or breakage.

In almost all cases (excluding the infected ones) implantation of a total condylar arthroplasty is the best means of treatment. Revision with a new unicondylar prosthesis has a very high failure rate and can only be used in case of early polyethylene wear.

Previous incisions might interfere with the most recent one. This should be kept in mind during the first operation. For revision surgery, we use a medial parapatellar incision for most of the medial but also the lateral unicondylar implants. The advantage lies in the opportunity to use the Insall snip for better exposure of the joint in case of severe scarring. It is necessary to use a lateral incision in case of severe valgus deformity, an osteotomy of the tibial tubercle is recommended.

Bone loss might be excessive, but it is normally located in only one compartment. Therefore, further surgery is generally easier than in TKA.

If there is minimal bone loss, a standard TKA may be used. The holes should be filled with autologous bone from the non-affected compartment. If there should be some doubt, a tibial stem may be used. Larger bone loss requires the use of stems. Defects might be reconstructed using autologous bone or cement reinforced by screws.

Ligament laxity sometimes requires the use of semi-constrained TKA types like posterior-stabilizing prostheses, ultracongruent plateaus in case of cruciate ligament laxity. Revision type prostheses are used for excessive collateral ligament laxity. Therefore, it is important to have a modular knee system in the operating room at the onset of surgery. As compared to revision after high tibial osteotomy, the results are much better. As compared to revision after total knee arthroplasty, the results are somewhat better but worse than in primary total knee arthroplasty.

Summary

In my opinion, UKA plays an important role in knee arthroplasty. It offers some advantages as compared to TKA, for example, much better proprioception of the knee, lower infection rate, and diminished bone loss in case of revision.

Since the implantation is technically more demanding, a longer learning curve can be expected. Good long-term results required correct alignment of the implant and undercorrection of the deformed axis. Since body weight has to mainly lie on the implant, polyethylene wear has to be considered. Optimized material both on the femoral and tibial components has to be chosen, as well as adequate thickness of the polyethylene plateau.

Keeping these principles in mind, UKA is a successful solution, especially for less active and normal weight patients over 55 years of age. UKA provides them with a knee with optimal biomechanics and an almost normal range of motion.

The problem of survival rates that are sometimes reduced in comparison to TKA should be diminished in time as materials, design and sugical technique improve rapidly.

References

1) Argenson J-N, O'Connor J-J: Polyethylene wear in meniscal knee replacement: A 1-9 year retrieval analysis of the Oxford knee. J. Bone Joint Surg., 74-B, 228-232, 1992.

2) Blunn G.W., Joshi A.B., et al.: Polyethylene wear in unicondylar knee prostheses: Acta Orthop. Scand (1992); 63(3) 247.

3) Böhler N.: Surface modification of the femoral component Orthopaedics (1995) 15, 6: 16.

4) Böhler N., Pastl K., Infanger A.: Uncemented unicompartmental knee arthroplasty. In Morscher: Endoprosthetics (1995) Springer, 368.

5) Bohnhorst J., Bartsch H., Mueller W.: Mittelfristige Ergebnisse bei sofortbelastung des zementfreien Böhler – Monocondylarschlittens, Orthop. Praxis (1996), Kongressband B. Baden: 96.

6) Carr A., Keyes G., Miller R, O'Connor J., Goodfellow J: Medial Unicompartmental Arthroplasty: A survival study of the Oxford knee. Clin Orthop., (1993); 295:205-13.

7) Cartier Ph, Cheaib S: Unicondylar knee arthroplasty: 2 to 10 years of follow-up evaluation. J. Arthroplasty, (1987); 2:157-162.

8) Cartier Ph Sanouiller J-L, Grelsamer R-P: Unicompartmental knee Arthroplasty Surgery. 10 Years minikum follow-up period. J Arthroplasty, (1996); 11,7;782-788.

9) Chesnut W.J: Preoperative diagnostic protocol to predict candidate for unicompartmental arthroplasty. Clin Orthop, (1991); 273:146-150.

10) Goodfellow J.W. Kershaw C.J, M.K, O'Connor J-J: The Oxford knee for unicompartmental osteoarthritis. J Bone Joint Surg (Br), (1988); 70:692-701.

11) Gunston F-H: Polycentric knee arthroplasty; prosthetic simulation of normal knee movement. J. Bone Joint Surg., (1971); 53A: 272-277.

12) Heck D.A., Marmor L.. et al.: Unicompartmental knee arthroplasty: a multicenter investigation with long-term follow-up evaluation. Clin. Orthop., 286, 154, 1993.

13) Hernigou Ph, Deschamps G. La prothèse unicompartimentale du genou-Symposium SOFCOT 95, Chir Orthop, (1996), 82, Suppl. I: 25-60.

14) Hodge WA, Chandler HP Unicompartmental knee replacement: comparison of constrained and unconstrained designs. J Bone Joint Surg. (1992) AM 74:877.

15) Insall JN, Aglietti P: A five to seven-year follow-up unicondylar arthroplasty. J Bone Joint Surg. (1980) 62:A, 1329.

16) Ivarsson I, Giliquist J: Rehabilitation after high tibial osteotomy and unicompartmental arthroplasty. Clin Orthop (1989) 266: 139.

17) Kisslinger E., Wessinghage D.: Langzeitergebnisse von 501 unikompartimentalen Schlittenprothesen des Kniegelenkes; Orthop. Praxis (1997); 33 (3) 152

18) Knight J.L, Atwater R.D., JIE Guo: Early failure of the porous coated anatomic cemented unicompartmental knee arthroplasty J. Arthroplasty (1997) 12, 1: 11.

19) Knutson K, Lewold S, Robertsson, Lidgren L: Swedish Orthopaedic Society. Prospective multicentre study of knee arthroplasties. Acta Orthop Scand, (1994); 65(4): 375:386

20) T.Koshino: Unicompartmental Arthroplasty of degenerative osteoarthritic knee with more than 10 – years follow-up – Cahiers d'enseignement de la Sofcot (1997) 61: 210.

21) Laurencin C.T., Zelicof S.B., Scott R.D., Ewald F.C.: Unicompartmental versus total knee arthroplasty in the same patient: a Comparative study. Clin Orthop (1991), 273: 151.

22) Macinthos, D.L.: Hemiarthroplasty of the knee using a space occupying prosthesis for painful varus and valgus deformities. J Bone Joint Surg. (1958) A, 40: 1431.

23) Marmor L: Result of single compartment arthroplasty with acrylic cement fixation. A minimum follow-up of two years. Clin Orthop (1977) 122: 181.

24) Marmor L: Marmor modular knee in unicompartmental desease. J Bone Joint Surg (1979) Am 61: 347.

25) Marmor L: Lateral compartment arthroplasty of the knee. Clin Orthop (1984), 186: 115.

26) Marmor L: Unicompartmental knee arthroplasty – Ten to 13 year follow-up study. Clinic. Orthop. (1988); 14-20.

27) Moller J-T: Unicompartmental arthroplasty of the knee. Cadaver study of the importance of the anterior cruciate ligament. Acta Orthop. Scand., (1985); 56:120-123.

28) Rosenberg T-D, Paulos L.E, Parker R.D, Coward D.B, Scott S.M: The forty-five-degree postero-anterior flexion weight bearing radiograph of the knee. J.Bone Joint Surg, (1988), 70-A: 1479 – 1483.

29) Scott R.D, Santore R.F: Unicondylar unicompartmental replacement for ostheoarthritis of the knee. J. Bone Joint Surg. (1981); 63-A: 536-544.

30) Scott R.D., Cobb A.G, McQuerary F.G, Thornhill T.S: Unicompartmental knee arthroplasty. 8 to 12 year follow-up evaluation with survivorship analysis. Clin orthop, (1991); 271:96-100.

31) Streicher R.M., Weber H., et al: – New surface modification for TI-TAR-7NB alloy: Oxygen diffusion hardening (ODH), Biomaterials (1991), 3, 125.

32) Streicher R.M., Weber H, Schoen R, Semlitsch MF: Wear resistant couplings for longer lasting articulating total joint replacements. (1992) Adv 10/179:186.

33) Stenström A., Lindstrand A., Lewold S.: Unicompartmental knee Arthroplasty with special reference to the knee – Arthroplasty Register in Cahiers d'enseignement de la SOFCOT 61 (1997), 159.

34) Swank M., Stulberg S.D., et al: - The natural history of unicompartmental Arthroplasty – Clin. Orthop. (1993), 286; 130.

35) Thornhill T.S, Scott R.D.: Unicompartmental total knee arthroplasty, Orthop Clin North (1989) Am, 20(2): 245

36) Wanivenhaus A., Gottsauner-Wolf F., et al: 2-to-4 year results of the cementless application of the PCA unicondylar knee prostheses- Z. Orthop. (1990) 128, 612.

37) Witvoet J, Peyrache M-D, Nizard R: Prostheses unicompartimental type Lotus dans le traitement des gonarthroses. Rev Chir Orthop, (1993); 79:565-576.

Chapter 11
The Posterior Cruciate Ligament and Total Knee Arthroplasty

Richard S. Laskin
Cornell University Medical College - New York

Over the past fifteen years, the question of whether to retain or sacrifice the posterior cruciate ligament during total knee replacement has been debated at most major total knee symposia. Many of the reasons given for one technique or the other have been anecdotal visceral, rather than scientific and reflective. It is, however, only by such scientific evaluation that one can hope to arrive at some meaningful conclusion regarding this important structure and its function in total knee replacement.

In this chapter, I will discuss the function of the ligament, its anatomy, and the surgical technique for performing a knee replacement with both its retention and its resection. Other areas of discussion will include the history of total knee arthroplasty as related to the posterior cruciate ligament, those situations in which the ligament should be routinely sacrificed, and the advantages of performing a total knee both with resection and retention techniques.

Anatomy and Function

In the normal knee, the posterior cruciate ligament aids in resisting posterior displacement of the tibia on the femur during flexion. Combined with the anterior cruciate ligament and the quadriceps and patellar tendons, it forms from the "four bar linkage" of the knee, which not only imparts stability but also guides femoral condylar rollback during flexion. As a consequence of this, it is obviously an important structure in the normal knee.

The posterior cruciate ligament is physically present as an intact structure in most arthritic knees.

Cloutier (4) and Scott (29) have both reported the presence of a posterior cruciate ligament in over 97% of their arthritic knees undergoing joint replacement. This is in contradistinction to the anterior cruciate ligament, however, which was absent in about 50% of the cases. There are probably many etiologies for these findings. The anterior cruciate ligament is more often damaged with torsional and angular injuries than is the posterior cruciate ligament, and once damaged it usually becomes rapidly atrophic. Furthermore, the posterior cruciate ligament has a richer blood supply than the anterior cruciate ligament and this may help in resisting minor injuries and the attendant damage from arthrosclerotic disease as the patient ages.

The posterior cruciate ligament has an abundant neurologic innervation. These nerve fibers are found primarily in the connective tissue between its main fascicular bundles. Gomez-Barena has demonstrated both Golgi-type and paciniform endings in the ligament, and these are most likely responsible for mediating its proprioceptive function, and Schultz (27) has demonstrated that cruciate ligaments have an abundant supply of mechanoreceptors.

Woo (35) has shown that in experimental animals the structure and innervation of ligaments changes with age, and this has been corroborated by Hollis and Lyon (13), Warren and Olankokun (34) and Kaplan (17). Despite this, neural endings can still be demonstrated in posterior cruciate ligaments from older osteoarthritic patients, the ones who would be undergoing knee replacement, and this suggests that the ligament does continue to have a proprioceptive function even in these cases.

The posterior cruciate ligament has its origin on the posteromedial aspect of the inter-condylar notch of the femur. Unlike the anterior cruciate ligament, whose insertion is on the surface of the tibia in the region of the tibial spines, the posterior cruciate ligament's tibial attachment is on the posterior aspect of the metaphysis extending as a broad band from approximately 3 mm below the articular surface to a level approximately 10 mm below the articular surface.

Since the ligament is physically present, retains innervation and blood supply, and has an important function in the normal knee, why is there any controversy regarding retaining it during a total knee arthroplasty? We surely do not have this same controversy regarding the medial or lateral collateral ligaments. A review of the history of knee replacement prostheses may help answer this question.

Historical Overview of Prosthesis Designs

Many of the early non-linked total knee designs (Modular (26), Cloutier (4, 5), Polycentric (11), and Geomedic (7)) allowed preservation of both the posterior and anterior cruciate ligaments in an attempt to "restore normal anatomy." If you preserve the anterior cruciate ligament, however, you cannot use a stem on the tibial component. Since a central stem aids in resisting loosening and subsidence, may of these resurfacing bicruciate retaining knees failed due to tibial component loosening.

In an attempt to enhance tibial component fixation, tibial components were then developed with a central stem. Obviously this required that the anterior cruciate ligament be sacrificed. Almost all of these initial stemmed tibial components had a cupped conforming articular surface with raised anterior and posterior polyethylene lips. This geometric configuration, combined with proper filling of the flexion space imparted anterior-posterior stability to the knee without requiring an intact PCL. For these knees, (Total Condylar (16), Freeman (9, 10)). the PCL was resected. The raised posterior lip, however, did not allow femoral rollback, so that maximum flexion was often limited to only 90°-100° (18).

There were a few prostheses that were designed with both a conforming cupped surface and a posterior cutout to allow retention of the posterior cruciate ligament.

Unfortunately this was not a bad compromise, it was worse. In these knees, (Duopatellar

(28)) the presence of the posterior cruciate ligament caused the femur to roll back on the tibia, while the cupped articular surface impeded this. The result was a condition called kinematic mismatch, a situation which often led to either rupture of the posterior cruciate ligament or a high level of polyethylene wear. As a result, these types of prostheses clinically failed early and gradually were abandoned.

The next phase of knee development progressed along two different tracks. Some designers began to study prostheses that would roll back and increase the potential for flexion. To do this, they developed tibial components, which were more flattened in an anteroposterior plane and had no posterior lip. Some of these prostheses were also flattened in the coronal plane (PCA (14), Kinematic (6)), while others maintained a more conforming surface in the coronal plane (Richard's Maximum (RMC)) (19)). It was hoped that this combination of implant design and a retained posterior cruciate ligament would give results that approached those in the normal knee.

Progressing along a completely different track, biomechanical scientists at the Hospital for Special Surgery in New York modified the original total condylar design. The posterior lip was flattened, and a central tibial polyethylene eminence was added to articulate with a cam on the femoral component. The concept was that as the knee flexed, the articulation between the polyethylene eminence and the femoral cam would guide roll back of the femur in a manner more like that in the normal knee, without having to rely upon any inherent function in the posterior cruciate ligament. The prototypical prosthesis of this design was the Insall-Burstein-I (15).

At present, most of the currently available knee prostheses have one of these three basic designs. There are prostheses with a partially conforming surface in the coronal plane but with a relatively flat anteroposterior surface that allow retention and functioning of the posterior cruciate ligament (Genesi II (20), Kinemax, Duracon, Natural Knee (12)). There are those knees with a central polyethylene peg eminence and femoral cam to replace the function of the posterior cruciate ligament (Insall Berstein II (31), Genesis II Posterior Stabilized, PFC stabilized). Finally, there are a few prostheses with a cupped articular surface in both planes and raised tibial anterior and posterior lips (Freeman-Samuelson, PFC Posterior Lipped, Natural Knee and Genesis II Deep Dished).

Surgical Technique for Retention of the PCL

It is possible to safely remove the proximal tibial surface in a manner so as not only to preserve but also not to damage an intact posterior cruciate ligament. To do this, we first resect the anteromedial portion of the tibial plateau. The saw blade is advanced to the inner portion of the posterior cortex and left in situ to protect the plateau. An osteotome is then used to vertically split the medial from the lateral tibial plateaus (Fig. 1). The posterior medial femoral cortex is then "fractured" using a small osteotome rather than with the saw. This helps prevent inadvertent posterior penetration with possible damage to the popliteal vascular structures. Finally, the saw blade is then rested on the cut medial surface and directed laterally to resect the lateral tibial plateau (Fig. 2). I have not routinely attempted to preserve a block of bone anterior to the posterior cruciate ligament, although this has been suggested (30) as a further way to avoid inadvertent damage to the ligament during resection of the tibia.

It has been alleged that proper exposure of the knee is not possible unless the posterior cruciate ligament is removed. Although there are reasons to remove the posterior cruciate ligament during knee replacement, exposure is not

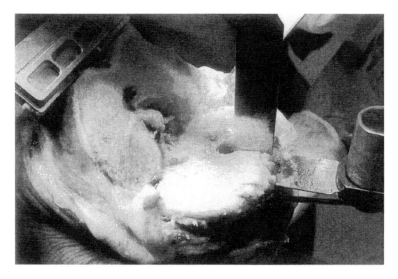

FIG. 1

one of them. If the soft tissues both medially and laterally are elevated to just beyond the mid coronal plane (Fig. 3), and the knee hyperflexed, the tibia can be easily subluxed anteriorly, even in the presence of an intact posterior cruciate ligament (22) (Fig. 4).

Prior to inserting the permanent components the surgeons should flex the knee with the trial implants in place. If the anterior portion of the tibial trial lifts off during flexion, or if the femoral condyle rolls back to the posterior half of the tibial plateau, the posterior cruciate ligament is too tight. This can be remedied by recessing the ligament. Several millimeters of the insertion of the ligament onto the posterior tibia can be elevated subperiosteally without damage to the entire ligament insertion. An alternative is to partially elevate the origin of the ligament from the femur. Either of these techniques will correct the tightness and allow proper tracking of the components without tibial component lift off.

Similarly, the surgeons should impart a posterior force on the tibia with the knee flexed 90°. If the posterior displacement is more than 3-5 mm, the posterior cruciate ligament is relatively loose, and a thicker bearing surface will be needed to obtain flexion stability.

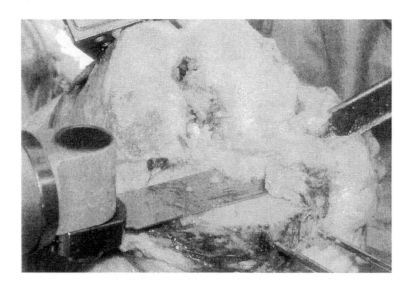

FIG. 2

FIG. 3

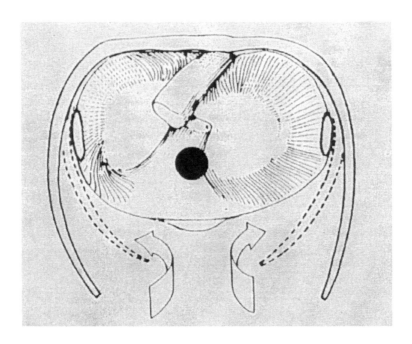

Using these two provocative tests, which Scott (30) has called POLO (pull out-lift off), the surgeon can ascertain that, at the completion of the arthroplasty, the posterior cruciate ligament is neither too tight nor too loose.

Surgical Technique for Resection of the PCL

There are several techniques for resection of the posterior cruciate ligament. The ligament may be simply released from either its proximal and distal end, or it may be excised in toto. Pro-ponents of the first technique allege that the released ligament will "reattach" to the posterior capsule and still continue to provide proprioceptive function to the knee. This has never been proven, however. Proponents of complete resection of the ligament have stated that a retained ligament that has been released at is origin or insertion may lead to a soft tissue impingement between the femoral and tibial components. Although this surely is not a common occurrence, we have revised two total knee prostheses in which this was the case. We have used all three techniques and have found that a release from the femur appears to be easiest in most cases. One should note, however, that there is often a small vessel in the posterior cruciate ligament adjacent to its femoral attachment and this should be cauterized at the time the ligament is released.

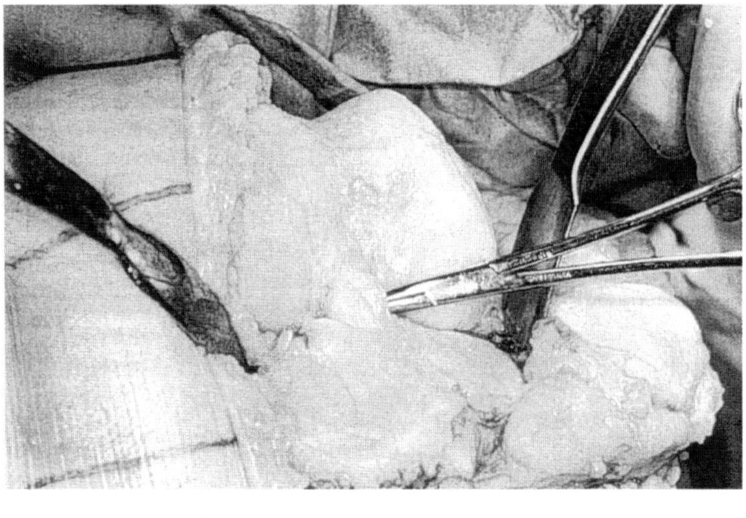

Special Indications for Resecting the Posterior Cruciate Ligament

It is obviously surgically possible to perform a total knee

FIG. 4

arthroplasty and still retain the posterior cruciate ligament. There are, however, situations in which retention of the ligament is inappropriate and detrimental.

1. Fixed flexion and Angular Deformities

In 1988 we performed a retrospective analysis of several groups of patients who had undergone total knee replacement. In some a posterior cruciate-retaining prosthesis had been used, while in others a posterior cruciate-substituting (PS) prostheses had been chosen (23). In the patients in whom the posterior cruciate ligament was retained, three types of implants were used: the RMC, the Tricon-M and the PCA. In actuality this represented only two articular geometries since the RMC and the Tricon-M had identical polyethylene surfaces and differed only in the method of fixation of the tibial component (cemented central stem in the RMC and uncemented lateral flanged pegs in the Tricon-M). The Insall Burstein prosthesis was used for those cases in which the posterior cruciate ligament was sacrificed. Although the study was neither specifically double-blinded nor randomized, the prosthetic choice for any individual patient was not based upon any specific knowledge, at that time, of the effect of the posterior cruciate ligament in the patient with a knee replacement.

There were 100 knees with a combined flexion and angular fixed deformity (varus or valgus) of less than 20°. Among them, there were 58 knees where a posterior cruciate-retaining prosthesis was used (Group A) and 42 knees in which a posterior-stabilized prosthesis was used (Group B). There were 11 knees with greater than 20° of fixed angular and flexion deformity. Among them there were 65 knees in which a posterior cruciate-retaining prosthesis was used (Group C) and 46 knees where a posterior-stabilized prosthesis was utilized (Group D).

All patients were evaluated at least 2 years after their arthroplasty. In Groups A and B (those with a combined angular and flexion deformity less than 20°), there was no statistical difference in the results either saving or substituting for the posterior cruciate ligament. However, for those with a combined angular and flexion deformity **greater than 20°**, patients with resection of the posterior cruciate ligament and insertion of a posterior-stabilized prosthesis (Group D) had better results than those in which the ligament was retained (Group C).

In Group C patients in whom the posterior cruciate ligament was retained there was a statistically significant decrease in the range of flexion (mean = 83°) to the Group D patients in whom the ligament was sacrificed (mean = 113°) (p<.01). Furthermore, mean residual flexion contracture in Group C was 11° while that in the posterior-stabilized group D patients was 3° (p<.001). The ability to obtain a tibiofemoral anatomical axis of an optimal 5°-7° of valgus occurred in 84% of the knees in Group D as compared to only 62% in Group C (p<.001). We felt that these inferior results were due to the fact that the posterior cruciate ligament was an integral part of the varus and flexion deformity, and, by not releasing it, the deformity could not be completely and properly corrected. As a result of this study, we suggested using posterior-stabilized prostheses for such patients with these types of fixed deformities.

We re-evaluated these patients 8-10 years later to see if there had been any change in these early outcomes (21). We continued to see a decreased flexion arc in those patients in whom a PCL retaining prosthesis had been used in the face of an initial severe deformity. We likewise found an increased incidence of radiolucent lines, medial knee pain, and revision in that group. The survivorship in that group was 72% compared to over 90% in the other groups. We observed that a large number of the patients in Group D had a postoperative wedge sign, as described by Sambakasis and Wilton. They felt that this sign represented the sequela of asymmetrical coronal stresses on the knee after the surgery. This would appear to corroborate our feeling that if the PCL was not released in a severe angular deformity, the deformity itself was not completely corrected.

2. Prior Patellectomy

Patellectomy continues to be a surgical option for patients with severely comminuted fractures of the patella as well as for a few patients with advanced patellofemoral degenerative disease. Many of these patients eventually require a total knee replacement for subsequent tibiofemoral arthrosis. We reviewed our patients who had undergone total knee replacement and who had undergone a prior patellectomy in an attempt to determine whether the prior surgery in some way compromised the result of the subsequent arthroplasty (25).

We segregated these patients into two groups. In Group I patients, a posterior-stabilized prosthesis was used, while in Group II a prosthesis with retention of the posterior cruciate ligament was inserted. In all cases, the knee was stable both anteroposteriorly and mediolaterally at the time of the index arthroplasty. When the patients were evaluated five years after the arthroplasty, however, those in whom the PCL had been spared had a statistically significant increase in anteroposterior instability as well as a statistically significant diminution in their ability to climb and descend stairs.

We further studied the patients who had undergone a patellectomy for trauma and compared them to the patients who had undergone a patellectomy for patellofemoral arthrosis. At five years after surgery, the results in the second group were definitely inferior, with a decreased flexion arc, and a higher proportion complaining of some pain with ambulation.

Finally, we compared the total knee patients who had undergone patellectomy for trauma and had been reconstructed with a posterior-stabilized prosthesis with a group of patients who were undergoing an index total knee replacement using a posterior-stabilized implant. The patients were matched for sex, age decade, and weight group. The results in the two groups were statistically similar (p< 1).

As a result of this study, we now recommend using a posterior-stabilized prosthesis for all patients who have undergone a prior patellectomy.

3. Rheumatoid Arthritis

As part of a study investigating the 5-7 year results of patients with rheumatoid arthritis who had undergone an uncemented total knee replacement, we discovered many knees which had exhibited good anteroposterior stability at the time of the index procedure, only to demonstrate moderate to severe instability at 7-8 years subsequently (21). Their X-rays were often normal, with no evidence of tibial subsidence. Many of these patients underwent revision surgery and in almost each case, the posterior cruciate ligament was not discernible as a distinct structure, although it had been present at the time of the index arthroplasty. In most of these cases a synovial biopsy revealed a Type I pattern, with moderate amounts of inflammatory cells. We have postulated that the synovitis in the joint led to the PCL dissolution in a manner analogous to its action on the transverse liga-

ment of the odontoid. As a result of these findings, we no longer recommend performing knee arthroplasty with posterior cruciate retention in patients with rheumatoid arthritis.

4. Prior High Tibial Osteotomy

As a consequence of a tibial osteotomy performed proximal to the tibial tubercle, there is posterior scarring that will involve the posterior cruciate ligament. Furthermore, the removal of a wedge of bone changes the length and orientation of the ligament. In a study presented at the Annual Meeting of the American Academy of Orthopaedic Surgeons in 1993, we reported that in over 70% of all the post-osteotomy patients undergoing total knee replacement, the posterior cruciate ligament was a fibrotic scarred band. In 27% of the patients it was not present at all at the time of the arthroplasty, It is for these reasons that in patients who are undergoing a knee replacement and who have had a prior tibial osteotomy, a posterior-stabilized implant should be used.

Posterior Cruciate-Retention Prostheses vs. Posterior-Stabilized Prostheses Advantages and Disadvantages

Proponents of retaining the posterior cruciate ligament during a total knee replacement cite several potential advantages. Andriachi (1, 2) has shown that retaining the ligament increases the potential for femoral roll back, and this results in a more normal gait especially when ascending or descending stairs. Retaining the ligament also allows for a tibial component that is not conforming, thereby allowing mixing of femoral and tibial components of different sizes.

Proponents of resecting the ligament and using a posterior-stabilized prosthesis state that it is extremely difficult to properly balance the ligament: if it is left too loose it is ineffectual, and if it is left too tight it can limit flexion, can increase polyethylene wear, and cause tibial component loosening. They state that the gait pattern with a posterior-stabilized implant is more normal and that rollback is more predictable if it is guided by the implant rather than by the posterior cruciate ligament.

In coming to these conclusion, most investigators have used at least two different types of prostheses with different articular surfaces. This adds other variables to their studies over and above the mere retention or sacrifice of the posterior cruciate ligament. The conclusions are therefore often invalid.

In an attempt to overcome this problem we began a study in 1991, in one hundred consecutive patients for whom a cruciate ligament-retaining prosthesis was not contraindicated. A prospective randomization was performed into two groups. In the first, the posterior cruciate ligament was retained and the standard cruciate-retaining prosthesis inserted. In the second group, the ligament was resected and the same prosthesis was used in these cases; a module with a cam was attached to the femoral component, and a tibial component polyethylene with a central eminence was used. Soft tissue balancing and bone resections were the same for both groups as was the postoperative physical therapy protocol. The range of motion of the patients in the two groups preoperatively was similar. The physical therapist was blinded as to which group each patient belonged to. The study had been evaluated and approved by the Institutional Review Board of the hospital, and each patient enrolled was carefully counseled as to the nature of the study and could elect whether to participate or not.

We found no statistical difference in the range of motion of the patients in these two groups both when evaluating the motion at the time of hospital discharge nor at two years subsequently. The rate of return of flexion while in the hospital was also similar in both groups, The rate of obtaining functional milestones while in the hospital was equal for both groups, There was no difference in the pain scores, stability, the overall Knee Society Score and Hospital for Special Surgery rating scores, and patient satisfaction scores between the two groups.

Equivalent motion using both PCL retaining and PS prostheses does not appear to be related to whether or not the tibial bearing surface is fixed or mobile. We have found this similar motion using a fixed bearing design, the Genesis II (24), and Stiehl (33) noted it using a mobile LCS prosthesis.

Since there appears to be no clinical difference between saving the posterior cruciate ligament and sacrificing it and using a posterior-stabilized implant for most primary total knee replacement patients (that is, those without a severe deformity, without a prior patellectomy or osteotomy, and those who do not have rheumatoid arthritis) are there other considerations which should be studied?

1. Removing Intercondylar Femoral Bone for a PS Femoral Design

To implant a posterior-stabilized femoral component a portion of the intercondylar bone of the distal femur must be resected. This potentially weakens the distal femur and may lead to fracture especially in the small, osteopenic patient.

Furthermore, if a revision of the implant is required, the amount of bone remaining for the revision is, in theory, less.

The severity of this problem is implant-related. It is specifically a problem if a femoral component design is chosen that requires an anterior-posterior resection of bone. We have developed a design, however, that requires reaming of the central bone of the intercondylar notch and allows retention of the anterior bridge (Fig. 6). In the laboratory we have shown that this technique does not significantly reduce the strength of the distal femur.

2. The Patellar Clunk Syndrome

Patellar clunk syndrome may be another consideration in deciding whether or not to use a posterior-stabilized implant. Patients with this syndrome have a palpable and audible clunk when the knee extends actively from approximately 30° of flexion.

Pathologically, it represents trapping of soft tissue in the intercondylar box of the implant as the knee extends. This incidence of this syndrome has been reported to be as high at 10% in patients undergoing the Insall Burstein II arthroplasty. This appears to represent a particular problem attendant to the shape of the intercondylar box in this implant since its incidence in other posterior-stabilized designs is significantly less. It has not been reported in posterior cruciate ligament-retaining femoral components.

3. Posterior-Stabilized Implants May Have Problems with Dislocation

All posterior-stabilized implants are not alike. The intercondylar eminence of the tibial component must be of the proper height and configuration in order to impart posterior stability to the knee. Furthermore, one cannot simply rely upon the eminence and cam for stability, but must balance the flexion space as carefully as one does in a posterior cruciate-retaining prosthesis. Failure to do this may result in subluxation of the tibial spine from the cam and possible actual dislocation and locking of the knee.

In an attempt to eliminate these potential problems with posterior-stabilized implants, Hoffmann has suggested the use of an ultra-congruent tibial component with raised anterior and posterior lips as an alternative to a posterior-stabilized implant with a central tibial eminence. Theoretically, however, such an implant should have an increased potential for contact with the patellar implant anteriorly and this may lead to abnormal polyethylene wear. Whether these theoretical considerations will be seen clinically has not yet been determined.

4. Congruency of the Bearing Surfaces

Many of the older tibial component designs that allowed posterior cruciate retention were less congruent than those that were posterior-stabilized. Biomechanically, decreased congruency leads to increase localized peak stresses in the polyethylene which can lead to an increase in wear and particle formation. This has been cited, therefore, as a reason for choosing a posterior-stabilized implant. However, many of the current third and fourth generation posterior cruciate-retaining designs have an articular geometry that is congruent so that this difference between the two types of prosthesis is becoming less of a consideration.

5. Joint Kinematics

Stiehl (32) Dennis (8) and Banks (3) have published a study of in vivo kinematics of knees after arthroplasty. They used digital fluoroscopic examination of the knee during a deep knee bend. Then by using a computer generated 3-D analysis they were able to superimpose the configuration of the specific implant used and determine the accurate contact areas between the femoral and tibial components.

They compared the results seen in patients in whom a knee replacement was performed with PCL retention and ones in whom a knee replacement was performed using a PS prosthesis. All the surgeries were performed by experienced knee surgeons with proper balancing of the flexion and extension spaces. For comparison, they also examined patients with normal knees, and sports medicine patients in whom there was an ACL deficiency.

In the normal knee, the contact point between the femur and tibia began approximately 5-10 mm anterior to the midline in full extension and gradually moved posteriorly as the knee flexed. In the knee in which a PS prosthesis had been inserted the contact point was in the midline in full extension but again proceeded posteriorly during flexion. These findings were fairly similar in all the normal and PS Prosthesis knees that were studied.

In the sports medicine patient with an ACL deficient knee the contact point was initially posterior to the mid coronal line in extension and then moved first anteriorly and then slightly posteriorly. This erratic paradoxical forward motion of the contact point was likewise seen in the patients in whom a PCL retaining prosthesis had been used.

Furthermore, the erratic pattern was different for each knee studied although all demonstrated this paradoxical roll forward. (Fig. 7)

Does this mean that despite proper balancing of the PCL motion and kinematics will be abnormal because of the absence of the ACL? Is indeed a knee in which the PCL is retained, merely an ACL deficient knee replacement knee? This evaluation is being studied now using normal gait patterns rather than a deep knee bend so as to further help us determine exactly what transpires with motion of the knee using a variety of prostheses.

6. Joint Proprioception

There is no unanimity as to whether the neurological innervation of the PCL assists in joint proprioception. The studies that have been performed are somewhat contradictory. If it does, however, this may be a further indication to retaining the ligament in clinical situations where it is possible.

Summary

Based upon the above studies, it is our current policy to attempt to retain the posterior cruciate ligament, if possible during a total knee arthroplasty. We pay particular care to balancing the flexion space and recessing the ligament when appropriate. We likewise routinely use a posterior stabilized implant in the patients with a fixed combined angular and flexion deformity 90°, in those with a prior high tibial osteotomy or patellectomy, and in those patients with inflammatory arthropathy. Using these guidlines, our results up to ten years after arthroplasty have been excellent both functionally and radiographically.

References

1) Andriacchi TP, Galante JO: Retention of the posterior cruciate ligament in total knee arthroplasty. J. Arthroplasty, 3: 13-19, 1998.
2) Andriacchi TP, Galante JO: Fermier RW: The influence of total knee replacement design on walking and stair climbing. J Bone Joint Surgery, 64A: 1328-1334, 1998
3) Banks S.A., Markovich G.D., and Hodge W.A.: In vivo kinematics of cruciate retaining and substituting knee arthroplasties. J. Arthroplasty, 12: 297-304, 1997.
4) Cloutier JM: Results of total knee arthroplasty with a nonconstrained prosthesis. J Bone Joint Surgery, 65A: 906-915, 1983.
5) Cloutier JM: Long term results after non constrained total knee arthroplasty. Cl.Orth., 273: 63-65, 1991.
6) Cobb AC, Ewald FC, Wright RJ, Sledge CB: The kinematic knee: survivorship analysis of 1943 knees. J Bone Joint Surgery, 72B: 542-546, 1990.
7) Coventry MN, Upshaw JE, Riley LJ, Finerman GAM, Turner RH: Geomedic total knee arthroplasty. Cl.Orth., 94: 171-184, 1973.
8) Dennis D., Komistek R,D,, Hoff W.A., Gabriel, S.M.: In vivo kinematics derived using an inverse perspective technique. Cl.Orth., 331:107-117, 1996.
9) Freeman MAR: A three to five year follow up of the Freeman Swanson arthroplasty of the knee. J Bone Joint Surgery, 59B: 64-71, 1977.
10) Freeman MAR, Todd RC, Bamert P, Day WH: ICLH arthroplasty of the hip. J Bone Joint Surgery, 60B: 339-344, 1978.
11) Gunston FH, Mackenzie RL: Complications of polycentric knee arthroplasty. Cl.Orth., 97: 120-127, 1976.
12) Hoffmann AA, Murdock LE, Wyatt RWB, Alpert JP: Total knee arthroplasty. A two to four year experience using an asymmetric tibial tray and a deep trochlear groove femoral component. Cl.Orth., 269: 78-84, 1991.
13) Hollis JM, Lyon RM, Marcin JP: Effect of age and loading axis on the failure properties of human ligaments. Transactions of the Orthopaedic Research Society, 13: 83, 1998
14) Hungerford D.S., Kenna RV, Krackow KA: The porous coated anatomical total knee. Orth. Clinic North Am. 13: 103-122, 1982.
15) Insall JN, Laschiewicz PF, Burstein AH: The posterior stabilized condylar prosthesis: a modification of the total condylar design. J Bone Joint Surgery, 64A: 1317-1323, 1982.
16) Insall JN, Ranawat CS, Aglietti P, Sshine J: A comparison of four models of total knee replacement prosthesis. J Bone Joint Surgery, 58A: 754-765, 1976.
17) Kaplan F.S., Nixon J.E., Reiz M.: Age-related changes in proprioception and sensation of joint position. Acta Ortho.Scand., 56: 72-74, 1985.
18) Laskin RS: Total condylar knee replacement in rheumatoid arthritis. J Bone Joint Surgery, 63: 42-49, 1981.
19) Laskin RS: RMC total knee replacement. A review of 166 cases. J. Arthroplasty, 1: 11-19, 1986.
20) Laskin RS: The Genesis modular total knee replacement with posterior cruciate retention. A three year follow up study. The Knee, 1: 146-153, 1994.
21) Laskin RS, O'Flynn H: Total knee replacement with posterior cruciate ligament retention in rheumatoid arthritis. Problems and complications. Cl.Orth., 345: 5-10, 1997.
22) Laskin RS, Rieger MA: The surgical technique for performing a total knee replacement arthroplasty. Orth. Clinic North Am., 20(1): 31-48, 1989.
23) Laskin RS, Rieger MA, Schob C, Turen C: The posterior stabilized total knee prosthesis in the knee with a severe fixed deformity. Am.J Knee Surgery, 1: 203 1998.
24) Laskin R.S.: Range of motion after total knee replacement. Orthopaedic Transaction, 1998. (In Press).
25) Laskin R.S. and Paletta G.: Total knee replacement in the patient who has undergone a patellectomy. J Bone Joint Surgery, 1995.
26) Marmor L: The modular knee. ClOrth., 94: 242-248, 1973.
27) Schultz R.A., Miller D.C., Kerr C.S.: Mechanoreceptors in human cruciate ligaments. A histologic study. J Bone Joint Surgery, 66A: 1072-1076, 1998.
28) Scott R: Duopatellar total knee replacement. The Brigham experience. Orth. Clinic North Am., 12: 89-102, 1982.
29) Scott R, Volatile TB: Twelve years experience with a posterior cruciate retaining total knee arthroplasty. Cl.Orth., 205: 100-107, 1986.
30) Scott R, Thornhill T.: Posterior cruciate supplementing total knee replacement using onforming inserts and cruciate recession: effect on range of motion and radiolucent lines. Cl.Orth., 309: 146-152, 1994.
31) Stern SH, Insall JN: Posterior stabilized prostheses. The results aftger a follow up of nine to twelve years. J. Bone Joint Surgery, 74A: 980-988, 1992.
32) Stiehl J.B., Komistek R.D., Dennis D.A., Paxson R.D.: Fluroscopic analysis of kinematics after posterior cruciate retaining knee arthroplasty. J. Bone and Joint Surgery, 77B: 884-889, 1998.
33) Stiehl J.B., Voorhorst P.E., Keblish P., Sorrels R.B.: Comparison of range of motion after posterior criciate ligament retention or sacrifice with a mobile bearing total knee arthroplasty. Am.J Knee Surgery, 10: 216-220, 1997.
34) Warren P.J., Olanlokun T.K. C.A.G.: Proprioception after total knee arthroplasty. The influence of prosthetic design. Cl. Orth., 297: 182-187, 1994.
35) Woo SLY, Buckwalter JA: Normal ligament. Structure, function and composition. In Injury and Repair of the Musculoskeletal Soft Tissues, pp.45-101. Edited by American Academy of Orthopaedic Surgeons. Park Ridge, Ill, American Academy of Orthopaedic Surgeons, 1987.

Chapter 12
Posterior Cruciate Ligament-Substituting Total Knee Arthroplasty: Rationale and Results

Mark W. Pagnano, Giles R. Scuderi, John N. Insall
Insall, Scott, Kelly Institute - New York

Introduction

Few controversies in orthopedic surgery have persisted for as long as the debate over the appropriate role of the posterior cruciate ligament (PCL) in total knee arthroplasty. Excellent long-term results have been obtained with cemented, condylar total knee components of the cruciate-sacrificing, cruciate-substituting and cruciate-retaining designs.

However, important new information in the areas of biomechanics (5, 14, 20, 29, 33), histology (17), gait-analysis (35), kinematics (7, 32) and the results from clinical trials (4, 6, 8, 9, 12, 13, 19, 22, 23, 30), have further strengthened our long-held belief that a posterior cruciate ligament-substituting total knee design is the implant of choice for most primary and revision total knee arthroplasties.

This chapter will review our rationale for favoring the posterior-stabilized knee design and present the published clinical results of posterior-stabilized total knee arthroplasty.

Historical Overview

Many current total knee implants were derived from the Total Condylar prosthesis which was introduced in 1974. That prosthesis is a cemented, cruciate-sacrificing, tri-compartmental prosthesis, with a relatively conforming tibiofemoral articulation (15).

The total condylar design relies on softtissue balance in flexion and extension and moderate conformity in the coronal and sagittal planes for stability because the posterior cruciate is excised but not substituted. In recent years the terms "total condylar" and "condylar" have become generic terms for any surface replacement knee design which accommodates patellar resurfacing and includes a one-piece tibial component with a central stem or keel.

To prevent posterior subluxation of the tibia and to improve both range of motion and stair-climbing ability, the total condylar prosthesis was modified to the posterior-stabilized (Insall-Burstein I) design in 1978 (16, 31) (Fig. 1).

A cam mechanism on the femoral component was designed to articulate with a central polyethylene peg rising from the tibial component. That post and cam mechanism acts as a functional substitute for the posterior cruciate ligament. The tibial components of the original total condylar and posterior-stabilized knees were of an all-polyethylene design. Metal backing was subsequently added to the tibial components and by late 1981 the metal-backed tibial component was used exclusively at the Hospital for Special Surgery.

In 1987 the posterior-stabilized design was modified to accommodate modular tibial inserts as well as metal wedges, stems and augments (Insall-Burstein II) (Fig. 2). The tibiofemoral articulation in both the posterior-stabilized (Insall-Burstein I) and the modular posterior-stabilized (Insall-Burstein II) designs has remained moderately conforming in both the coronal and sagittal planes (31).

Design modifications that provide specific right and left femoral components and that improve patellofemoral tracking are part of the latest iteration of the posterior stabilized knee (Legacy) (Fig. 3).

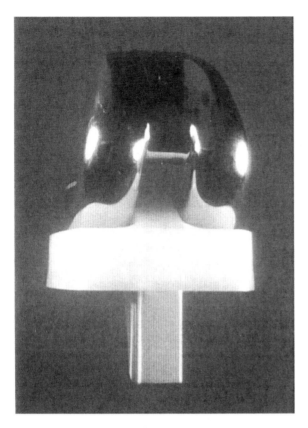

FIG. 1 - The Insall-Burstein posterior-stabilized knee was a modification of the Total Condylar knee design. The post and cam mechanism of the posterior-stabilized knee limits posterior translation of the tibia and improves range of motion by promoting femoral rollback.

et al. used fluoroscopy to study the invivo kinematics of 5 normal knees and 47 cruciate retaining total knees of 5 different designs (32). In contrast to the normal knees, the cruciate-retaining total knees demonstrated a tibiofemoral contact point which was posterior in extension and translated anteriorly with knee flexion (7). While the normal knees in that study moved smoothly during the flexion cycle, the cruciate-retaining total knees demonstrated a discontinuous or skidding motion.

Dennis et al. have also shown that cruciate-retaining designs demonstrate paradoxical anterior femoral translation with knee flexion. Those authors expressed concern that anterior femoral translation may promote premature polyethylene wear in cruciate-retaining total knees. The posterior-stabilized total knees studied by Dennis et al. more closely reproduced normal knee kinematics but neither the posterior-stabilized nor the cruciate-retaining designs fully duplicated normal femoral rollback.

A biomechanical study by Mahoney et al. has suggested that both posterior-stabilized and cruciate-retaining total knees result in less femoral rollback and less quadriceps muscle efficiency than the normal knee (20) (Fig. 5 and 6). That study did find, however, that the posterior-stabilized design produced more rollback and better quadriceps efficiency than the cruciate-retaining knees. Those authors were

Kinematics

Summary: The in vivo kinematics of the posterior-stabilized knee are more predictable than those of the cruciate-retaining knee.

Retention of the posterior cruciate ligament was introduced as a way to improve total knee arthroplasty kinematics, preserve anatomic femoral rollback, and to increase knee range of motion. Recent work, however, suggests that the in vivo kinematics of the cruciate-retaining knee are unpredictable (7, 32) (Fig. 4). The kinematics of the posterior-stabilized knee, meanwhile, appear more reproducible and are governed by the interaction of the femoral cam and tibial post. Stiehl

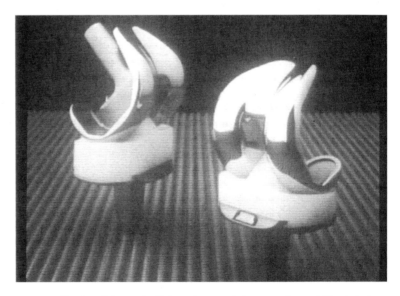

FIG. 2 - The Insall-Burstein II knee is a modular posterior-stabilized design. That design allows for modular tibial inserts as well as metal augmentation wedges and stems.

disappointed at the consistent loss of extensor mechanism efficiency that was seen with the cruciate-retaining knees.

Range of Motion

Summary: The posterior-stabilized knee reliably and reproducibly results in mean maximum flexion of 110 to 115 degrees.

The original cruciate-sacrificing total condylar design produced a mean maximum flexion of 90 to 95 degrees (15). That amount of flexion is near the theoretic limit for a total knee lacking femoral rollback. The introduction of the posterior-stabilized design allowed flexion to improve to a mean of 105-115 degrees. With the cruciate-retaining total knees, recent emphasis has been placed on balance, by selective partial release, of the posterior cruciate ligament (26). In conjunction with the technique of posterior cruciate balancing, several large series of cruciate-retaining total knees report mean maximum flexion of 110 to 115 degrees (26). One prospective series of 242 total knee arthroplasties compared cruciate-retaining, cruciate-sacrificing, and posterior-stabilized knee designs (13). The posterior-

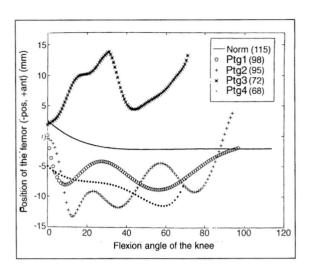

FIG. 4 - The in vivo kinematics of posterior-cruciate retaining total knees are unpredictable. Each of the four cruciate-retaining knee designs shown here demonstrate a tendency to translate anteriorly with flexion (so-called roll-forward) as compared with the normal knee that will roll-back (from Stiehl et al. (32).

stabilized knees in that study demonstrated a mean range of motion (112 degrees) that was significantly greater than the cruciate-retaining knees (104 degrees). In addition, the posterior-stabilized knee group was the only group in which the 95 percent confidence limit for motion was above 90 degrees.

Wear

Summary: Clinically significant polyethylene wear is rare in cemented posterior-stabilized total knee arthroplasty.

Most reports in the literature regarding marked polyethylene wear in total knee arthroplasty involve cruciate-retaining knee designs. Most often those cruciate-retaining knees have a flat-on-flat tibiofemoral articulation, thin tibial inserts, and / or heat-pressed tibial polyethylene. Leaving the posterior cruciate ligament too tight in flexion has also been implicated in the etiology of posteromedial polyethylene wear in cruciate-retaining total knees. Cruciate-retaining total knee designs that have a moderately conforming tibiofemoral articulation in both the coronal and sagittal planes have had few problems with excessive polyethylene wear (6).

Polyethylene wear has not proven to be a major clinical problem in the posterior-stabilized total knee arthroplasty. The posterior-sta-

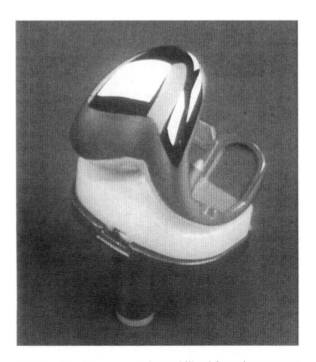

FIG. 3 - The Legacy posterior-stabilized knee incorporates design modifications to improve patellar tracking and includes specific right and left femoral components.

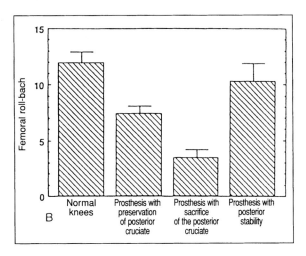

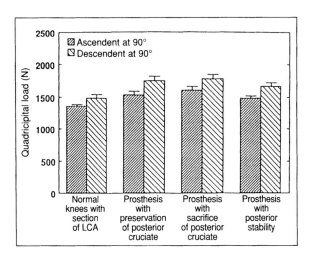

FIG. 5 - Femoral roll-back during stair climbing is markedly better with a posterior-stabilized knee design than with either a cruciate-retaining or cruciate-sacrificing knee design (from Mahoney et al. (20)).

FIG. 6 - Quadriceps load with various prosthesis types is illustrated. Posterior-cruciate retention does not significantly improve extensor efficiency compared to posterior-cruciate substitution (from Mahoney et al. (20)).

bilized design includes moderate conformity of the tibiofemoral articulation in both the coronal and sagittal planes. That conformity results in very favorable wear characteristics. At 10 to 14 years follow-up, Colizza et al. observed no evidence of marked polyethylene wear in a consecutive series of 165 posterior-stabilized total knees.

Loosening

Summary: Aseptic loosening of the tibial or femoral component is rare following cemented posterior-stabilized total knee arthroplasty.

In the posterior-stabilized knee, the interaction of the femoral cam with the tibial post results in a net compressive force directed down the shaft of the tibia. Bone cement is well suited to withstand those compressive forces. Clinical results confirm that the bone cement interface beneath the tibial component of a posterior-stabilized total knee is durable. With the use of a cemented, metal-backed tibial component the posterior-stabilized prosthesis has demonstrated a 14 year survivorship of 98.1 percent (12). In the cruciate-retaining knee the intact posterior cruciate ligament may be able to resist shear stresses that occur at the prosthesis interface. That theoretical resistance to shear stress has not resulted in a survivorship advantage for the cruciate-retaining knees. At 10 to 15 years follow-up there is little in the litera-

ture to suggest a clinical difference between the durability of the bone-prosthesis-cement interfaces of cruciate-retaining and posterior-stabilized knee designs inserted with cement (24, 28, 30, 34).

Proprioception

Summary: Contemporary tests for proprioception are unable to consistently demonstrate an advantage for either cruciate-retaining or posterior-stabilized knee designs.

Mechanoreceptors have been identified in both the anterior and posterior cruciate ligaments. It had been suggested that preservation of the posterior cruciate would improve proprioception following total knee arthroplasty. Recent work, however, suggests that marked neurologic degeneration occurs within the posterior cruciate ligament as part of the arthritic process (17). Warren et al. observed that proprioception improved after total knee arthroplasty with either a cruciate-retaining or posterior-stabilized knee design (33). Those authors suggested that greater improvement occurred after the cruciate-retaining total knees. In contrast, Simmons et al. noted that in patients with severe arthritis better postoperative proprioception was obtained with a posterior-stabilized total knee arthroplasty (29). Becker et al. have compared bilateral paired cruciate-retaining and posterior-stabilized knees (4). Fifty percent of the patients were unable to express a preference for one knee or the other. The other fifty percent were equally divided between those who preferred the cruciate-retaining knee and those who preferred the posterior-stabilized knee.

Gait Analysis

Summary: Comprehensive gait analysis with isokinetic muscle testing reveals no significant differences between posterior-stabilized total knees and age-matched normal knees.

The gait studies published by Andriacchi et al. suggested that patients with posterior cruciate-retaining total knees had more normal stair climbing ability than patients with a posterior stabilized knee (2). Those authors also found that all patients with a total knee arthroplasty demonstrated gait abnormalities during normal walking that included: shorter stride length, reduced mid-stance flexion, and abnormal mechanics of the knee as reflected in the flexion and extension moments at the knee. Using comprehensive gait analysis and isokinetic muscle testing, Wilson et al. have recently studied 16 patients with posterior-stabilized total knees and compared them to 32 age-matched control subjects (35). (Fig. 7) Wilson et al. found no significant differences between the posterior-stabilized knees and normal knees in regard to spatio-temporal gait parameters. No difference was seen in knee range of motion during stair climbing or in isokinetic muscle strength. When compared to historical controls Wilson et al. judged the posterior-stabilized total knees to be equivalent to the cruciate-retaining designs and superior to the cruciate-sacrificing total condylar knee. Those authors have subsequently performed a matched study of bilateral total knee arthroplasties with a posterior-stabilized knee on one side and a cruciate-retaining knee on the opposite side. With the same comprehensive gait analysis, no difference was seen in gait parameters or stair climbing ability between the cruciate-retaining and posterior-stabilized knees.

Correction of Deformity

Summary: In the knee with a fixed angular deformity, ligament balancing is technically easier with a posterior-stabilized total knee than with a cruciate-retaining knee.

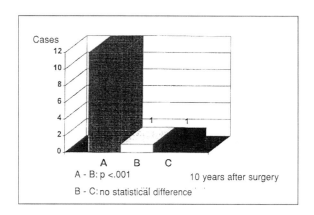

Fig. 7 - For combined preoperative deformities of varus and flexion greater than 15 degrees, the loosening rate of the cruciate-retaining knee (Group A:12 of 65 loose) is markedly higher than the rate for the posterior-stabilized knee (Group B:1 of 50 loose) and higher than the rate for cruciate-retaining knees without preoperative deformity (Group C:1 of 46 loose) (from Laskin) (19).

Many authors, including some who routinely choose to utilize cruciate-retaining knee designs, have reported that the correction of fixed angular deformities of the knee and subsequent balance of the medial and lateral collateral ligaments is more difficult when the posterior cruciate is retained (3). Laskin has reported the results of total knee arthroplasty in patients with a preoperative varus deformity of more than 15 degrees (19). At 10 years follow-up, the 65 knees with a cruciate-retaining knee had more pain, more radiolucencies beneath the prostheses, less range of motion, and a lower survivorship when compared to 50 posterior-stabilized total knees (Fig. 8). If a surgeon chooses to implant a cruciate-retaining knee in the patient with a fixed angular deformity then partial release of the posterior cruciate has been recommended by Ritter et al. (25). While retention of the posterior cruciate may be technically possible in the patient with a fixed deformity, it is technically more demanding and may compromise the long term results of the total knee arthroplasty when compared to cruciate substitution with a posterior-stabilized knee.

Bone Loss

Summary: No studies have suggested that bone loss from the intercondylar region after primary posterior-stabilized total knee arthroplasty is clinically important.

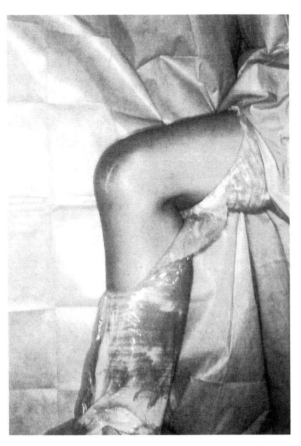

FIG. 8 - A posterior cruciate-retaining knee with flexion instability may demonstrate a marked posterior sag sign at 90 degrees of flexion.

The post and cam mechanism of the posterior-stabilized knee requires the resection of additional bone from the intercondylar region of the distal femur. Some authors have expressed concern that removal of that intercondylar bone would lead to marked bony deficiency at the time of revision total knee arthroplasty. To our knowledge, no studies to date have suggested that intercondylar bone loss associated with posterior-stabilized knee designs compromises the results of revision total knee arthroplasty. Mintzer et al. have demonstrated that pronounced stress shielding occurs beneath the anterior femoral flange of both cruciate retaining and posterior stabilized knees (21). That suggests that whatever bone remains in the notch region of cruciate-retaining knees is of poor quality. Most surgeons choose to implant a posterior-stabilized knee at the time of revision knee arthroplasty and thus bone loss from the intercondylar notch is often inconsequential.

Stability

Summary: So-called flexion instability is now a recognized cause of poor results following cruciate-retaining total knees. Balance of the flexion and extension gaps has long been recognized as critical to the success of posterior-stabilized total knees.

Several recent biomechanical studies have shown that it is difficult to reproduce the normal strain pattern in the posterior cruciate ligament after a cruciate-retaining total knee. In 8 knees, Incavo et al. found the posterior cruciate was too tight in 3 knees and too loose in 3 knees (14). Mahoney et al. tested 8 knees using several different cruciate-retaining knees and found that over-tightening the posterior cruciate occurred frequently (20). Those authors reported that when the posterior cruciate ligament was tight there was either a loss of flexion or the ligament would rupture. Recent clinical reports have suggested that delayed rupture of the posterior cruciate can cause pain and problems after cruciate-retaining total knee arthroplasty. Pagnano et al. have reported on 25 painful, posterior cruciate-retaining total knee replacements treated at the Mayo Clinic for so-called flexion instability (22). Those knees were all well-aligned and well-fixed with no evidence of medial-lateral laxity, infection, loosening or reflex sympathetic dystrophy. Those patients presented with a typical constellation of symptoms including: a sense of knee instability without true giving way episodes, recurrent knee effusion, and generalized soft-tissue tenderness around the knee. All of those patients had an unbalanced flexion gap as demonstrated by a posterior sag sign at 90 degrees of flexion or a positive posterior drawer test (Figs. 9 and 10). At the time of revision total knee arthroplasty, Pagnano et al. found that the posterior cruciate was grossly incompetent in each of those cases. Those authors reported that revision of the cruciate-retaining total knee to a posterior-stabilized knee with appropriate balance of the flexion and extension spaces was a reliable treatment for flexion instability.

The Young and Active Patient

Summary: The results of posterior-stabilized total knee arthroplasty in patients with degenerative arthritis under the age of 55 have been very encouraging.

The disappointing results of early cemented total hip arthroplasties in the young and active patient has made many surgeons slow to expand the indications for total knee arthroplasty to patients under age 55. Several authors have suggested that the benefits of posterior cruciate ligament retention would be most apparent in the young, active patient. Several studies from the 1980s suggested favorable 3 - 5 year results with both cruciate-retaining and cruciate-sacrificing total condylar knees in patients under the age of 55. The majority of patients in those studies had a preoperative diagnosis of rheumatoid arthritis. A recent report by Diduch et al. presented an average 8 year follow-up of 114 posterior-stabilized total knees in patients under the age of 55 years (8). All of the patients in that series had a diagnosis of degenerative arthritis and the mean age was 51 years. Polyethylene wear, loosening, and osteolysis were not commonly seen in this group of young and active patients. Twenty-four percent of the patients in that series regularly participated in activities such as tennis, skiing, bik-

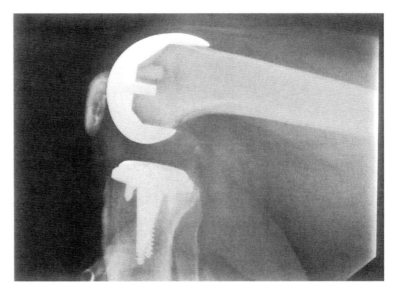

FIG. 9 - Lateral radiograph demonstrates a positive posterior drawer test in a cruciate-retaining knee with flexion instability.

ing, or heavy farm or construction work. The cemented posterior-stabilized total knees in that series appeared to be reliable in relieving pain and improving function and appeared to be durable at a mean of 8 years follow-up (Figure 11).

Clinical Results of Posterior-Stabilized Total Knee Arthroplasty

Insall et al. initially reported the 2 to 4 year results of 118 posterior-stabilized knees in 1982 (16) (See Table I). In that report, 88 percent of the knees were rated excellent; 9 percent were good or fair; and 3 percent were poor. A subsequent study at 5 to 8 years follow-up revealed 79 percent excellent; 17 percent good; and 4 percent poor results. Aglietti and Buzzi have obtained similar results at 3 to 8 years of follow-up with 90 percent excellent and good results.[1] In addition, Scott et al. demonstrated 98 percent excellent and good results with the posterior-stabilized knee at 2 to 8 years (27).

Nine to twelve year follow-up of 194 cemented posterior-stabilized knees with an all-polyethylene tibial component was reported by Stern and Insall in 1992 (30). In that study 61 percent excellent, 25 percent good, 6 percent fair, and 7 percent poor results were calculated with the Hospital for Special Surgery rating

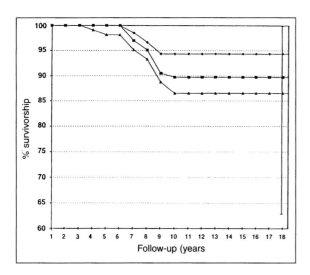

FIG. 10 - Survivorship of the cemented posterior-stabilized total knee in patients under 55 years of age with a diagnosis of osteoarthritis. Endpoints: femoral or tibial revision (diamonds); femoral or tibial or patellar revision (squares); and any re-operation (triangles). I-bars indicate 95 percent confidence interval (from Diduch et al.) (8).

Table I

Clinical Results of Posterior Stabilized Total Knee Replacement

Autor	Reference	F/U	Design	Knees	Flexion	% G/E	Survivorship
Aglietti	J Arthro 3,1988	5.5 aa.	Insall-Burstein	73	96	93	
Emmerson	JBJS 78-B, 1996	12.7 aa.	Kinematic stabilizer	109	98	–	95% at 10 years 87% at 13 years
Font Rodriguez	AAOS, 1996	survival	Insall-Burstein	265(all poly)	–	–	94% at 16 years
				2036 (metal)	–	–	98% at 14 years
Hanssen	JBJS 70-A, 1998	3 aa.	Kinematic stabilizer	79	101	85	
Hirsch	CORR 309, 1994	2.7 aa.	Insall-Burstein II	85	112		
Insall	JBJS 64-A, 1982	2-4 aa.	Insall-Burstein	118	115	97	
Insall	CORR 192, 1985	3.5 aa.	Insall Burstein	303	112	94	
Rand	JBJS 73-A, 1991	survival	Multiple designs	–	–		97% at 5 years
Ranawat	JBJS 79-A, 1997	4.8 aa.	Press Fit Condylar	125	111	93	97% at 6 years
Stern	JBJS 74-A, 1992	10 aa.	Insall-Burstein	289	–	86	94% at 13 years

system. Survivorship analysis revealed an average annual failure rate of 0.4 percent and a 13 year survival of 94 percent. A recent survivorship analysis has confirmed that metal backing of the tibial component has enhanced fixation and reduced the rate of aseptic loosening of the tibia (12). Font-Rodriguez et al. have reported a 94 percent 16 year survival using the posterior-stabilized prosthesis with an all-polyethylene tibia and a 98 percent 14 year survival with a metal-backed tibial component (12). Ranawat et al. found 93 percent excellent and good results and a 97 percent 6 year survival with a modular posterior-stabilized design using metal-backed tibial components (23). Emmerson et al. reported 95 percent 10 year survival with another posterior-stabilized knee design (9).

Conclusions

Arguments that suggested that retention of the posterior cruciate ligament during total knee arthroplasty would allow better range of motion, better joint stability, more normal gait

and enhanced prosthetic longevity have not been supported by the latest clinical and basic science research. In the United States there has been a marked increase recently in the use of posterior-stabilized prostheses for primary total knee arthroplasty. That shift toward the pos-

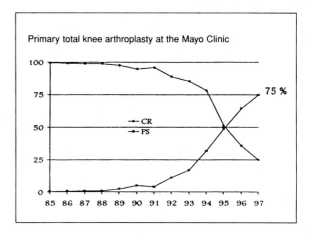

FIG. 11 - The percentage of cruciate-retaining and posterior-stabilized knee implants used for primary total knee arthroplasty at the Mayo Clinic. Note the marked shift toward use of a posterior-stabilized implant in the 1990s.

terior-stabilized knee is reflected in the experience of one of the largest orthopedic centers, the Mayo Clinic. In 1990 less than ten percent of all primary total knees at the Mayo Clinic were of a posterior-stabilized design. By 1997 the posterior-stabilized design was used in 75 percent of all primary total knee replacements (Fig. 12).

The range of motion after posterior-stabilized total knee arthroplasty averages 112 - 115 degrees in several large series and motion greater than 90 degrees is more reliably attained with a posterior-stabilized knee. While occasional instances of dislocation do occur after posterior-stabilized knee arthroplasty, it is now apparent that flexion instability can be problematic in the cruciate-retaining knee as well. Recent gait analysis studies do not support a difference between posterior-stabilized and cruciate-retaining knees in regard to stair climbing ability. Finally, the durability of the cemented posterior-stabilized total knee has been well established and represents the gold standard in regard to prosthetic longevity. We recommend the use of a cemented, posterior-stabilized total knee arthroplasty as the implant of choice for primary total knee arthroplasty.

References

1) Aglietti P., Buzzi R.: Posteriorly stabilized total-condylar knee replacement.Three to eight years' follow-up of 85 knees. J Bone Joint Surg 70-B: 211-216, 1988.

2) Andriacchi, T.: Gait analysis and total knee replacement. In Current Concepts in Primary and Revision Total Knee Arthroplasty, eds. JN Insall, WN Scott, and GS Scuderi. Philadelphia: Lippincott, 1996.

3) Barnes C. L., Sledge C. B.: Total knee arthroplasty with posterior cruciate ligament retention designs. In Surgery of the Knee, ed. J N Insall. 2nd ed., 815-827. New York: Churchill Livingstone, 1993.

4) Becker M. W., Insall J. N., Faris P. M.: Bilateral total knee arthroplasty: one cruciate retaining and one cruciate substituting. Clin Orthop 271: 122-124, 1990.

5) Cash, R. M.; Gonzalez, M. H.; Garst, J.; Barmada, R.; Stern, S. H.: Proprioception after arthroplasty: role of the posterior cruciate ligament. Clin Orthop 331: 172-178, 1996.

6) Colizza, W.; Insall, J. N.; Scuderi, G. R.: The posterior stabilized knee prosthesis. Assessment of polyethylene damage and osteolysis after a minimum ten-year follow-up. J Bone and Joint Surg 77-A: 1713-1720, 1995.

7) Dennis, D.; Komistek, R.; Hoff, W.; Gabriel: In vivo knee kinematics derived using an inverse perspective technique. Clin Orthop 331: 107-117, 1996.

8) Diduch, D. R.; Insall, J. I.; Scott, W. N.; Scuderi, G. R.; Font-Rodriguez, D. F.: Total Knee Replacement in Young, Active Patients. J Bone Joint Surg 79-A: 575-582, 1997.

9) Emmerson, K. P.; Moran, C. G.; Pinder, I. M.: Survivorship analysis of the kinematic stabilizer total knee replacement: a ten to fourteen year follow-up. J Bone Joint Surg 78-B: 441-445, 1996.

10) Fehring, T. K., Valadie, A. J.: Knee instability after total knee arthroplasty. Clin Orthop 299: 157-163, 1994.

11) Firestone, T. P.; Krackow, K. A.; Davis, J. D.; Teeny, S. M.; Hungerford, D. S.: The management of fixed flexion contractures during total knee arthroplasty. Clin Orthop 284: 221-227, 1992.

12) Font-Rodriguez, D. E.; Insall, J. N.; Scuderi, G. R.: Survivorship of cemented total knee arthroplasty. American Academy of Orthopaedic Surgeons-Annual Meeting 1996.

13) Hirsch, H. S.; Lotke, P. A.; Morrison, L. D.: The posterior cruciate ligament in total knee surgery: save, sacrifice, or substitute. Clin Orthop 309: 64-68, 1994.

14) Incavo, S. J.; Johnson, C. C.; Beynnon, B. D.; Howe, J. G.: Posterior cruciate ligament strain biomechanics in total knee arthroplasty. Clin Orthop 309: 88-93, 1994.

15) Insall, J. N.; Hood, R. W.; Flawn, L. B.; Sullivan, D. J.: The total condylar prosthesis in gonarthrosis. A five to nine year follow-up of the first one-hundred consecutive replacements. J Bone Joint Surg 65-A: 619-628, 1983.

16) Insall, J. N.; Lachiewicz, P. F.; Burstein, A. H.: The posterior stabilized condylar prosthesis. A modification of the total condylar design. Two to four-year clinical experience. J Bone Joint Surg 64-A: 1317-1323, 1982.

17) Kleinbart, F. A.; Bryk, E.; Evangelista, J.; Scott, W. N.; Vigorita, V. J.: Histologic comparison of posterior cruciate ligaments from arthritic and age matched knee specimens. J Arthroplasty 6: 726-731, 1996.

18) Landy, M. M., Walker, P. S.: Wear of ultra-high molecular weight polyethylene components of 90 retrieved knee prostheses. J Arthroplasty 3: S73-S85, 1988.

19) Laskin, R. S.: Total knee replacement with posterior cruciate ligament retention in patients with a fixed varus deformity. Clin Orthop 331: 29-34, 1996.

20) Mahoney, O. M.; Noble, P. C.; Rhoads, D. D.; Alexander, J. W.; Tullos, H. S.: Posterior cruciate function following total knee arthroplasty: a biomechanical study. J Arthroplasty 9: 569-578, 1994.

21) Mintzer, C. M.; Robertson, D. D.; Rackemann, S.; Ewald, F. C.; Scott, R. D.; Spector, M.: Bone loss in the distal anterior femur after total knee arthroplasty. Clin Orthop 260: 135-143, 1990.

22) Pagnano, M.W.; Hanssen, A.D.; Stuart, M.J.; Lewallen, D.G.: Flexion instability after primary posterior cruciate retaining total knee arthroplasty. In Proceedings of the Knee Society 1998. Clin Orthop (in press).

23) Ranawat, C. S.; Luessenhop, C. P.; Rodriguez, J. A.: The press-fit condylar modular total knee system: four to six year results with a posterior-cruciate-substituting design. J Bone Joint Surg 79-A: 342-348, 1997.

24) Rand, J. A., Ilstrup, D. M.: Survivorship analysis of total knee arthroplasty. J Bone Joint Surg 73-A: 397-409, 1991.

25) Ritter, M. A.; Faris, P. M.; Keating, E. M.: Posterior cruciate ligament balancing during total knee arthroplasty. J Arthroplasty 3: 323-326, 1988.

26) Scott, R. D., Thornhill, T. S.: Posterior cruciate supplementing total knee replacement using conforming inserts and cruciate recession: effect on range of motion and radiolucent lines. Clin Orthop 309: 146-149, 1994.

27) Scott, W. N.; Rubinstein, M.; Scuderi, G. R.: Results after knee replacement with a posterior cruciate-substituting prosthesis. J Bone Joint Surg 70-A: 1163-1173, 1988.

28) Scuderi, G. R.; Insall, J. N.; Windsor, R. E.; Moran, M. C.: Survivorship of cemented knee replacements. J Bone Joint Surg 71-B: 798-803, 1989.

29) Simmons, S.; Lephart, S.; Rubash, H.; Pifer, G. W.; Barrack, R.: Proprioception after unicondylar knee arthroplasty versus total knee arthroplasty. Clin Orthop 331: 179-184, 1996.

30) Stern, S. H., and Insall, J. N.: Posterior stabilized prostheses. Results after follow-up of nine to twelve years. J Bone Joint Surg 74-A: 980-986, 1992.

31) Stern, S. H., Insall, J. N.: Total knee arthroplasty with posterior cruciate ligament substitution designs. In Surgery of the Knee, ed. J N Insall. 2nd ed., 829-867. New York: Churchill Livingstone, 1994.

32) Stiehl, J. B.; Komistek, R. D.; Dennis, D. A.; Paxson, R. D.; Hoff, W.: Fluoroscopic analysis of kinematics after posterior cruciate retaining knee arthroplasty. J Bone Joint Surg 77-B: 884-889, 1995.

33) Warren, P. J.; Olanlokun, T. K.; Cobb, A. G.; Bentley, G.: Proprioception after knee arthroplasty: the influence of prosthetic design. Clin Orthop 297: 182-187, 1993.

34) Weir, D. J.; Moran, C. G.; Pinder, I. M.: Kinematic of condylar total knee arthroplasty: 14 year survivorship analysis of 208 consecutive cases. J Bone Joint Surg 78-B: 907-911, 1996.

35) Wilson, S. A.; McCann, P. D.; Gotlin, R. S.; Ramakrishnan, H. K.; Wootten, M. E.; Insall, J. N.: Comprehensive gait analysis in posterior stabilized knee arthroplasty. J Arthroplasty 11: 359-367, 1996.

Chapter 13
Meniscal-Bearing Knee Arthroplasty

Frederick F. Buechel
New Jersey Medical School - New York

History and Development of Mobile Bearings

Human joint replacements have been developed with the specific bioengineering requirements to provide normal kinematics, maintain fixation and minimize wear. Lowering contact stresses to within the reported medical load limit of 5 MP (22) while allowing kinematically acceptable motion provides a meniscal bearing surface that is resistant to fatigue wear and has demonstrated normal abrasive wear behavior over a 20 year period as seen in both clinical, simulator, and retrieval studies, (17, 18, 27, 33, 44).

The first complete systems approach to total knee replacement using meniscal bearings was developed in 1977 and reported in 1986 (20). Unicompartimental, bicompartimental and tricompartimental disease were managed with a variety of primary and revision components that allowed retention of both cruciates, only the posterior cruciate or no cruciate ligaments. Additionally, the first metal-backed, rotating-bearing patellar replacement was developed in 1977 to provide mobility with congruity in patellofemoral articulation. This New Jersey Low-Contact-Stress (LCS) total knee system, initially used with cement in 1977, was expanded to non-cemented use in 1981 with the availability of sintered-bead, porous-coating (48) and remains the only knee system in the United States to have undergone formal FDA-IDE Clinical Trials in both cemented and cementless application before being released for general clinical use (16, 23, 25) (Figure 1).

The kinematic tibiofemoral motion requirements dictate the use of spherical upper tibial bearing surfaces and a flat undersurface to accommodate the variety of movements in the most congruent way. The Oxford meniscal knee (33) uses matching spherical surfaces for the femoral component and the upper meniscal-bearing surface and a flat surface to match a flat tibial component. This preferred geometry appears to work well as a medial unicompartmental replacement (26), but has had dislocation problems in other applications (32), most likely caused by a larger than normal single radius of curvature of the femoral component, which under the pull of the posterior cruciate ligament in flexion moves the bearing too far posteriorly.

A design solution to the Oxford problem in the presence of cruciate ligaments is seen in the New Jersey Low Contact-Stress (LCS) (18) femoral component which uses the same spherical surface of revolution in the medial-lateral plane but decreases the radius of curvature from extension to flexion, thus maintaining full area contact on the upper meniscal-bearing surface from 0 to 45 degrees where walking loads are encountered and maintaining at least spherical line contact, at flexion angles. This surface geometry allows a more central femoral component position in flexion by reducing the posterior cruciate ligament tension, which tends to pull the femur posteriorly when over-stretched. Another design solution to prevent meniscal-bearing dislocation is the use of radial tracks on the LCS tibial components. These tracks allow axial rotation and controlled A-P translation, which impedes direct dislocation by means of the cruciate bone bridge posteriorly and the patellar tendon anteriorly. When combined with stable flexion and

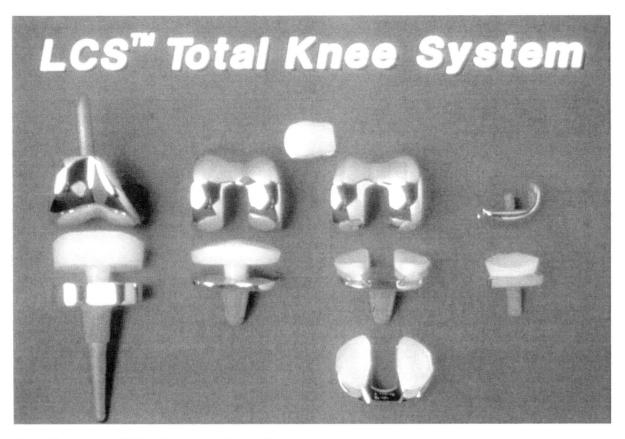

FIG. 1 - New Jersey LCS Knee Replacement System Components.

extension gaps at surgery, the LCS meniscal bearing can be safely used when both cruciate ligaments are intact or if only the posterior cruciate ligament is intact.

In the event of a non-functional or absent posterior cruciate ligament, central stability with the ability to axially rotate is essential. The long-term survivorship studies of Scuderi (53) and Ranawat (49) have demonstrated that a centrally-stabilized total condylar knee replacement is predicted to last for 15 years in over 90% of cases, when used in elderly patients with low-loading demands. These important studies prove that cruciate function is not essential for successful long-term fixation and function in low demand situations.

Since wear increases as the loads and demands increase, it seem most appropriate to utilize the proven fixation and central-stabilizing concepts of the total condylar device and provide a more wear resistant and dislocation-resistant bearing surface to achieve better long

term survivorship and reduce wear-related failures. These concepts led to the development of a rotating-platform total knee device, which employs the same spherical surface geometry as the meniscal bearings.

The patellofemoral design process, like the tibiofemoral design process, seeks to provide proper motion and maintain contact stresses below 5MP during walking, stair climbing and deep knee bending. Button or non-rotating anatomical type patellar replacements suffer from either high point or line contact stresses or from overconstraint. High contact stress will cause early wear failure (50), while overconstraint will cause early loosening failure (3). For these reasons a rotating-bearing patellar replacement was developed to maintain spherical area contact on the medial and lateral facets while congruently matching the surface of revolution of the deep-sulcus femoral groove. Rotating-bearing patellar replacement of the LCS design greatly improves upon the contact stress seen in other configurations (22).

Wear Properties of Mobile Bearings and Fixed Bearings

Retrieval analysis of the tibiofemoral and patellofemoral bearing surfaces have demonstrated a high clinical wear rate of non-conforming fixed-bearing knee replacement (28, 29, 31, 40, 47). Similar retrieval analysis of meniscal bearings, rotating platform bearings and rotating patellar bearings demonstrated significantly less wear than fixed-bearings (16). Although, mobile-bearings allow reduced contact stress, they can be overloaded to failure by excessive weight, excessive activity, mal-alignment, or a combination of these factors. Additionally, poor quality polyethylene and inferior sterilization methods can contribute to increased wear-related failures.

The overall failure rate of bicruciate-retaining meniscal bearing TKR as a result of fracture, dislocation or bearing wear-through has 3 out of 95 TKR's or 3.2% in my personal series of primary and multiply operated knee replacements followed for 2 to 19 years, mean 8.5 years.

The overall failure rate of posterior cruciate-retaining meniscal-bearing TKR as a result of fracture, dislocation or bearing wear-through has 3 out of 178 TKR's or 1.7% in my personal series of primary and multiply-operated knee replacements followed for 2 to 12 years, mean 5 years.

The overall failure rate of rotating-platform TKR's due to bearing dislocation has been out of 294 TKR's or 0.6% in my personal series of primary and multiply operated knee replacements followed for 4 to 18 years, mean 10 years. Two rotating-platform bearings (0.6%) developed severe wear requiring revision; no fractured bearings were seen.

Failure Modes of Rotating-bearing Patellar Replacements

Failure of the rotating-bearing patella have been rare (24,39) and usually associated with displaced patellar fractures, malposition, subluxation or excessive, repetitive hyperflexion loads.

The overall complications of rotating-bearing patellar replacements that required revision

surgery in 515 knees originally followed for 6 months to 11 years (24) and now followed for 8 to 19 years, mean 12.5 years was 4/515 or 0.8%. Long-term rotating-patella replacement retrievals have demonstrated continued mobility and minimal wear.

Fixation of Mobile Meniscal Bearings

Methyl methacrylate bone cement was the initial adjunctive method of bony attachment for the first New Jersey LCS unicompartmental meniscal bearing used in 1977, (5) and for subsequent bicompartmental and tricompartmental devices.

The tibial fixation surface of the LCS Unicompartmental knee replacement employs a flat, tibial loading plate and a short angled stem to resist tipping and shear loads. Bicruciate-retaining LCS tibial components use three short fixation fins for anchorage, while posterior cruciate-retaining LCS meniscal bearing and LCS rotating-platform tibial components utilize a short, conical metaphyseal fixation stem centered in the proximal tibia. All femoral components utilize shallow cement locking pockets and centralized femoral fixation pegs.

The rotating-bearing patellar replacement utilizes a cruciform fin geometry for fixation. This geometry reinforces the thin metal-plate against torsional failure and reinforces the patellar remnant against fractures while engaging the patellar bone stock sufficiently to prevent loosening.

Cementless fixation with sintered-bead Co-Cr-Mo porous coating on the Co-Cr-Mo, substrate (Porocoat, DePuy, Indiana) using the same articulating and fixation geometries of the New Jersey LCS knee system (Deppuy, Warsaw, Indiana) was first used clinically in 1981. Bicruciate-retaining and rotating-platform tibial components were developed with 4 screw holes and speherical seats. These implants used 6.5 mm cancellous bone screws to augment fixation.

Our concerns over fretting corrosion, screw breakage, osteolysis and potential neurovascular injuries from screw penetration led us away from screw fixation later in the same year. These early concerns are now complications that have been documented by several authors (28, 47, 51).

Press fit, non-screw fixed, LCS knee replacements with porous coating have been in clinical use since late 1981.

Ten year survivorship studies have demonstrated a 96.5% overall survivorship using non-screw-fixed, press-fit, porous-coated, cementless fixation, thereby justifying its continued use (5,6,7,8). The specifics of individual component survivorship will be presented later in this chapter.

Clinical Application of Mobile, Meniscal Bearings Unicompartmental Knee Replacement

The first LCS meniscal-bearing knee replacement used clinically in 1977 was a cemented medial, unicompartmental device New Jersey LCS knee, implanted in a 64 year old, 82 Kg, post-meniscectomy osteoarthritic man who maintained an excellent clinical result until his death from cardiac failure 10 years after surgery.

Unicompartmental meniscal bearings are well-adapted for knee replacement, since they allow retention of both cruciate ligaments and allow the normal forward and backward translational movement of the femur on the tibia as well as axial rotation and varus-valgus movement with excellent congruity of the bearing surfaces. The Oxford meniscal-bearing unicompartmental device has had excellent success when used as a medial unicompartmental replacement (26), but has functioned less consistently as a lateral compartment replacement because of significant dislocation problems (32).

The Cementless LCS unicompartmental was approved by the FDA Orthopaedic advisory panel in August 1991 and released for general use by the FDA in November 1992 after successful completion of an FDA-IDE clinical trial. Good or excellent results using a strict scoring scale (4) were seen in 98.4% of 122 patients followed for 2 to 6 years mean 3.3 years. One bearing fractured following trauma, and one tibial component loosened in a patient with post-traumatic, osteoporotic bone deficiency. Progressive disease in the opposite knee compartment was an additional cause for revision. Such disorders represent current failure mechanisms for this device and are now considered contraindicated.

Bicompartmental Knee Replacement

The articulating geometry of the femoral component is critical to the success or failure of the patellar component. A bispherical, continuous-surface of revolution-femoral-groove matching a bispherical, congruently-tracking, patellar component will provide a long service for the patellar bearing. This same femoral groove can match the anatomical patellar geometry and can allow retention of the natural patella, with highly predictable results (38). Keblish (37) has reported no difference between bicompartmental (retention of natural patella) and tricompartmental (replaced patella) knee replacements using the unique femoral groove of the LCS design (19) with a 10 year clinical series of patients in whom one patella was replaced and the other patella was retained (37).

Such predictability can allow patella retention in patients such as farmers or laborers who require repetitive squatting loads that may increase patellar component wear. Additionally, patella retention in conditions such as patella infera, alta or hypoplasia can facilitate central tracking without fear of early knee replacement failure (12). Lastly, those patients with previous patellectomies can undergo a patella tendon bone grafting (11) and enjoy a well functioning bicompartmental replacement with improvement in both quadriceps leverage and tibiofemoral dislocation resistance.

Tricompartmental Knee Replacement/Bicruciate-retaining Meniscal Bearing TKR

The concept of retaining both viable cruciate ligaments is appealing, since normal knee kinematics depend upon the anterior-posterior translation of the femur on the tibia which is under the direct control of these intact structures (54). Ligament loads greater than body weight have been recorded for all knee ligaments.

Thus, in theory at least, in the absence of each ligament structure these loads would need to be carried by the remaining ligaments and perhaps transferred to the prosthesis itself. As such, retention of all load bearing ligaments would be ideal, if normal kinematic knee motion were allowed.

Based on these concepts, the bicruciate-retaining, LCS meniscal-bearing knee replacement was developed and successfully tested in FDA-IDE clinical trials (16).

The use of 3 fixation fins, rather than a central conical peg, has led to a greater incidence of tibial component loosening with this device than with central conical peg devices (15). Also, reports from Hamelynck in Holland have determined that loosening of these tri-finned components is increased in patients with previous high tibial osteotomies or proximal tibial fractures (34). Such conditions appear to alter blood flow and impede osteointegration in cementless bicruciate-retaining knees and as such remain contraindications to their cementless use. Additionally, early or late rupture of the anterior cruciate ligament degrades the arthroplasty to the level of an ACL deficient knee in many cases and raises doubts as to whether ACL retention should be attempted in other than circumstances of youth, good bone stock, and a perfect ACL, which is a rare situation at best. Still in all, those knees with intact ACL's, excellent bone stock and solid fixation of components represent the best possible TKR's as they function and act as normal knees (7).

Posterior Cruciate-Retaining Meniscal Bearing

Retention of the posterior cruciate ligament has been reported to improve quadriceps leverage, increase extension torque and improve flexion over cruciate-sacrificing design (45). In fixed-bearings, this increased motion and function is related to increased posterior roll-back on the incongruent tibial-bearing surface, which increases wear over cruciate-sacrificing, fixed-bearing designs (30). A meniscal-bearing device allows more congruent roll-back in flexion to improve wear resistance over fixed-bearing designs.

The Oxford meniscal knee, however, functioned poorly with only an intact PCL. As such, the Oxford knee developers did not recommend using the Oxford device in any ACL deficient knee and cautioned against the use of any meniscal-bearing device in the absence of the ACL. With this in mind, the significant dislocation rate of 9,3% reported by Bert in 1990 (2) using rotating-platform and posterior cruciate-retaining LCS knee replacements would tend to support this concept. However, as was pointed out in rebuttal to the Bert article (9), meniscal or rotating bearings require adequate control of the flexion and extension gaps during surgery to maintain contact stability of the prosthesis. As such, failure to maintain flexion and extension gap stability will compromise the results of any mobile-bearing knee replace-

ment, whether both, one or no cruciates ligaments are preserved.

The successful FDA-IDE cementless clinical trial of the posterior cruciate-retaining, meniscal-bearing LCS knee replacement documented the ability to retain only the posterior cruciate ligament and maintain long-term stability and function with a meniscal-bearing device (23,43).

Tibial component loosening and dislocations were seen in knees with poor flexion stability and were noted to be technique-rather than implant-related as noted similarly in the Bert Study (9). Early or late posterior cruciate ligament instability remains a concern for this arthroplasty. Intraoperative diligence to avoid any release of this ligament attachment is desirable and if PCL compromise is noted, then replacement to a centrally-stabilized, rotating-platform is advisable for long-term stability and function.

Cruciate-sacrificing, Rotating-platform

Cruciate sacrifice is often desirable in certain conditions such as fixed-flexion, fixed-valgus and in some severe fixed-varus deformities. It is often unavoidable in conditions where significant trauma, rheumatoid arthritis or inflammatory osteoarthritis have destroyed these structures. In such cases, a centrally-stabilized device with long-term fixation and excellent wear properties would be most desirable. The cemented total condylar knee replacement has been used in such cases of elderly patients over a 10 to 15 year period with exceptionally good results and reported 90% survivorship, using revision as an end point. (53).

Considering these results to represent the standard for future design comparison, any cemented or cementless cruciate-sacrificing design should demonstrate at least a 90% 10 year survivorship and have contact stresses less than the total condylar device to merit any attention (21).

Additionally, since total condylar range motion was only considered to be fair (85 to 90 degrees) and reported dislocations fairly frequent, any new design should improve upon motion and dislocation resistance.

The LCS rotating-platform knee replacement represents an improvement over the total condylar device in concept and in clinical performance. Conceptually, the deeper engagement of the rotatable, spherically congruent surfaces allow lower contract stresses during normal walking, namely 25 Mpa for total condylar and 4.9 Mpa for LCS. (46). This deeper engagement also improves dislocation resistance over the total condylar device. The LCS device utilizes a conical central tibial component stem which approximates the successful total condylar stem. Thus, similar fixation is achieved with rotational relief of shear stresses to tibial fixation with the rotating-platform design.

FDA-IDE Clinical Trials have demonstrated long-term safety and efficacy of the rotating-platform in a wide variety of primary and multiply operated cases in both cemented and cementless applications. The FDA orthopaedic advisory panel recommended approval of the cemented LCS Rotating platform device in 1984 (16) and of the cementless device in 1991 (25), making the rotating-platform the first, and currently, the only total knee device in the United States to be approved for both cemented and cementless applications by means of an FDA-IDE clinical trial.

Revision Total Knee Replacement

Aseptic, failed knee replacement surgery is usually accompanied by a loss of bone stock and a loss of the cruciate ligaments. In such cases, a centrally-stabilized, rotating-platform device with intramedullary stems can be used to successfully salvage a wide variety of complex pathologies. These stems can be fixed to the femoral or tibial components or be modular constructs with the ability to increase or decrease diameter as well as length similar to that found in current revision hip replacements (14).

Attention to surgical technique, in regard to flexion-extension stability, as well as varus-valgus ligamentous balancing remains crucial to revision success. In those few cases in which AP stability continued to be a problem, the use of a high, central-post, posterior-stabilized prosthesis the Total Condylar III design (41) or a rotating-hinge is preferred.

Survivorship Analysis of Cemented and Cementless Meniscal-bearing Knee Replacements

Surgical estimates of at least 90% at the 10 year interval using an endpoint of revision of any component for any reason, has been recommended as the standard for primary total knee replacement (21). Any knee replacement failing to achieve this level of success should not be routinely used until design improvements can clearly demonstrate advantages over other standard designs to warrant further clinical use.

Meniscal-bearing knee replacements have demonstrated this high level of survivorship in several designs. The Oxford meniscal knee has been specifically indicated for medial, unicompartmental, non-inflammatory arthritis and in such conditions, when both cruciate ligaments are intact, has a reported 99.1% survivorship at the 10 year interval when used with methacrylate bone cement (27). Cementless, long-term use of the Oxford device has not been reported and its use in bicompartmental and lateral unicompartmental applications is not recommended.

The cemented, LCS unicompartmental meniscal knee replacement has a reported 91% survivorship at the 10-year interval when used for either the medial or lateral compartments in conjunction with intact cruciate ligaments and non-inflammatory degenerative arthritic conditions. The cementless, LCS unicompartmental replacement has a reported 98% survivorship at the 10-year interval when indicated for the same conditions as the cemented device. Inflammatory conditions such as rheumatoid arthritis, severe osteoporosis and ACL deficiency are contraindicated for LCS meniscal bearing unicompartmental replacement and have been a documented source of failure in such cases (13).

The cemented LCS bicruciate-retaining, meniscal-bearing total knee replacement has a reported 90% survivorship at 10 years and the cementless device has a 95% survivorship at the same time interval. Undersizing the tibial component in the cemented group and previous high tibial osteotomy or tibial plateau fracture in the cementless group were causes for failure and are now contraindicated for these devices. Additionally, it is not recommended to use the bicruciate device when the ACL has been disrupted or is deficient, but rather the centrally-stabilized, posterior cruciate-retaining meniscal-bearing or A-P glide tibial components are preferred.

The cementless LCS posterior cruciate-retaining meniscal-bearing total knee replacement has a 97% survivorship over the initial 10 year interval. It was released for clinical use in 1984 and remains the most popular meniscal-bearing knee replacement worldwide at the present time. Flexion instability (2,9) and late rupture of the PCL can compromise the long-term results with this device. It is important to be sure of PCL integrity and balanced flexion-extension gaps at surgery (10) for reproducible long term results with this implant.

The cemented LCS rotating-platform total knee replacement used for cruciate ligament deficiency has a reported 97% survivorship at 10 years and the cementless device has a 98% survivorship at the same time interval. Flexion instability has been identified as the unusual but main problem with this device. The successful cemented and cementless survivorship of this implant represents a new standard for successful total knee replacement to which future designs should be compared.

Future Directions of Meniscal-bearing Knee Replacement

Meniscal bearings represent the logical approach for future development of human knee joint replacements. This fact is supported by long-term survivorship and contact stress studies, which favor mobile bearings over fixed-bearings in a wide variety of clinical applications varying from unicompartmental to tricompartmental arthroplasty (1, 15, 18, 22, 27, 29, 35, 36, 42, 52, 55). As such, it is important to explore alternative bearing geometries and biomaterials to optimize future designs.

Improved ceramic biomaterials such as aluminum oxide, zirconium oxide and titanium nitride appear to offer improved wear resistance over polished metal surfaces. Bulk ceramics such as alumina and zirconia, however, have mechanical limitations, in that they are notch and impact sensitive, which precludes their use in thin shell applications. Polished, titanium nitride ceramic, on the other hand, has the ability to be applied by a physical vapor deposition process (26) as a thin film on a metallic substrate to offer both impact and wear resistance.

Thin-film, polished titanium nitride ceramic surfaces against UHMWPe offer wear resistance of more than 3 times over similar polished-Co-Cr-Mo surfaces, thus offering a strong potential as a bearing material for more active patient use.

This material has been developed and used clinically in active patients undergoing cementless meniscal-bearing knee joint replacement with no clinical difference in performance-outcome over a 7/year interval compared to similar cementless Co-Cr-Mo meniscal-bearing knee replacements.

With documented improvement of wear resistance of such ceramics on polyethylene meniscal bearings, it is reasonable to presume that athletic performance, in terms of running or jumping, may be possible and predictable with these improved bearing materials. Such patients are currently being closely monitored for athletic performance using these devices.

Future meniscal-bearing knee joint development will undoubtedly rely on some of the basic principles presented in this chapter. It is of utmost importance for orthopaedic surgeons and mechanical engineers to work together in this important area of implant design, to insure that our future joint replacement developments remain practical improvements over past misadventures.

References

1) Bartel, D.L., Bicknell, V.L., Wright, T.M.: The effect of conformity, thickness, and material on stress in ultra-high molecular weight polyethylene components for total joint replacement. J. Bone Joint Surg., 68A: 1041-1051, 1986.

2) Bert, J.M.: Dislocation/subluxation of meniscal elements after New Jersey Low-Contact Stress total knee arthroplasty. Clin. Orthop. 254: 211-215, 1990.

3) Bourne, R.B., Goodfellow, J.W., O'Connor, J.J.: A functional analysis of various knee arthroplasties. Transactions of the 24th Annual Meeting of The Orthopaedic Research Society, Dallas, Texas, 21-23, 1978, p. 156.

4) Buechel, F.F..: A simplified evaluation system for the rating of knee function. Orthop. Rev.: 97-101, 1982.

5) Buechel, F.F.: Cementless LCS endoprostheses: Concepts and 10 year evaluation. Presented at the 4th World Bio Materials Congress. Berlin, Germany, April 27,1992.

6) Buechel, F.F.: Cementless meniscal bearing TKA. Presented at the Eight Annual Current Concepts in Joint Replacement Symposium. Orlando, Florida, December 18, 1992.

7) Buechel, F.F.: Cementless mobile bearing TKR: 10 years results. Presented at the Seventh Annual Joint Replacement Symposium. Palm Beach, Florida, October 23, 1992.

8) Buechel, F.F.: Fourteen year survivorship analysis of mobile bearing total knee arthroplasties. Presented at The State of the Art in Total Joint Replacement Symposium. Phoenix, Arizona, November 24, 1992.

9) Buechel, F.F.: Letters to the Editor. Re: Dislocation/subluxation of the LCS Knee Replacement. Clin. Orthop. 264:309, 1991.

10) Buechel, F.F., Sorrels, B.: New Jersey LCS Milestone Surgical Procedure. Depuy Division of Boeringer Mannheim Corp., Warsaw, Indiana, 1995.

11) Buechel, F.F.: Patella tendon bone grafting for patellectomized patients undergoing knee replacement. Clin. Orthop. 271: 72-78, 1991.

12) Buechel, F.F.: Treatment of the patella in revision total knee surgery using a rotating-bearing patellar replacement. Orthop. Rev. Supp. 76-82, 1990.

13) Buechel, F.F., Keblish, P.K., Pappas, M.J., et al: New Jersey LCS Unicompartimental Knee replacement: clinical, radiographic, statistical and survivorship analyses of 106 cementless cases performed by 7 surgeons. Food and Drug Administration Panel Presentation. Rockville, Maryland, August 16, 1991.

14) Buechel, F.F. Pappas, M.J: Efficacy and application of modular Stem in THR. Presented at the Combined Meeting of the Orthopaedic Associations of the English Speaking World. Toronto, Canada, june 21-26, 1992. (Poster Exhibit)

15) Buechel, F.F., Pappas, M.J.: Long-term survivorship analyses of cruciate sparing versus cruciate sacrificing knee prostheses using meniscal bearings. Clin. Orthop. 260: 162-169, 1990.

16) Buechel, F.F., Pappas, M.J.: New Jersey integrated total knee replacement system: Biomechanical analysis and clinical evaluation of 918 cases. FDA Panel Presentation, Silver Spring, Maryland, July 11, 1984.

17) Buechel, F.F., Pappas, M.J.: New Jersey LCS Knee replacement system biomechanical rationale and comparison of cemented and non-cemented results (A two to five follow-up). Contemp. Orthop., 1984.

18) Buechel, F.F., Pappas, M.J.: New Jersy LCS Knee replacement system: 10 year evaluation of meniscal bearings. Orthop. Clinic N.A., 20: 147-177, 1989.

19) Buechel, F.F., Pappas, M.J.: New Jersey Meniscal Bearing Knee U.S. Patent No. 4,340,978, July 27, 1982.

20) Buechel, F.F., Pappas, M.J.: The New Jersey Low Contact Stress knee replacement system: Biomechanical rationale and review of the first 123 cemented cases. Arch. Orthop. Trauma Surg. 105:197-204, 1986.

21) Buechel, F.F., Pappas, M.J., Greenwald, A.S.: Use of survivorship and contact stress analyses to predict the long term efficacy of new generation joint replacement designs: A model for FDA device evaluation. Orthop. Rev., 20: 50-55, 1991.

22) Buechel, F.F., Pappas, M.J., Makris, G.: Evaluation of contact stress in metal-backed patellar replacements: a predictor of survivorship. Clin. Orthop., 273: 190-197, 1991.

23) Buechel, F.F., Pappas, M.J., Peoples, S., Davenport, J.M., Friddle, N.M.: New Jersey LCS Posterior cruciate Retaining Total Knee Replacement: Clinical, radiographic, statistical, and survivorship analyses of 395 cementless cases performed by 13 surgeons. Food and Drug Administration Panel Presentation. Rockville, Maryland, June 1, 1990.

24) Buechel, F.F., Rosa, R.A., Pappas, M.J.: A metal-backed, rotating-bearing patellar prosthesis to lower contact stress: an 11 year clinical study. Clin. Orthop. 248: 34-49, 1989.

25) Buechel, F.F., Sorrels, B., Pappas, M.J.: New Jersey Rotating Platform total knee replacement: Clinical, radiographic, statistical, and survivorship analyses of 346 cases performed by 16 surgeons. Food and Drug Administration Panel Presentation. Gaithersburg, Maryland, November 22, 1991.

26) Coll, B.F., Jacquot, P.: Surface modification of medical implants and surgical devices using TiN Layers. Surface Coating Technology. 36:867-878, 1988.

27) Carr, A.J., Keyes, G., Miller, R.K.: Medial unicompartmental arthroplasty: A survival study of the Oxford Meniscal Knee. Presented at The Ninth Combined Meeting of the Orthopaedic Association of the English-speaking World. Toronto, Canada, June 21-26, 1992, (Poster Exhibit).

28) Collier, J.P., Mayor, M.B., Surprenant, B.A., et al. The Biomechanical problems of polyethylene as a bearing surface. Clin. Orthop. 261: 107-113, 1990.

29) Engh, G.A., Dwyer, D.A., Hanes, C.K.: Polyethylene wear of metal-backed tibial components in total and unicompartmental knee prosthesis. J.Bone Joint Surg. 74B: 9-17, 1992.

30) Ewald, F.C., Jacobs, M.A., Miegel, R.E., et al: Kinematic total knee replacement. J. Bone Surg. 66A: 1032, 1984.

31) Freeman, M.A.R., Railton, G.T.: Should the posterior cruciate ligament be retained or resected in condylar non-meniscal knee arthroplasty? The case for resection. J Arthrop., Suppl., 53-62, 1988.

32) Goodfellow, J.W., O'Connor, J.: Clinical Results of the Oxford Knee surface arthroplasty of the tibio-femoral joint with a meniscal bearing prostheses. Clin. Orthop. 205: 21-42, 1986.

33) Goodfellow, J., O'Connor, J. The mechanics of the knee and prosthesis design. J Bone joint Surg. 60B: 358, 1978.

34) Hamelynck, K.: Results of 106 Cementless Bi-Cruciate Retaining meniscal bearing knee replacements in osteoarthritis. Personal Communication 1991.

35) Huang, C.H., Lee, Y.M., Su, R.Y., et al: Clinical results of the New Jersey Low Contact Stress knee arthroplasty with two to five years follow-up. J. Orthop. Surg. ROC 8:295-303, 1991.

36) Huson, A., Spoor, C.W., Verbout, A.J.: A model of the human knee derived from Kinematic principles and its relevance for endoprosthesis design. Acta Morphal. Neerl. Scand. 270:45, 1989.

37) Keblish, P.A.: Patella retention vs. re-surfacing. Presented at The Issues in Orthopaedic Implant Technology Symposium Rancho Mirage, California. November 10-15, 1992.

38) Keblish, P.A., Greenwald, S.A.: Patella retention versus patella resurfacing in total knee arthroplasty. Presented at the 58th Annual Meeting of the American Academy of Orthopaedic Surgeons, March 7-12, 1991. (Scientific Exhibit).

39) Keblish, PA., Pappas, M.J.: Rationale and selection of prosthetic types in mobile bearing total knee arthroplasty. Presented at The 59th Annual American Academy of Orthopaedic Surgeons. Washington, D.C. February 20-25, 1992. (Scientific Exhibit).

40) Landy, M., Walker, P.A.: Wear in condylar replacement knees. A.10 year follow-up. Trans. Orthop. Res. Soc. 10:96, 1985.

41) Lombardi, A.V., Mallory, F.J., Vaughn, B.K., et al: the Total Condylar III prosthesis in complex primary total knee arthroplasty: A three to ten year clinical and radiograph evaluation. Presented at The combined Meeting of The Orthopaedic Associations of the English Speaking World.

42) Moran, C.G., Pinder, I.M., Lee, T.A., et al: Survivorship analysis of the uncemented porous coated Anatomic knee replacement. J. Bone Joint Surg. 73A: 848-857, 1991.

43) New Jersey Low contact Stress Posterior Cruciate Retaining Cementless Total knee Replacement Approval for United States Distrubution. Letter to Depuy, Warsaw, Indiana, from Food and Drug Administration, Rockville, Maryland, October 2, 1990.

44) O'Connor, J., Goodfellow, J., Biden, E.: Designing the human knee. In Stokes, I.A.F. (ed).: Mechanical Factors and the skeleton. London, John Libbey, 1981.

45) Oshner, J.L., Dorr. L.D., Gronley, J., at al.: Prospective Comparison of Posterior Cruciate-Retaining Versus Cruciate Sacrificed Total Knee Arthroplasty. Presented at the 55th Annual Meeting of The American Accademy of Orthopaedic Surgeons. Atlanta, Georgia, February 4-9, 1988.

46) Pappas, M.J., Makris, G., Buechel, F.F.: Biomaterials for hard tissue applications. In Pizzoferrato, A., Marchetti, P.G., Ravaglioli A., Lee, A.J.C. (eds): Biomaterials and Clinical Applications: Evaluation of Contact Stresses in Metal-Plastic Replacements. Amsterdam, Elsevier, 1987, pp. 259-264.

47) Peter, P.C., Engh, G.A., Dwyer, K.A.: Osteolysis after total knee arthroplasty without cement. J. Bone Joint Surg. 74A: 864-876, 1992.

48) Pillar, R.M., Cameron, J.U., Welsh, R.P., et al: Radiographic and morphologic studies of load-bearing porous-surfaced implants. Clin. Orthop. 156:249-57, 1981.

49) Ranawat, C.S., Flynn, W.F., Saddler, S., et al. Long-term results of the Total Condylar knee arthroplasty. A 15 year survivorship study. Presented at The Ninth Combined Meeting of The Orthopaedic Association.

50) Rose, R.M., M.D., Paul, I.L., et al: Wear of the tibial component of the knee prosthesis. Transactions of the 28th annual Orthopaedic Research Society, New Orleans, Lousiana, January 19-21, 1982, Vol. 7p. 252.

51) Schatzer, J., Horne, J.G., Summer-Smith, G.: The effect of movement on the holding power of screws in bone. Clin. Orthop. III: 257-262, 1975.

52) Schlepckow, P.: Three dimensional Kinematics of total knee replacement system. Arch. Orthop. Trauma Surg. III: 204-209, 1992.

53) Scuderi, G.R., Insall, J.N., Windsor, R.E., et al: Survivorship of cemented knee replacements. J Bone Joint Surg. 71B:798-803, 1989.

54) Tria, A.J., Klein, K.S.: An illustrated guide to the Knee Biomechanics. Chapter 2, pp. 31-38 Churchill Livingstone, New York.

55) Nielsen, P.T., Hansen, E.B., and Rechnagel K.: Cementless total knee arthroplasty in unselected cases of osteoarthritis and rheumatoid arthritis: A 3 year folllow-up study of 103 cases. J. Arthrop., 7:137-143, 1992.

Chapter 14
Total Internal Constraint Prosthesis

Giorgio Fontanesi, Roberto Rotini

Rizzoli Orthopaedic Institute - Bologna

Treatises on knee replacement surgery often recall so-called constraint prostheses as models of great historical value because of the poor clinical results obtained. In recent years, the increase in cases of knee replacement to be submitted to revision, and the development of "less rigid" prosthetic designs, have brought these models back to the lime light. Thus, it is the purpose of this chapter to evaluate the relevance of prostheses with greater articular mechanical constraint, paying particular attention to the technical features of new models and to their indications.

The definition of total internal constraint prosthesis (TIC), as compared to the traditional definition of the constraint prosthesis, makes the classification of new models more correct (7, 21).

TIC models include ones that, by completely substituting the function of the ligaments, totally control the stability of the neo-articulation.

The variability of the internal constraint system allows for the subdivision of models into those with a fixed hinge, a rotating hinge, or hingeless (Fig. 1).

Classification

1) Fixed hinge models are characterized by an absolute interprosthetic constraint with a central pivot that locks the tibial component to the femoral one.

The forerunner of these models is the Walldius prosthesis (1951), followed by the Shiers model (1954): both of these models were characterized by the presence of long intramedullary stems that by self-centering in the canal made implantation technically easy. Subsequently, the G.u.e.p.a.r. prosthesis was frequently used (1970), designed with a more posterior rotation center and to be applied using acrylic cement. All of these models were abandoned because of the high incidence of mobilization and rupture caused by the excessive rigidity of the implant (15).

The few models with a fixed hinge that are still in use today require the presence of polyethylene inserts at the tibial level, and of polyethylene washers inserted in the central horizontal pivot, making the system less rigid (1, 2).

Blauth with his prosthesis (Fig. 2) characterized by a femoral component with 6° valgus, by a tibial component with a central stem, and by four antirotational pivots, reports a ten-year survival rate with an 89% incidence, a 3% incidence of infections, a 1.2% incidence of aseptic detachment, and a 13% incidence of patellar subdislocation (1).

2) Rotating hinge models were introduced in the seventies (Herbert 1972, Trillat 1973, Bliert 1974).

The model that has had the most success in Europe is the Endomodel Rotating devised at the Endoclinik of Hamburg (5). The cross-shaped joint allows for 165° flexion and 20-25° tibial rotation per side. The femoral stem, with 6° of valgus, presents diaphyseal centralizers that guarantee effective cortical hold and accurate recovery of the mechanical axis. Alongside the standard model, one with a trochlea is available, indicated in revision surgery, and recently, a version with cementless modular stems has been introduced (Fig. 3). Out of 1075 Endomodel Rotating replacements reviewed after 2-7 years, Engelbrecht reports a 90% success rate, a 1.3% incidence of infections, and a 0.6% incidence of aseptic detachments.

In the USA, the rotating hinge model used most is the Hinge Kinematic Rotating (17), char-

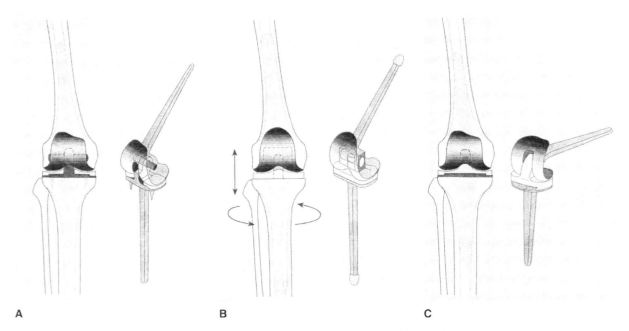

FIG. 1 - Illustrations of three different types of TIC models: a) with a fixed hinge, b) with a rotating hinge, c) hingeless.

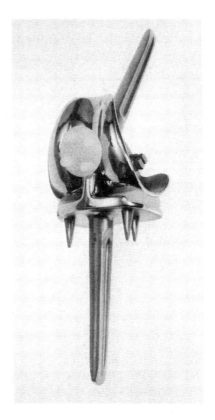

FIG. 2 - Blauth prosthesis: TIC with a fixed hinge.

acterized by a tibial component with two elements, the first of which is constrained to the femoral component and inserted with a rotating peg on the second one fixed to the bone surface (Fig. 4).

The recently introduced S-ROM Rotating Hinge model is similar for its double prosthetic constraint (Fig. 5). The modular system includes a complex prosthetic assembly to obtain more metaphyseal hold even when there is severe loss of bone substance (13).

3) Models without a hinge involve a central fit system with a varyingly shaped pivot that stabilizes the prosthesis on all levels.

In 1973, Gschwend, Scheier, and Bahler presented the G.S.B. prosthesis, whose main feature is the presence of a central tibial pivot with rounded end that is articulated with a semilunate intercondylar fissure surfaced with polyethylene (Fig. 6). A recent review of 638 G.S.B. prostheses reported a 90% success rate over a ten-year period, a 3.7% incidence of infection, and a 0.87% incidence of aseptic mobilization (9).

This group includes the Total Condylar III prosthesis (T.C.III); devised in 1977 at the Hospital for Special Surgery, it constitutes the total internal constraint prosthesis used most in the United States (3, 4, 10, 18, 19, 20). This model is characterized by a rectangular prominence that emerges from the tibial plate that is fitted into the intercondylar notch, producing mid-lateral and anteroposterior stability. By associating the four main series on T.C.III out of a total of 114 cases, a 73% incidence of positive cases, a 5.2% incidence of infections, and a 2.3% incidence of asep-

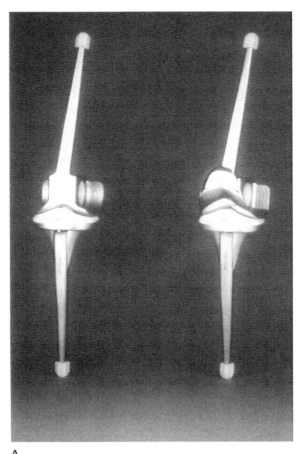
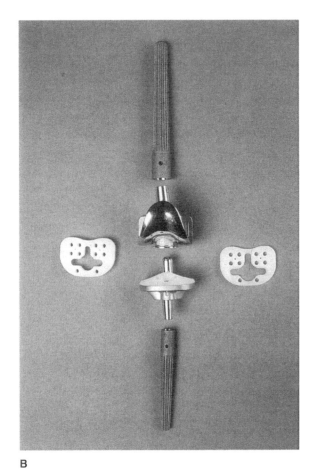

A   B

FIG. 3 - Endomodel Rotating Model: TIC with rotating hinge: a) Models with or without trochlea to be used with cement. b) Cement-less modular model.

tic detachment may be observed (3, 4, 10, 18).

One of the models developed from the T.C. III is the Constrained Condylar Knee (C.C.K.) currently available with cementless modular intramedullary stems (12) (Fig. 7). From the first reports, the results obtained with this model are comforting, as well (87% positive cases), considering that it has been reserved for complex prosthetic knee replacements (14).

This group can also include the Dual Articular prosthesis, characterized by a tibial insert provided with a large pivot articulated with the femoral box and a bi-helicoidal base that can rotate on a metal plate (8) (Fig. 8).

Indications

TIC prostheses are indicated to be used in primary and revision surgery. In 1986, Insall (11)

FIG. 4 - Kinematic Rotating Hinge model: TIC with rotating hinge.

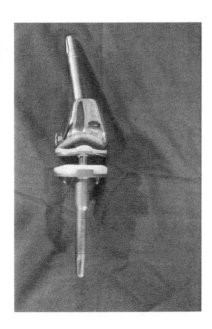

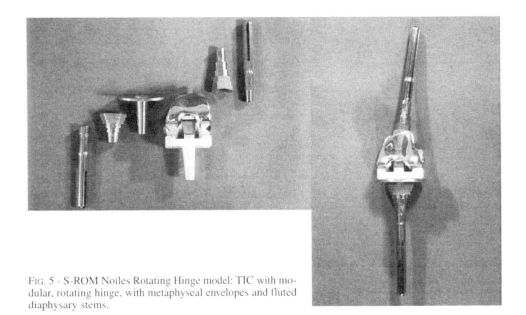

Fig. 5 - S-ROM Noiles Rotating Hinge model: TIC with modular, rotating hinge, with metaphyseal envelopes and fluted diaphysary stems.

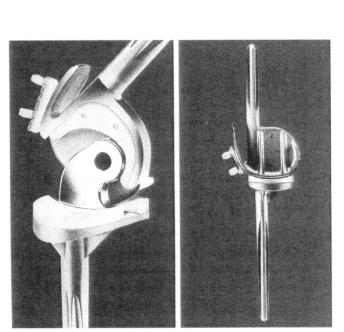

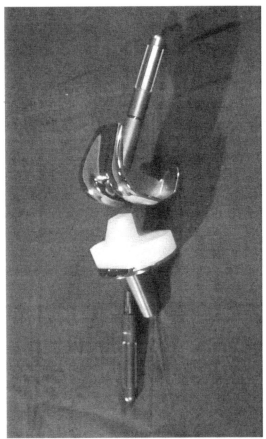

FIG. 6 - G.S.B. model: TIC without hinge.

FIG. 7 - C.C.K. model: TIC without hinge.

believed that the use of constrained prostheses was limited to 1-10% of prosthetic pathologies of the knee, and considered this model to be "an ace up the sleeve" available to the surgeon in case of need, particularly when revision was required. Certainly, in primary implants, models with a minor or intermediate internal constraint are to be preferred (6), as when severe deformity is present, correct alignment of the mechanical axis and good stability with suitable ligament balancing may be obtained. A loss of bone substance is not a contraindication to the use of these models, as bone grafts or metal thicknesses and components with intramedullary pegs may be used.

In our opinion, the use of TIC in primary implant surgery should be limited to cases with severe deformity, in which multidirectional laxity is associated, preferably in patients of advanced age and more often in rheumatoid arthritis rather than osteoarthritis. Other elective indications are represented by severe joint stiffness that calls for an extensive capsuloligamentous release prosthetic implant (Fig. 9) and by tumor surgery that requires extensive joint demolition (Fig. 10).

TIC models are more indicated in pathologies for which revision surgery is performed, particularly in cases where bone substance loss and ligament injury are more extensive. An elective indication is represented by the failure of the implant as a result of ligamentous laxity (Fig. 11).

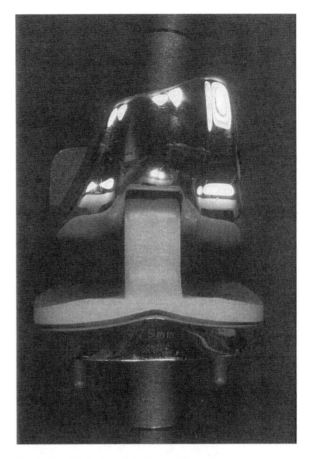

FIG. 8 - Dual Articular model: TIC without hinge.

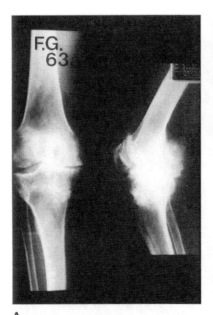
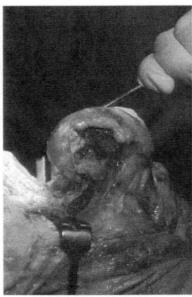
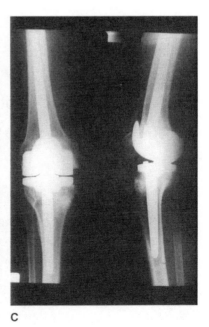

A   B   C

FIG. 9 - a) X-ray of patient aged 63 years with rigid arthritic knee. b) Extensive peripheral capsuloligamentous release makes the use of a TIC prosthesis necessary. c) X-ray of the same case with TIC prosthesis with a rotating hinge and cementless stems.

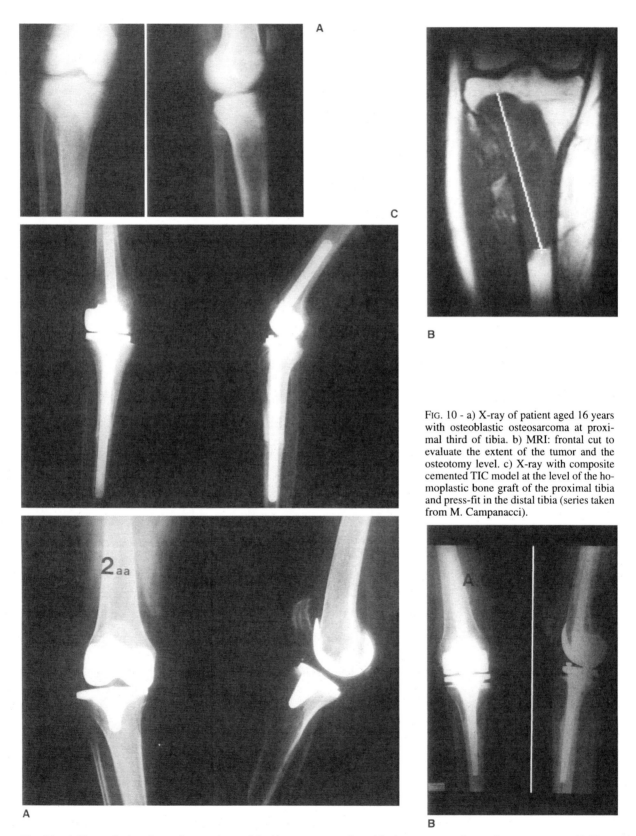

FIG. 10 - a) X-ray of patient aged 16 years with osteoblastic osteosarcoma at proximal third of tibia. b) MRI: frontal cut to evaluate the extent of the tumor and the osteotomy level. c) X-ray with composite cemented TIC model at the level of the homoplastic bone graft of the proximal tibia and press-fit in the distal tibia (series taken from M. Campanacci).

FIG. 11 - a) X-ray of minor internal constraint model with severe posterolateral laxity two years after replacement surgery. b) X-ray with revision model TIC with cemented rotating hinge and tibial spacer.

The Experience at the Rizzoli Orthopaedic Institute

At the Rizzoli Institute, from the very first experiences by Paltrinieri-Trentani (16) in degenerative pathologies, unlike tumor surgery, prosthetic models with minor internal constraint (MIC) or intermediate internal constraint (IIC) have always been preferred (Table I).

The main hesitation in using these implants that require long intramedullary pegs because of

TAB. I - Knee prostheses used at the Rizzoli Institute (1990-1997).

	Degenerative Pathologies	Tumor Pathologies
MIC Prosthesis	n° 753	n° 0
IIC Prosthesis	n° 142	n° 1
TIC Prosthesis	n° 19	n° 229

the narrow joint constraint of the two components, is the fear of infection occurring. In cases such as these, in addition to the higher risk of explantation as compared to standard models, infection is more difficult to eliminate and fusion may often be difficult to carry out (Fig. 12).

It is also important to not overlook the possibility of using cementless stems that, if on one hand may reduce the risk of infection and the difficulties of explantation, on the other, by obtaining diaphyseal press-fit, expose the patient to the risk of intra- and postoperative fractures (Fig. 13).

The TIC prosthetic model most used by us is the Endomodel Rotating prosthesis.

Surgery includes preparation of the femoral canal with rasps of increasing caliber to receive the resection guide equipped with intramedullary stem with centralizer equal in size to the last rasp used. The saw blade is placed on the guide to make bone resections in the intercondylar region. The guide is inserted in the intercondylar space and the femoral condyles are

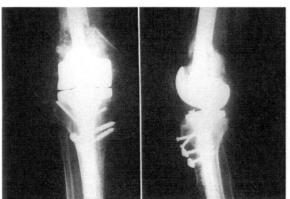
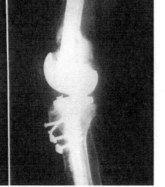

A

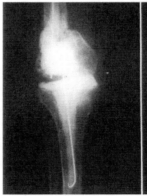
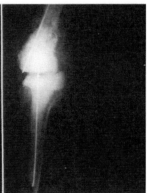

B

C

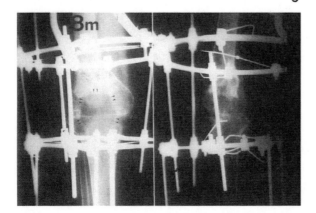

FIG. 12 - a) X-ray of TIC model implanted on the sequelae of unconsolidated fracture of the distal femur complicated by infection. b) Removal of the model and application of spacer cement with antibiotic. c) Fusion with Ilizarov apparatus; after 8 months fusion is obtained at the level of the condylar regions with the presence of central fistulized osteolytic area.

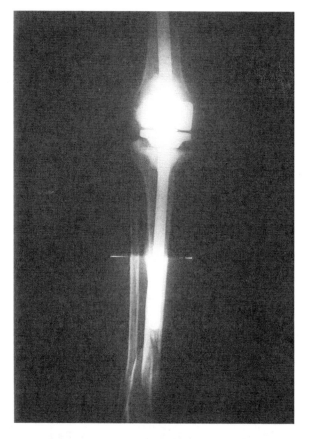

FIG.13 - X-ray of TIC prosthesis with fracture of the tibia at the level of the apex of the cementless stem that occurred during postoperative rehabilitation.

shaped on the form of the internal profile of the prosthesis (Fig. 14a).

The tibial stage begins with the preparation of the canal and with the use of an aligner-resecter with an intramedullary stem (Fig. 14b). Proximal resection is carried out, and a triflangiate rasp is inserted in the canal corresponding to the shape of the tibial stem. Based on the size of the prosthesis chosen, trial assembly is carried out.

Three different sizes are available with or without femoral trochlea (for primary or revision respectively), with a standard or anti-dislocating polyethylene insert and tibial thicknesses to be reserved for cases with bone loss.

When cementless intramedullary stems are used, cement is limited to the support surface (Fig, 14c).

Conclusions

Improvements obtained in the biomechanics of the TIC prosthesis and the increase in knee

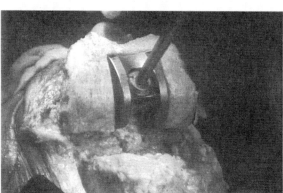

A

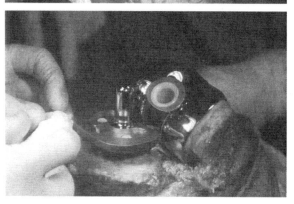

C

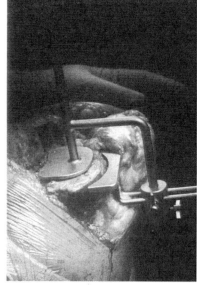

B

FIG.14 - Surgical stages of TIC model with a rotating hinge: a) femoral preparation; b) tibial preparation; c) lodging of prosthetic components limiting the use of cement to the support surface.

prostheses to be submitted to revision surgery will in the years to come lead to a greater diffusion of these models. An up-dating of the classification provides a more accurate knowledge of current prosthetic models. Indications for TIC prostheses must be carefully selected for cases with greater laxity and bone deformity because if on one hand the new generations of this model strongly guarantee results, some doubts do exist as to the higher incidence of septic complications and their resolution.

To this purpose, a useful innovation was the introduction of cementless intramedullary stems.

Although our experience with these models is not consolidated, we believe that they are very useful in primary implant surgery to treat particularly complex cases with degenerative pathology, and especially when tumor pathology is present. They constitute a solution for prosthetic loosening when reimplantation is required in cases with multidirectional ligamentous laxity.

Without a doubt, the possibility currently offered by numerous prosthetic systems to choose among different solutions of internal constraint with the same implant base represents the best possible condition for the surgeon.

References

1) Blauth W., Hassenpflug J.: Are uncostrained components essential in total knee arthroplasty. Long-term results of the Blauth knee prosthesis. Clin. Orthop.1990, 258, 86-94.

2) Capanna R., Campanacci D.A., Del Ben M., Caldora P., Morris H.G. : Rimodellamento periprotesico negli steli non cementati ad ancoraggio diafisario nelle protesi da revisione. Min. Ortop. Traum. 1993, 44, 943-949.

3) Chotivichit A.L., Cracchiolo A., Chow G. H., Dorey F.:Total knee arthroplasty using the Total Condylar III knee prosthesis. J. Arthroplasty, 1991, 6, 341-356.

4) Donaldson W. F., Sculco T. P., Insall J.N., Ranawat C. S.:Total condylar III prosthesis: long-term follow-up study.Clin. Orthop., 1988, 226, 21-28.

5) Engelbrecht E., Nieder E., Strickle E., Keller A.:Intra-condylare kniegelenksendo-prosthese mit rotationsmoglichkeit Endo-model. Chirurg, 1981, 52, 368-375.

6) Fontanesi G., Costa P., Rotini. R, Pignedoli P.:Artroprotesi totali di ginocchio P.C.A.. Giorn. It. Ortop. e Traum. 1988, 14, 43-50.

7) Fontanesi G. : Classificazione delle protesi totali di ginocchio. Chir.Organi Mov. 1997, 82, 1-6.

8) Goddard N.J. : Experience with the Dual-Articular Knee. Second Symposium of Revision Surgery, Zell am See, Austria, 1993.

9) Gschwend N., Siegrist H.: Das GSB-Kniegelenk. 1991, Orthopade, 20, 197-205.

10) Hohl M.W., Crawford E., Zelicof S.B., Ewald F.C.: The Total Condylar III prosthesis in complex knee reconstruction. Clin. Orthop.; 1991, 273, 91-97.

11) Insall J.N.:Artroplastica totale del ginocchio.In:Chirurgia del ginocchio. Roma. Verduci Editore.1986. 621-734.

12) Insall J.N.: Revisione dei fallimenti asettici delle artroprotesi di ginocchio.In: Insall J.N. (Ed.) Chirurgia del ginocchio. Roma. Verduci Editore. 1995, 893-913.

13) Jones R.E. : Management of complex revision problems with a Modular Total Knee System. Orthopedics; 1996, 19, 802-804.

14) Lachiewicz P.F., Falatyn S.P.:Clinical and radiographic results of the total condylar and costrained condylar total knee artrhroplasty. J. Arthroplasty.1996. 11. 916-922.

15) Morgan E.L., Rand J.A.: Results of total knee arthroplasty using older constrained implant designs. In: Rand J.A. (Ed.) Total knee arthroplasty. New York. Raven press. 1993, 177-191.

16) Paltrinieri M., Sandrolini S., Trentani C.: L'artroprotesi di ginocchio. Chir. Organi Mov. 1971, 60, 613-621.

17) Rand J.A., Chao E.Y.S., Stauffer R.N.: Kinematic Rotating Hinge total knee arthroplasty. J.Bone Joint Surg. (A) 1987, 69, 489-497.

18) Rand J.A.: Revision total knee arthroplasty using the Total Condylar III prosthesis. J. Arthroplasty. 1991, 6, 1-6.

19) Rosemberg A.G., Verner J.J. Galante J.O.: Clinical results of total revision using the Total Condylar III prosthesis. Clin. Orthop. 1991, 273, 83-90.

20) Sculco T.P.: Total Condylar III prosthesis in ligament instability. Orthop. Clin. North Am. 1989, 20, 221-226.

21) Tooms R.E.: Artroplastica della tibiotarsica e del ginocchio. In: Crenshaw A.H. (Ed.) Chirurgia ortopedica di Campbell, Bologna, Grasso Editore, 1991, 1161- 1227.

Section 4

COMPLICATIONS

Chapter 15

Wound Complications
in Total Knee Arthroplasty

Douglas A. Dennis

Colorado School of Mines, Rose Musculoskeletal Research Laboratory - Denver

Primary wound healing is critical for the success of any total knee arthroplasty (TKA). Any delay in wound healing risks infection and arthroplasty failure (1). Prevention of soft-tissue problems through the proper selection of skin incision, an understanding of vascular anatomy and patient risk factors, and prompt management should wound problems arise, is imperative to achieve desired results.

Vascular Anatomy

The blood supply to the soft tissues of the anterior aspect of the knee is completely random, with contributions from multiple vessels (2-8). This blood supply arises predominantly from the terminal branches of the peripatellar anastomotic arterial ring. This anastomotic ring has numerous contributing arterial branches, including the medial and lateral superior genicular arteries, the medial and lateral inferior genicular arteries, the supreme genicular artery, the anterior tibial recurrent artery, and a branch of the profunda femoris artery (Fig. 1). In contrast to the skin circulation of the thigh proximal to the knee, there is no underlying muscle or intermuscular septa directly anterior to the knee to provide a direct pathway for arterial perforators (2-5). Skin circulation in this area is dependent on the dermal plexus, which originates directly from arterioles traveling within the subcutaneous fascia. Any surgical dissection performed superficial to this subcutaneous fascia disrupts the arterial supply to the skin and increases the possibility of skin necrosis. Elevation of skin flaps about the anterior aspect of

the knee requires dissection deep to the subcutaneous fascia to preserve the perforating arteriolar network between the subcutaneous fascia and dermal plexus (2).

Choice of Skin Incision

Analysis of vascular anatomy about the knee suggests that choice of a midline skin incision is less disruptive to the arterial network (2). Medial peripatellar skin incisions are undesirable, because they create a large, laterally based skin flap, which has been associated with higher wound complication rates (2). Transcutaneous oxygen measurements, both before and after skin incisions about the knee, have demonstrated reduced oxygenation of the lateral skin region (9, 10) The further medially the skin incision is made, the larger the lateral skin flap. A larger lateral skin flap has a lower oxygen tension, which increases the risk of wound complications. Placement of the skin incision slightly lateral to the midline will assist in eversion of the patella, particularly in obese patients in whom a large and bulky lateral skin flap resists patellar eversion.

For patients in whom a previous skin incision is present, utilization of the previous skin incision is generally recommended. Although it is usually safe to ignore previous short medial or lateral peripatellar skin incisions, one should beware of wide scars with thin or absent subcutaneous tissue, as damage to the underlying dermal plexus is likely, increasing the risk of wound necrosis (2). Problems with placement of a longitudinal incision crossing

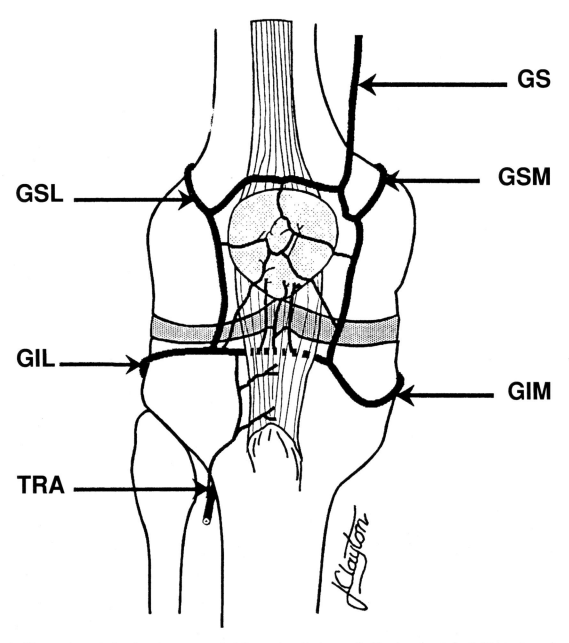

FIG. 1 - Diagram demonstrating the extraosseous peripatellar anastomotic ring supplied by six main arteries (LSG lateral superior genicular; MSG medial superior genicular; MIG medial inferior genicular; LIG lateral inferior genicular; SG supreme genicular; ATR anterior tibial recurrent). (Reproduced with permission from Dennis DA: Patellofemoral complications in total knee arthroplasty: A literature review. *Am J Knee Surg* 1992; 5:156-166).

a transverse incision previously used for high tibial osteotomy are uncommon (11, 12).

If long parallel skin incisions exist, choice of the lateral-most skin incision is favorable to avoid a large lateral skin flap which has been previously compromised at the time of the initial lateral skin incision. In complex situations, such as knees with multiple skin incisions or previously burned or irradiated skin, consideration of plastic surgical consultation is wise, both for the design of the upcoming skin incision as well as for consideration of preoperative muscle flap procedures if the risk of skin necrosis is substantial. In selected complex situations, wound problems can be reduced by using a staged technique. A "pre-revision" skin incision to the depth of the subcutaneous fascial layer is made and is then closed. If this incision heals without difficulty, one can later proceed with TKA through this incision with much greater confidence.

Soft-tissue expansion techniques have been used successfully in cases of contracted soft tissues from previous skin incisions or exposure of the skin to irradiation or burns (13-18). These techniques involve implantation, usually subcutaneously, of an expandable reservoir, into which saline can be intermittently injected to expand the surface area of the skin. Studies have shown that this technique maintains epidermal thickness. Although some dermal thinning is encountered, actual dermal collagen synthesis is increased. Complications with soft-tissue expansion have been minimal and include hematoma formation, reservoir deflation, infection, and skin necrosis from overly vigorous soft-tissue expansion.

Technical Factors

A thorough preoperative vascular examination of the limb is necessary to minimize the risk of wound-healing difficulties. The skin incision for TKA should be of adequate length to avoid excessive tension on the wound edges, particularly when the knee is in extremes of flexion. Gentle retraction of the skin edges is necessary to avoid disruption of perforating arterioles originating in the subcutaneous fascial layer. It is best to attempt to avoid undermining large areas of skin. If undermining of skin flaps is required, it must be done in the subfascial plane to preserve the blood supply to the skin, which originates in the dermal plexus (2,5). Numerous studies have demonstrated that a lateral retinacular release decreases lateral skin oxygenation and increases the subsequent risk of wound complications (19-22). If a lateral retinacular release is required, attempts should be made to preserve the lateral superior geniculate artery. Meticulous wound hemostasis is required to avoid postoperative hematomas. Routine use of suction drainage will reduce pain and postoperative ecchymosis. Lastly, wound closure without tension is imperative to minimize the risk of skin necrosis.

Patient Risk Factors

Numerous reports suggest an increased incidence of wound-healing difficulties in patients who chronically use corticosteroids (2, 23-30). Corticosteroid use has been shown to decrease fibroblast proliferation, which is necessary for proper wound healing (24). Chronic corticosteroid use also reduces collagenase clearance from the healing wound, which results in diminished collagen accumulation at the wound healing site and a subsequent decrease in wound tensile strength (23, 29, 30). An increased incidence of wound complications in patients with rheumatoid arthritis has been well documented. Although the specific cause of this association is not known, it may be related to the increased long-term use of corticosteroids in many of these patients (31-36).

Patients with substantial obesity demonstrate increased wound complication rates (26, 35, 37, 38). Extreme obesity can create exposure difficulties in TKA, necessitating more vigorous retraction of skin flaps and the subsequent risk of soft-tissue devascularization. Additionally, in heavier patients with a thick adipose layer, the skin is less adherent to its underlying vascular supply, which increases the risk of separation of the dermis from the subcutaneous layer during skin retraction (2).

Malnutrition, represented by albumin levels less than 3.5 g/dl and total lymphocyte counts less than 1500 cells/mm^3, has been associated with poor healing of Syme amputation stumps and may play a role in wound healing following TKA (38, 39). The damaging effects of cigarette smoking have been well documented and are related to the systemic vasoconstriction resulting from nicotine use (40-44).

While the exact relationship is unclear, the increased frequency of wound problems in patients with diabetes mellitus may be secondary to delayed collagen synthesis and delayed wound tensile strength. Early capillary ingrowth into the healing wound is also reduced (2, 38, 45-47). Use of high-dose nonsteroidal anti-inflammatory drugs inhibits the acute inflammatory response, which is an important step in the early phases of wound healing. Inhibition of this early, acute inflammatory response may exacerbate wound healing difficulties (48). Patients on chemotherapy may be similarly at risk for delayed wound healing. The routine need to discontinue methotrexate in preoperative patients with rheumatoid arthritis is unclear. Bridges and associates (49) found a slight increase in the incidence of infection in ten patients treated with methotrexate when compared with patients with rheumatoid arthritis in whom methotrexate had been discontinued more than 1 month preoperatively. Other larger comparison studies have demonstrated no increase in wound-healing complications with continuance of methotrexate perioperatively in patients with rheumatoid arthritis (50, 51).

Adequate hydration is necessary for satisfactory wound healing. Hypovolemia can delay wound healing due to reduced oxygen delivery to the healing soft tissues (2). Reduction in transcutaneous oxygen levels has been documented to increase wound healing complications following lateral retinacular release in TKA (20) and to decrease wound healing after soft-tissue flap transfers (52). Use of continuous passive motion beyond 40° has been shown to reduce transcutaneous oxygen tension measured in the healing wound edges, especially during the initial 3 days following TKA. Continuous passive motion should be limited to less than 40° in the early postoperative period (53, 54). Additional risk factors for wound complications following TKA include those knees in which the anterior skin has previously been irradiated or suffered severe scarring from previous burns.

Wound Complication Management

Various types of wound complications can occur, including prolonged postoperative drainage, superficial soft-tissue necrosis, and full-thickness soft-tissue necrosis, in which the prosthetic components are usually exposed. All three types of wound problems require immediate attention, as delay in treatment risks deep infection and subsequent failure of the TKA.

Prolonged Serous Drainage

If the TKA wound is chronically draining yet the wound does not exhibit substantial erythema or purulence, immobilization and local wound care can be attempted. In the author's experience, if drainage persists beyond 5 to 7 days despite immobilization and local wound care, spontaneous cessation of drainage is unlikely and surgical debridement is indicated. Subcutaneous hematomas or large intra-articular hemarthroses are commonly encountered in

cases of persistent wound drainage. Hematomas threaten the wound by increasing soft-tissue tension, releasing toxic breakdown products of hemoglobin, and serving as a healthy medium for bacterial growth (2)

Scientific data are lacking to clearly support surgical drainage rather than observation of the nondraining hematoma. We recommend treating the nondraining hematoma nonsurgically through close observation as long as no signs of impending skin necrosis from excessive soft-tissue tension are present. An additional consideration for surgical drainage is a large hematoma that substantially limits of knee range of motion. Drainage procedures should be performed in the operating theater with perioperative antibiotic prophylaxis.

The incidence of prolonged drainage in patients who eventually develop culture-proven infected TKA ranges from 17% to 50% (55-57). Weiss and Krackow (55), in a retrospective review of 597 TKA procedures, found eight patients (1.3%) with persistent wound drainage. All were treated with surgical irrigation and debridement and parenteral antibiotics. All cases healed without infection despite the fact that two patients (25%) had positive cultures at the time of irrigation and debridement. The authors suggest that prompt surgical management in these cases may prevent chronic drainage problems from becoming established infections.

Superficial Soft-Tissue Necrosis

Necrotic tissue generally requires surgical debridement. Small necrotic areas less than 3 cm in diameter may heal with local wound care or delayed secondary closure (28). Larger areas of superficial necrosis should be debrided and covered by split-thickness skin grafting or fasciocutaneous flaps (58, 59).

Full-Thickness Soft-Tissue Necrosis

Full-thickness soft-tissue necrosis is usually associated with exposed prosthetic components and requires immediate, aggressive debridement. Simple secondary closure procedures are often unsuccessful, and some type of flap reconstruction is usually required. Various types of flaps have been used, including cutaneous (60), fasciocutaneous (58, 59), and myocutaneous flaps (60-67). Bengtson and associates (61) reported on treatment of ten TKAs with full-thickness skin loss and exposed prosthetic components. Delayed closure failed in six of six cases in which it was attempted. Split thickness skin grafting failed in both cases in which it was tried. In contrast, coverage with gastrocnemius myocutaneous flaps proved successful and was recommended as the treatment of choice in these cases. Gerwin and associates (67) reviewed 12 patients with full-thickness skin necrosis and exposed prostheses, six of whom had positive deep cultures. All patients were treated with aggressive debridement and closure with medial gastrocnemius myocutaneous flaps. Eleven of 12 patients (92%) obtained excellent results, with ten (82%) retaining their prosthetic components or having a successful reimplantation.

The medial head of the gastrocnemius muscle is often the preferred type of flap reconstruction. It is both larger and 2 to 3 cm longer than the lateral gastrocnemius muscle. Furthermore, because it does not have to traverse the fibula, it therefore has a larger arc of rotation. It provides excellent soft-tissue coverage in the region of the patella and tibial tubercle, the area where the incidence of skin necrosis is the highest. Free myocutaneous flaps may also be used (2, 68), but they are reserved for cases with full-thickness necrosis which cannot be covered with gastrocnemius or other local flap reconstructions.

Antibiotic Use

Parenteral antibiotics are often required in cases with persistent drainage and wound necrosis, but they should not be used indiscriminately. Unnecessary use of antibiotics risks alteration of bacterial flora and sensitivities, should deep infection occur (2). Joint aspiration for culture is suggested before initiation of antibiotic therapy in order to maximize culture results. Cultures of superficial drainage are often spurious with little correlation with deep infecting organisms (2, 28, 69).

Summary

Wound problems are a dreaded complication following TKA and the ideal is to avoid them. Preventive measures include proper choice of the skin incision, gentle handling of the soft tissues, meticulous hemostasis, and wound closure without excessive tension. Should persistent wound drainage or soft-tissue necrosis occur, early intervention is imperative, because delay risks deep infection and failure of the TKA. Cases associated with full-thickness soft-tissue necrosis often require transfer of well-vascularized tissue, such as a medial gastrocnemius myocutaneous flap reconstruction.

References

1. Poss R, Thornhill TS, Ewald FC, et al: Factors influencing the incidence and outcome of infection following total joint arthroplasty. Clin Orthop 1984;182:117–126.
2. Klein NE, Cox CV: Wound problems in total knee arthroplasty. In Fu FH, Harner CD, Vince KG, et al (eds): Knee Surgery. Baltimore, MD, Williams & Wilkins, 1994, vol 2, pp 1539–1552.
3. Müller W (ed): The Knee: Form, Function and Ligament Reconstruction. Berlin, Germany, Springer–Verlag, 1983, pp 158–167.
4. Scapinelli R: Studies on the vasculature of the human knee joint. Acta Anat 1968;70:305–331.
5. Craig SM: Soft tissue considerations in the failed total knee arthroplasty. In Scott WN (ed): The Knee. St. Louis, MO, Mosby-Year Book, 1994, vol 2, pp 1279–1295.
6. Abbott LC, Carpenter WF: Surgical approaches to the knee joint. J Bone Joint Surg 1945;27:277–310.
7. Björkström S, Goldie IF: A study of the arterial supply of the patella in the normal state, in chondromalacia patellae and in osteoarthrosis. Acta Orthop Scand 1980;51:63–70.
8. Waisbrod H, Treiman N: Intra–osseous venography in patellofemoral disorders: A preliminary report. J Bone Joint Surg 1980;62B:454–456.
9. Johnson DP: Midline or parapatellar incision for knee arthroplasty: A comparative study of wound viability. J Bone Joint Surg 1988;70B:656–658.
10. Johnson DP, Houghton TA, Radford P: Anterior midline or medial parapatellar incision for arthroplasty of the knee: A comparative study. J Bone Joint Surg 1986;68B:812–814.
11. Ecker ML, Lotke PA: Wound healing complications. In Rand JA (ed): Total Knee Arthroplasty. New York, NY, Raven Press, 1993, pp 403–407.
12. Windsor RE, Insall JN, Vince KG: Technical consideration of total knee arthroplasty after proximal tibial osteotomy. J Bone Joint Surg 1988;70A:547–555.
13. Mahomed N, McKee N, Solomon P, et al: Soft-tissue expansion before total knee arthroplasty in arthrodesed joints: A report of two cases. J Bone Joint Surg 1994;76B:88–90.
14. Argenta LC, Marks MW, Pasyk KA: Advances in tissue expansion. Clin Plast Surg 1985;12:159–171.

15. Manders EK, Oaks TE, Au VK, et al: Soft-tissue expansion in the lower extremities. Plast Reconstr Surg 1988;81:208–219.

16. Manders EK, Schenden MJ, Furrey JA, et al: Soft-tissue expansion: Concepts and complications. Plast Reconstr Surg 1984;74:493–507.

17. Radovan C: Tissue expansion in soft-tissue reconstruction. Plast Reconstr Surg 1984;74:482–492.

18. Riederman R, Noyes FR: Soft tissue skin expansion of contracted tissues prior to knee surgery. Am J Knee Surg 1991;4:195–198.

19. Clayton ML, Thirupathi R: Patellar complications after total condylar arthroplasty. Clin Orthop 1982;170:152–155.

20. Johnson DP, Eastwood DM: Lateral patellar release in knee arthroplasty: Effect on wound healing. J Arthroplasty 1992; 7(suppl):427–431.

21. Kayler DE, Lyttle D: Surgical interruption of patellar blood supply by total knee arthroplasty. Clin Orthop 1988; 229:221–227.

22. Scuderi G, Scharf SC, Meltzer LP, et al: The relationship of lateral release to patella viability in total knee arthroplasty. J Arthroplasty 1987;2:209–214.

23. Craig SM: Soft tissue considerations. In Scott WN (ed): Total Knee Revision Arthroplasty. Orlando, FL, Grune & Stratton, 1987, pp 99–112.

24. Green JP: Steroid therapy and wound healing in surgical patients. Br J Surg 1965;52:523–525.

25. McNamara JJ, Lamborn PJ, Mills D, et al: Effect of short-term pharmacologic doses of adrenocorticosteroid therapy on wound healing. Ann Surg 1969;170:199–202.

26. Nelson CL: Prevention of sepsis. Clin Orthop 1987; 222:66–72.

27. Petty W, Bryan RS, Coventry MB, Peterson LF: Infection after total knee arthroplasty. Orthop Clin North Am 1975; 6:1005–1014.

28. Sculco TP: Local wound complications after total knee arthroplasty. In Ranawat CS (ed): Total Condylar Knee Arthroplasty:Technique, Results, and Complications. New York, NY, Springer–Verlag, 1985, pp 194–196.

29. Wahl LM: Hormonal regulation of macrophage collagenase activity. Biochem Biophys Res Commun 1977; 74:838–845.

30. Werb Z: Biochemical actions of glucocorticoids on macrophages in culture: Specific inhibition of elastase, collagenase, and plasminogen activator secretion and effects on other metabolic functions. J Exp Med 1978; 147:1695–1712.

31. D'Ambrosia RD, Shoji H, Heater R: Secondarily infected total joint replacements by hematogenous spread. J Bone Joint Surg 1976;58A:450–453.

32. Garner RW, Mowat AG, Hazleman BL: Wound healing after operations on patients with rheumatoid arthritis. J Bone Joint Surg 1973;55B:134–144.

33. Grogan TJ, Dorey F, Rollins J, et al: Deep sepsis following total knee arthroplasty: Ten-year experience at the University of California at Los Angeles Medical Center. J Bone Joint Surg 1986;68A:226–234.

34. Thomas BJ, Moreland JR, Amstutz HC: Infection after total joint arthroplasty from distal extremity sepsis. Clin Orthop 1983;181:121–125.

35. Wilson MG, Kelley K, Thornhill TS: Infection as a complication of total knee-replacement arthroplasty: Risk factors and treatment in sixty-seven cases. J Bone Joint Surg 1990; 72A:878–883.

36. Wong RY, Lotke PA, Ecker ML: Factors influencing wound healing after total knee arthroplasty. Orthop Trans 1986; 10:497.

37. Cruse PJ, Foord R: A five-year prospective study of 23,649 surgical wounds. Arch Surg 1973;107:206–210.

38. Ecker ML, Lotke PA: Postoperative care of the total knee patient. Orthop Clin North Am 1989;20:55–62.

39. Dickhaut SC, DeLee JC, Page CP: Nutritional status: Importance in predicting wound-healing after amputation. J Bone Joint Surg 1984;66A:71–75.

40. Craig S, Rees TD: The effects of smoking on experimental skin flaps in hamsters. Plast Reconstr Surg 1985; 75:842–846.

41. Benowitz NL, Kuyt F, Jacob P III: Influence of nicotine on cardiovascular and hormonal effects of cigarette smoking. Clin Pharmacol Ther 1984;36:74–81.

42. Mosely LH, Finseth F, Goody M: Nicotine and its effect on wound healing. Plast Reconstr Surg 1978;61:570–575.

43. Rees TD, Liverett DM, Guy CL: The effect of cigarette smoking on skin-flap survival in the face lift patient. Plast Reconstr Surg 1984;73:911–915.

44. Kaufman T, Eichenlaub EH, Levin M, et al: Tobacco smoking: Impairment of experimental flap survival. Ann Plast Surg 1984;13:468–472.

45. Goodson WH III, Hunt TK: Studies of wound healing in experimental diabetes mellitus. J Surg Res 1977; 22:221–227.

46. Goodson WH III, Hunt TK: Wound healing and the diabetic patient. Surg Gynecol Obstet 1979;149:600–608.

47. McMurry JF Jr: Wound healing with diabetes mellitus: Better glucose control for better wound healing in diabetes. Surg Clin North Am 1984;64:769–778.

48. McGrath MH: The effect of prostaglandin inhibitors on wound contraction and the myofibroblast. Plast Reconstr Surg 1982;69:74–85.

49. Bridges SL Jr, Lopez Mendez A, Tracy I, et al: Should methotrexate be discontinued prior to total joint arthroplasty in rheumatoid arthritis patients? Arthritis Rheum 1989; 32(suppl 4):543.

50. Kasden ML, June L: Postoperative results of rheumatoid arthritis patients on methotrexate at the time of reconstructive surgery of the hand. Orthopedics 1993;16:1233–1235.

51. Perhala RS, Wilke WS, Clough JD, et al: Local infectious complications following large joint replacement in rheumatoid arthritis patients treated with emthotrexate versus those not treated with methotrexate. Arthritis Rheum 1991; 34:146–152.

52. Achauer BM, Black KS, Litke DK: Transcutaneous PO₂ in flaps: A new method of survival prediction. Plast Reconstr Surg 1980;65:738–745.

53. Goletz TH, Henry JH: Continuous passive motion after total knee arthroplasty. South Med J 1986;79:1116–1120.

54. Johnson DP: The effect of continuous passive motion on wound-healing and joint mobility after knee arthroplasty. J Bone Joint Surg 1990;72A:421–426.

55. Weiss AP, Krackow KA: Persistent wound drainage after primary total knee arthroplasty. J Arthroplasty 1993; 8:285–289.

56. Bengtson S, Knutson K, Lidgren L: Treatment of infected knee arthroplasty. Clin Orthop 1989;245:173–178.

57. Insall J, Aglietti P: A five to seven-year follow-up of unicondylar arthroplasty. J Bone Joint Surg 1980; 62A: 1329–1337.

58. Hallock GG: Salvage of total knee arthroplasty with local fasciocutaneous flaps. J Bone Joint Surg 1990; 72A: 1236–1239.

59. Lewis VL Jr, Mossie RD, Stulberg DS, et al: The fasciocutaneous flap: A conservative approach to the exposed knee joint. Plast Reconstr Surg 1990;85:252–257.

60. Lian G, Cracchiolo A III, Lesavoy M: Treatment of major wound necrosis following total knee arthroplasty. J Arthroplasty 1989;4(suppl):S23–S32.

61. Bengtson S, Carlsson A, Relander M, et al: Treatment of the exposed knee prosthesis. Acta Orthop Scand 1987; 58:662–665.

62. Eckardt JJ, Lesavoy MA, Dubrow TJ, et al: Exposed endo-prosthesis: Management protocol using muscle and myocu-taneous flap coverage. Clin Orthop 1990;251:220–229.
63. Greenberg B, LaRosa D, Lotke PA, et al: Salvage of jeop-ardized total-knee prosthesis: The role of the gastrocnemius muscle flap. Plast Reconstr Surg 1989;83:85–89;97–99.
64. Hemphill ES, Ebert FR, Muench AG: The medial gastroc-nemius muscle flap in the treatment of wound complications following total knee arthroplasty. Orthopedics 1992; 15:477–480.
65. Salibian AH, Anzel SH: Salvage of an infected total knee prosthesis with medial and lateral gastrocnemius muscle flaps: A case report. J Bone Joint Surg 1983;65A:681–684.
66. Sanders R, O'Neill T: The gastrocnemius myocutaneous flap used as a cover for the exposed knee prosthesis. J Bone Joint Surg 1981;63B:383–386.
67. Gerwin M, Rothaus KO, Windsor RE, et al: Gastrocnemius muscle flap coverage of exposed or infected knee prosthe-ses. Clin Orthop 1993;286:64–70.
68. Gordon L, Levinsohn DG: Versatility of the latissimus and serratus anterior muscle transplants in providing cover for exposed hardware and endoprostheses. Orthop Trans 1992; 16:68.
69. Insall J, Scott WN, Ranawat CS: The total condylar knee prosthesis: A report of two hundred and twenty cases. J Bone Joint Surg 1979;61A:173–180.

Chapter 16
Mechanical Loosening of Total Knee Arthroplasty

Paul Lombardi, Alexander Miric, Thomas P. Sculco

The Hospital for Special Surgery - New York

Patient Factors

In the process of evaluating possible risk factors for failure of total knee arthroplasty, multiple studies have attempted to identify patient characteristics that may predispose one to a poor result. During this process, a number of such characteristics have been suggested to affect the outcome of total knee arthroplasty, and evidence has been presented to support and refute each one of these assertions. In general, these patient characteristics can be divided into two broad categories: a) those related to patient demand, and b) those related to the quality of the bone. Factors studied in regard to patient demand on the prosthesis include the patient's age, weight, and activity level. Factors studied in regard to the bone quality include the patient's primary diagnosis, medical condition, sex and degree of preoperative joint deformity.

Patient Demands

Since failure at the bone/cement interface constitutes a large portion of mechanical failures after total knee arthroplasty, it stands to reason that increased stress at this interface may be associated with an increase in the rate of implant loosening. The activity level of the patient has been referred to by a number of authors as an important consideration prior to performing a total knee arthroplasty. However, difficulties with quantifying a specific patient's activity level have limited the amount of data collected with respect to the effect of this variable on arthroplasty outcome. Consequently, there is little in the literature directly addressing this assertion. Mintz, et al., after an arthroscopic evaluation of worn polyethylene components, noted the influence of activity level on wear rates. However, no evaluation of the patient's level of activity is mentioned. In fact, one study that attempted to correlate outcome with a preoperative ambulation rating failed to find any relation between the two.

More often, age has been used as an indicator for level of activity. In a review of 32 knee arthroplasty revisions, Tsao, et al. cited decreased age as a significant predictor of an increased risk of failure. Although this view has been shared by others (1), it is not shared by all (4). Ahlberg and Lunden (6), for example, failed to find a link between age and risk of revision in their review of revised knee arthroplasties. While it would seem self-evident that younger patients would place higher demands on a prosthetic knee, in turn, leading to earlier failure, it is not clear that such a direct relationship exists.

Since a patient's body weight is related to the joint reactive forces transmitted through the weight bearing joints, it has been studied as a possible factor in the failure of a knee arthroplasty. This factor is especially significant in light of the number of obese patients undergoing total knee arthroplasty. Bostman reported a 27% rate of obesity among patients admitted for total knee arthroplasty. Weight has been implicated by a number of authors as a factor in the failure of a total knee (2, 3, 5, 8, 9). Among these authors, Healy et al. reported a significantly greater weight among patients suffering from patellofemoral complications. The data from other studies, however, often fails to illustrate such a clear association. Weight may lead to increased wound problems and possibly infection.

In a review of 257 total knee arthroplasties, Stern and Insall reported a significantly greater incidence of patellofemoral symptoms among moderately and severely obese patients. However, they failed to find any discernible difference in survival or overall scores among the different weight groups. In contrast, Kaufer et al. (4) did not find an association between weight and patellar symptoms, while others have reported no association between weight and any marker of poor outcome (1). A more sedentary lifestyle among obese patients has been offered as one of the possible reasons that a clear association between weight and arthroplasty failure is often not uncovered (11).

Bone Quality

While many authors have tried to delineate the effects of increased stress on the bone/cement interface, others have attempted to study the effects of bone quality on this interface. Poor bone quality may lead to a reduction in the strength of this interface which, in turn, may precipitate mechanical failure of the implant. While concerns about the bone quality among patients with rheumatoid arthritis has lead to comparisons between patients diagnosed with rheumatoid arthritis and those diagnosed with osteoarthritis, the findings have often proven surprising. Ahlberg and Lunden (6) reported a disproportionately higher percentage of revision knee arthroplasties among patients with osteoarthritis. Furthermore, the five year survival of revision implants has been reported to be significantly higher among patients diagnosed with rheumatoid arthritis (9). Other studies have suggested no difference in outcome among between patients with different diagnoses (4, 13). Due to the higher incidence of osteoporosis among elderly women, it has been postulated that sex may influence the outcome of total knee arthroplasty. However, more than one study has failed to show a significant difference in outcome between men and women (4, 6). Malalignment associated with poor bone quality is a common source of tibial bone collapse and loosening (Fig. 1).

The medical history of a patient has also been studied as a possible factor related to outcome. While an increased rate of infection has been described among patients with diabetes, this study did not report a higher rate of mechanical failure among these patients. Other

studies have also failed to uncover a difference in rates of loosening based on the patient's past medical history, although previous history of surgery on the same knee has been associated with a higher rate of revision (6).

While perhaps not directly related to bone quality, the effect of preoperative deformity on arthroplasty failure has also been studied. Windsor et al. reported a higher rate of femoral loosening among patients with a preoperative valgus deformity, and attributed this to aggressive lateral releases leading to devascularization of the lateral femoral condyle. While Kaufer et al. (4) report a higher incidence of hematoma formation, delayed wound healing and peroneal nerve palsy among patients with a preoperative valgus deformity, they noted a higher rate of loosening among patients with a

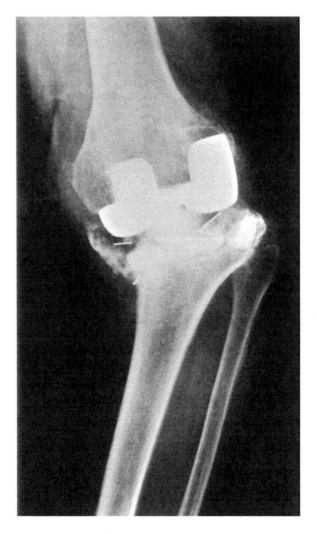

FIG. 1

significant varus deformity. It was noted by the authors that the majority of these failures remained in varus after the arthroplasty. It is here that the true association between varus position and early failure may lie.

For each patient characteristic studied, authors have reported evidence that supports and refutes an association with failure of the prosthesis. Rarely is a clear association between a single factor and mechanical loosening revealed. It is more likely that these factors act in concert with each other and with those related to the prosthesis and the procedure itself. Such a relationship would help explain the widely divergent and often contradictory data collected with regard to patient characteristics.

The Patella

The patellofemoral joint has proven to be one of the most problematic aspects of modern knee arthroplasty (10). Problems with instability, maltracking, patella infera and patella baja have typically been attributed to component malposition. However, there are a series of patellofemoral complications that can occur in spite of the best surgical technique. These complications can be broadly seperated into those due to the patellar implant, the patellofemoral articulation and those due to the patella itself.

The Patellar Implant

The majority of patellar resurfacing has employed an all-polyethylene component in conjunction with polymethylmethacrylate fixation. In general excellent results have been obtained with this method, and loosening rates are typically below 2% (10, 16) (Fig. 2). However, during the 1980s, two concepts were introduced that led to alterations in patellar design. One concept was that by stiffening an all-polyethylene component by adding a metal backing, joint contact loads were distributed over a larger area of bone, reducing the chances of bone failure and subsequent implant loosening. The second concept involved the ability of achieving biologic fixation of implant components by the ingrowth of bone into porous layers of the component surface. The development of these two concepts led to the introduction of metal-backed and porous-coated patellar components. However, these designs, in turn, lead to two unexpected results: increased generation of wear debris and increased rates of implant loosening.

The influence of thickness on polyethylene stresses became highlighted after the introduction of metal-backed patellar components. The metal backing was often included at the expense of polyethylene thickness, resulting in even greater stresses on the polyethylene. This has lead to significant increases in the rates of wear and dissociation when compared to those of the pure polyethylene component (10). In addition to increased polyethylene wear, other described mechanisms of metal-backed patellar component failure include exposure of the metal backing, fracture of the polyethylene and fracture of the fixation pegs from the metal baseplate (27). The aforementioned complications have led to surgeons largely abandoning the use of metal-backed patellar components. Use of all polyethylene components in conjunction with methylmethacrylate fixation have

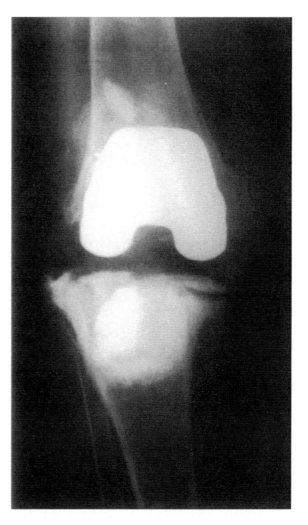

Fig. 2

combined to once again lower rates of mechanical complications.

The Patellofemoral Articulation

The patella, in some patients, may encounter a mechanical obstruction to smooth tracking within the femoral notch. The patient will often complain of catching, clicking and, in some instances, the sensation of a clunk. The mechanical obstruction is due to tissue that catches between the patella and femoral component and its location has been described to be on the anterior femur just superior to the femoral component or on the quadriceps tendon immediately superior to the patella. With deep knee flexion, this fibrosynovial mass becomes entrapped in the intercondylar femoral notch. As the knee is extended, the nodule is pulled out of the notch, producing the aforementioned mechanical symptoms.

One of the etiologic factors described is the abrupt change in the radius of curvature of certain femoral components. (Fig. 3) This occurs almost exclusively among posterior cruciate ligament substituting designs in which an abrupt anterior transition is necessary to accommodate the peg-in-box stabilizer. It is believed that the quadriceps tendon may rub over the anterosuperior edge of the intercondylar notch, irritating the tendon and leading to the production of reactive, fibrous tissue. A second mechanism described involves proximal placement of the patellar prosthesis, leading, once again, to irritation of the quadriceps tendon and the production of reactive tissue.

Conservative treatment, including a quadriceps strengthening program, is occasionally successful. However, debridement of this fibrous tissue is sometimes necessary. This can be performed either arthroscopically or through open debridement of the nodule and has proven quite effective (32).

The Patella

The prevalence of patellar fractures after total knee arthroplasty is reported to range from 0.1% to 8.5%. They represent the most common type of extensor mechanism disruption. There appears to be an optimal level of patellar bone resection for prosthetic resurfacing, leaving at least 15 mm of residual bone. Excessive bone resection may significantly weaken the remaining portion. This loss of strength, in com-

bination with the disruption of the patellar blood supply that frequently follows the medial capsulotomy and possible lateral release, may predispose the patella to fracture. Other technical factors, such as the creation of a large central defect or violation of the anterior patellar cortex, may create an area of stress concentration, leaving the patella further vulnerable to fracture.

Design effects

Metal Backing

Tibial component fixation follows several general principles: compressive load bearing, broad surface coverage and protection with a central stem. However, fixation of the tibial component without metal backing to distribute the loads into the tibial bone does not give ade-

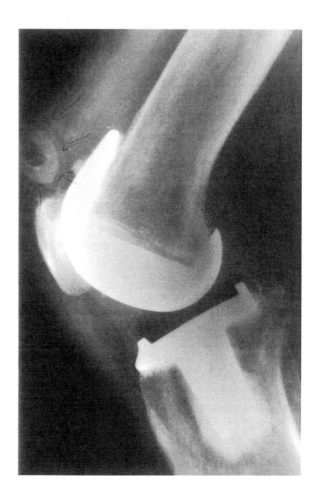

FIG. 3

quate support to the polyethylene, and allows high levels of micromotion between the cement and the upper tibial surface. The flexible polyethylene fails to provide adequate rigidity between the stem and the articular surface, leading to an eccentric load that overloads the cancellous trabeculae and deforms the polyethylene. In addition, metal-backing the tibial tray greatly diminishes the peak stresses between the arthroplasty surfaces and the cancellous surface. This was initially predicted by finite element analysis, as metal distributes loads more evenly over the proximal tibia. Clinical results suggest that long-term survivorship is, indeed, closely related to this feature. However, the initial use of metal-backed tibial components was not nearly as successful.

Because of the rapid loss of tibial bone strength as the osteotomy is performed more distal, a minimal tibial resection has been stressed. While such a minimal resection helps to maintain the strength of the proximal tibia, it can also limit the space available for the tibial component. The limited space along with the advent of metal-back designs lead to the proliferation of thin polyethylene components. Within a few years, however, the accelerated failure of these components was noted (44). The need for a minimal thickness for the tibial polyethylene had already been described. However, with the advent of metal-backing, this issue has once again re-emerged. In a study with 27 tibial prostheses retrieved from knee replacements, the wear rate of high-density polyethylene at least 6 mm thick was 0.025 mm/year. Despite this data, 8 mm has generally been accepted as the minimum thickness for the polyethylene portion of the tibial component. Polyethylene wear debris in total knee replacement generates larger particles because of the reduced joint congruity compared to total hip replacement.

Osteolysis is therefore much less common after total knee replacement. Catastrophic polyethylene failure is seen after poor design, particularly in flat polyethylene surfaces.

Tibial resection constraints also led to the design and development of thinner tibial metal trays that are more at risk to fracture. While this has remained a relatively rare problem, several factors have been identified as contributing to this failure. Tray thickness, tray material, manufacturing techniques, in situ loading and tray design/shape have all been noted to influence the strength of a tibial tray.

Similar difficulties have been encountered with metal-backed patellar components. This is covered in detail elsewhere in this chapter.

Component Geometry

Component goemetry has long been known to be a contributing factor to the mechanical failure of knee arthroplasties. Component loosening was a much greater problem during the advent of knee replacement. To maintain stability and resurface both the tibia and femur, constrained prostheses were designed and used. Many of these designs were linked or hinged. Fixation and stability was provided by intramedullary stems. However, loosening at the stem interface was soon apparent and this quickly became an issue. Even the introduction of polymethylmethacrylate fixation did not significantly alter this problem of premature failure.

Subsequent design changes have sought to decrease reliance on mechanical constraint and increase reliance on the soft-tissue envelope around the knee. For the most part, these newer designs have been found to have a lower incidence of loosening and, consequently, higher survival rates. Today, most total knee designs fall into one of four categories. These categories include the condylar replacement (e.g., Total Condylar design), the stabilized condylar replacement (e.g., Insall-Burstèin design), superstabilized condylar replacement (e.g., Constrained Condylar Knee), and the rotating or fixed linked hinge. While linked hinge prostheses continue to be plagued by higher rates of loosening, relatively low rates of failure have been reported for condylar and stabilized condylar designs. Only slightly greater rates have been reported for superstabilized condylar designs.

Currently, discussions regarding component

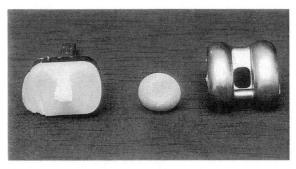

FIG. 4

geometry frequently center around the shape of the femoral component. As loosening of the components has significantly decreased in incidence, the patellofemoral articulation has proven to be a new source of complications. The geometry of the femoral component has been shown to have far reaching effects on the tracking of the patellofemoral articulation. This design requires consideration of three important factors: range of motion, kinematics and long-term performance. Adequate functional performance requires a range of motion of at least 100 degrees. The patella must also provide an adequate lever arm and appropriate protection to the quadriceps tendon as it traverses the knee joint. Lastly, the implant design must also provide long-term stable fixation.

Range of motion of a total knee design is generally controlled by the shape of the femorotibial articulation. The need for a large range of motion leads to the patella articulating with the femur almost through a significant portion of the femoral intercondylar area. Through this path, the patella must encounter significant changes in the articulating geometries and contact forces.

Ignoring the above requirements can lead to loss of strength and premature failure. The groove of the femoral component should correspond to the depth of the groove of the femur (2). Prostheses with relatively shallow grooves may force the patella too far anteriorly, decreasing the range of motion and adversely affecting the kinematics of the knee. This may also increase the probability of lateral patellar subluxation or dislocation.

Prostheses also have been produced with varying heights for the lateral femoral condyle. The prominance of the lateral condyle probably helps to prevent lateral subluxation of the patella. The higher the lateral anterior femoral condyle, the less likely it is the patella will sublux or dislocate (2). However, a large prosthetic lateral condyle may also contribute to impingement of the soft tissues in the lateral portion of the knee. This, in turn, may lead to decreased range of motion and pain. The size of this condyle must be a compromise of these two constraints.

References

1) Scott, RD, Joyce, MJ, Ewald, FC, Thomas, WH. McKeever metallic hemiarthroplasty of the knee in unicompartmental degenerative arthritis. J Bone and Joint Surg 67A: 203-207, 1985.
2) Moreland, JR. Mechanisms of failure in total knee arthroplasty. Clin Orthop Rel Res 226: 49-64, 1988.
3) Mintz, L, Tsao, AK, McCrae, CR, Stulberg, SD, Wright, T. The arthroscopic evaluation and characteristics of severe polyethylene wear in total knee arthroplasty. Clin Orthop Rel Res 273: 215-222, 1991.
4) Kaufer, H, Matthews, LS. Spherocentric arthroplasty of the knee. Clinical experience with an average four-year follow-up. J Bone Joint Surg 63A: 545-559, 1981.
5) Tsao, A, Mintz, L, McRae, CR, Stulberg, SD, Wright, T. Failure of the porous-coated anatomic prosthesis in total knee arthroplasty due to severe polyethylene wear. J Bone Joint Surg 75A: 19-26, 1993.
6) Ahlberg, A, Lunden A. Secondary operations after knee joint replacement. Clin Orthop Rel Res 156: 170-174, 1981.
7) Bostman, OM. Prevalence of obesity among patients admitted for elective orthopaedic surgery. Int J Obesity 18: 709-713, 1994.
8) Thornhill, TS, Dalziel RW, Sledge CB. Alternatives to arthrodesis for the failed total knee arthroplasty. Clin Orthop Rel Res 170: 131-140, 1982.
9) Rand, JA, Peterson, LFA, Bryan, RS, Ilstrup, DM. Revision total knee arthroplasty. Instr Course Lect 35: 305-318, 1986.
10) Healy, WL, Wasilewski SA, Takei, R, Oberlander, M. Patellofemoral complications following total knee arthroplasty. J Arthroplasty 10: 197-201, 1995.
11) Stern, SH and Insall JN. Total knee arthroplasty in obese patients. J Bone Jont Surg 72A: 1400-1404, 1990.
12) Mont, MA, Mathur, SK, Krackow, KA, Loewy, JW, Hungerford, DS. Cementless total knee arthroplasty in obese patients: A comparison with a matched control group. J Arthroplasty 11: 153-156, 1996.
13) Jigante, JJ, Goldstein, WM, Williams, CS. A comparison of the perioperative morbidity in total joint arthroplasty in the obese and nonobese patient. Clin Orthop Rel Res 289: 175-179, 1993.
14) Serna, F, Mont, MA, Krackow, KA, Hungerford, DS. Total knee arthroplasty in diabetic patients: Comparison to a matched control group. J Arthroplasty 9: 375-379, 1994.
15) Windsor, RE, Scuderi, GR, Moran, MC, Insall JN. Mechanisms of failure of the femoral and tibial components in total knee arthroplasty. Clin Orthop Rel Res 248: 15-19, 1989.
16) Lynch, AF, Rorabeck, CH, Bourne, RB. Extensor mechanism complications following total knee arthroplasty. J Arthroplasty 2: 135-140, 1987.
17) Leblanc JM. Patellar complications in total knee arthroplasty. A literature review. Orthop Rev 18: 296-304, 1989.
18) Goldberg, VM, Figgie, MP, Figgie, HE III, Sobel, M. The results of revision total knee arthroplasty. Clin Orthop Rel Res 226: 86-92,1988.
19) Goldberg, VM, Figgie, HE, III, Figgie, MP. Technical considerations in total knee surgery. Management of patella problems. Orthop Clin North Am 20: 189-199, 1989.
20) Rae, PJ, Noble J, Hodgkinson, JP. Patellar resurfacing in total condylar knee arthroplasty. Technique and results. J Arthroplasty 5: 259-265, 1990.
21) Doolittle, KH, Turner, RH. Patellofemoral problems following total knee arthroplasty. Orthop Rev 17: 696-702, 1988.

22) Bartel, DL, Burstein, AH, Santavicca, EA, Insall, JN. Performance of the tibial component in total knee replacement. J Bone Joint Surg 64A: 1026-1033, 1982.

23) Engh, CA, Bobyn, JD. Biologic fixation in total hip arthroplasty. Thorofare, N.J., Slack, 1985.

24) Bartel, DL, Wright, TM, Edward, D. The effect of metal backing on stresses in polyethylene. In: Hungerford, DS, ed. The hip. St. Louis: CV Mosby, 1983: 229-239.

25) Brick, GW, Scott, RD. The patellofemoral component of total knee arthroplasty. Clin Orthop Rel Res 231: 163-178, 1988.

26 Rand, JA, Gustilo, RB. Technique of patellar resurfacing in total knee arthroplasty. Tech Orthop 133: 57, 1988.

27) Stulberg, SD, Stulberg, BN, Hamati, Y, Tsao, A. Failure mechanisms of metal-backed patellar components, Clin Orthop Rel Res 236: 88-105, 1988.

28) Bayley, JC, Scott, RD. Further observations onmetal-backed patellar component failure. Clin Orthop Rel Res 236: 82-87, 1988.

29) Bayley, JC, Scott, RD, Ewald, FC, Holmes, GB, Jr. Failure of the metal-backed patellar component after total knee replacement. J Bone Joint Surg 70A: 668-674, 1988.

30) Rosenberg, AG, Andriacchi, TP, Barden R, Galante, JO. Patellar component failure in cementless total knee arthroplasty. Clin Orthop Rel Res 236: 106-114, 1988.

31) Hozack, WJ, Rothman, RH, Booth, RE, Jr, et al. The patellar clunk syndrome. A complication of posterior stabilized total knee arthroplasty. Clin Orthop Rel Res 241: 203-208, 1989.

32) Vernace, JV, Rothman, RH, Booth, RE, Jr, et al. Arthroscopic management of the patellar clunk syndrome following posterior stabilized total knee arthroplasty. J Arthroplasty 4: 179-182, 1989.

33) Ritter, MA, Campbell, ED. Postoperative patellar complications with or without lateral release during total knee arthroplasty. Clin Orthop Rel Res 219: 163-168, 1987.

34) Scott, RD, Turoff, N, Ewald, FC. Stress fracture of the patella following duopatellar total knee arthroplasty with patellar resurfacing. Clin Orthop Rel Res 170: 147-151, 1982.

35) Reuben, JD, McDonald, CL, Woodard, PL, Hennington, LJ. The effect of patella thickness on patella strain following total arthroplasty. J Arthroplasty 6: 251-258, 1991.

36) Clayton, ML, Thirupathi, R. Patellar complications after total condylar arthroplasty. Clin Orthop Rel Res 170: 152-157, 1982.

37) Josefchak, RG, Finlay, JB, Bourne, RB, Rorabeck, CH. Cancellous bone support for patellar resurfacing. Clin Orthop Rel Res 220: 192-199, 1987.

38) Scott, RD. Duopatellar total knee replacement: the Brigham experience. Orthop Clin North Am 13: 89-102, 1992

39) Bargren, J, Blaha, J, Freeman, M. Alignment in total knee arthroplasty. Clin Orthop Rel Res 173: 178-183, 1983.

40) Walker, PS, Reilly, D, Ben-Dove, M. Load transfer in the upper tibia before and after tibial component attachment. Trans ORS 26: 164, 1980.

41) Walker, PS, Hsu, HP, Zimmerman, RA. A comparative study of uncemented tibial components. J Arthroplasty 5: 245-253, 1990.

42) Askew, MJ, Lewis, JL, Keer, LM. The effect of post geometry, material and location on interface stress levels in tibial components of total knee. Trans Orthop Res Soc 25: 97, 1979.

43) Murase, K, Crowninshield, RD, Pedersen, DR, Chang, T. An analysis of tibial component design in total knee arthroplasty. J Biomech 16: 13-22, 1982.

44) Bartel, DL, Bicknell, VL, Wright, TM. The effect of conformity, thickness and material on stresses in ultra-high-molecular-weight components for total joint replacement. J Bone Joint Surg 68A: 1041-1051, 1986.

45) Bartel, DL, Burstein, AH, Toda, EA, et al. The effect of conformity and plastic thickness on contact stresses in metal-backed plastic implants. J Biomech Eng 107: 193, 1985.

46) Rand, JA, Ilstrup, DM. Survivorship analysis of total knee arthroplasty. J Bone Joint Surg 73A: 397-409, 1991.

47) Wright, TM, Bartel, DL. The problem of surface damage in polyethylene total knee components. Clin Orthop Rel Res 205: 67-74, 1986.

48) Engh, CA. Failure of the polyethylene bearing surface of a total knee replacement within four years. J Bone Joint Surg 70A: 1093-1096, 1988.

49) Wright, TM, Rimnac, C, Stulber, D, et al. Wear of polyethylene in total joint replacements: Observations from retrieved PCA knee implants. Clin Orthop Rel Res 276: 126-134, 1992.

50) Plante-Bordeneuve, P, Freeman, MA. Tibial high density polyethylene wear in conforming tibiofemoral prostheses. J Bone Joint Surg 75B: 630-636, 1993.

51) Engh, GA, Kimberly, AD. Mechanical failure: Implant breakage and loosening, In: Fu, FH, Harner, CD, Vince, KG, eds. Knee Surgery. Baltimore: Williams and Wilkins, 1994: 1507-1527.

52) Brady, TA, Garber, JN. Knee joint replacement using the Shiers knee hinge. J Bone Joint Surg 56A: 1610-1614, 1974.

53) Grimer, RJ, Karpinski, MRK, Edward, AN. The long term results of stanmore total knee replacements. J Bone Joint Surg 66B: 55-62, 1984.

54) Walker, PS. Biomechanics and design of artificial knee joints. In, Morrey, FB, ed. Reconstructive surgery of the joints. New York, Churchill Livingstone, 1996: 1371-1388.

Chapter 17
Treatment of the Infected Total Knee Arthroplasty

Russell E. Windsor
The Hospital for Special Surgery - New York

Infection after total knee arthroplasty represents perhaps the worst complication of this operation that a surgeon must treat. Only through identification of various risk factors and development of prophylactic regimens has the incidence of infection decreased. Successful treatment depends on a team approach, with cooperation of an orthopaedic surgeon, plastic surgeon, and an infectious disease specialist.

Incidence of Infection

The incidence of infection after total knee replacement ranges from 1.1% to 12.4% (1, 2, 3, 4, 5). The Mayo Clinic reported a 1.2% incidence of infection out of 3,000 primary total knee replacements (6). Higher infection rates were reported with cemented linked hinges, such as the GUEPAR prosthesis (1). Patients with rheumatoid arthritis, who often are immunologically suppressed, have a greater infection risk (7). Wilson et al. (5) studied 4,171 total knee arthroplasties, 67 of which became infected. The risk of infection increased in men with rheumatoid arthritis, in patients with skin ulceration, and in patients having undergone prior knee operations. Skin infections were the most common source of infection (8). In addition, infection was associated with obesity, recurrent urinary tract infections, and oral corticosteroid use, although the correlation did not achieve statistical significance (9).

Prevention of Infection

Tooth extraction causes a bacteremia, which may hematogenously seed a total knee replacement (10). Antibiotic prophylaxis in dental procedures is universally recommended, but is still debated. Prospective reports have shown the risk of hematogenous seeding of bacteria around prosthetic joints. Although antibiotic prophylaxis in dental procedures is universally recommended, it is still debated (11). However, the current standard of care in this regard is to protect the patient undergoing dental procedures with prophylactic antibiotics. Currently, it is recommended that during the first 2 years after surgery, patients receive antibiotic prophylaxis 1 hour before the dental manipulation. It is no longer recommended to repeat the dose 6 hours later, as was defined in the past. Although it is relatively safe to discontinue prophylaxis 2 years after total knee replacement for dental procedures, antibiotics are still recommended when other operations on the urinary tract or bowel are undertaken (12).

Patients with chronic renal insufficiency and neoplasm requiring chemotherapy are at risk for infection due to chronic neutropenia and, in some cases, compromised immunity. Diabetes mellitus may pose an increased risk of infection due to the increased risk of wound-healing problems. Superficial wound necrosis may at times communicate with the deeper tissues of the knee and lead to deep infection (13). Psoriatic ulcerations may be difficult to sterilize and it is generally recommended to avoid making an incision through these areas.

The surgeon may influence the infection rate, not only by technique but also by prosthetic design selection. For example, surface replacements have an overall infection rate of less than 1%. However, metal-on-metal constrained hinge designs, such as the GUEPAR prosthesis, have a reported infection rate which approaches 14%. Many of these infections occur late, sometimes several years after implantation. The reason for this high incidence is not altogether clear, but is probably related to the presence of metallic debris, which in turn causes the formation of a membranous sac containing fluid and debris around the prosthesis (14, 15). Impregnation of the bone and soft tissues with metallic fragments and the large bone-cement interface may become factors, especially if the implant is loose. Constrained prostheses with metal-on-plastic bearing surfaces also demonstrate a higher infection rate. For example, the stabilocondylar prosthesis had an 8.3% infection rate in a small series of 36 cases. Consequently, constrained hinged prostheses with cemented intramedullary stems have become largely obsolete in the United States. For most clinical situations, a non- or semiconstrained surface total knee replacement will perform well and reduce the potential for infection.

The use of preoperative antibiotics is now common for total knee replacement. The use of laminar air flow and surgical hoods with panel enclosures contributes to decrease the infection rate at the time of initial surgical intervention. Current in-hospital infection rates should be <1% utilizing these methods and careful, aseptic technique.

Skin necrosis with secondary deep extension may lead to a deep infection. Incisions placed at one side of the knee, for open fracture reduction and internal fixation, may predispose to skin necrosis. These incisions are generally insufficient to use for gaining exposure during total knee replacement, which ordinarily requires a midline, longitudinal incision. Although previous incisions should be used as much as possible during any knee replacement, it is sometimes necessary to use a separate longitudinal incision to gain proper exposure despite the risk of creating an island of devascularized skin between the new incision and the healed old one. Preserving at least a 7 centimeter distance between incisions can minimize the risk of skin necrosis. If wound necrosis appears, the knee should be immobilized until spontaneous separation of the eschar occurs. Early and aggressive debridement may lead to deep contamination that might otherwise have been avoidable. Very large necrotic areas, however, should be handled aggressively, utilizing appropriate skin grafts as needed. If the surgeon suspects that the wound may not heal ap-

propriately, a delay procedure or use of tissue expanders may help avoid unnecessary skin necrosis. The delay procedure involves placement of an incision about two weeks before the proposed date for total knee replacement. The incision is taken down to the extensor mechanism and medial and lateral skin flaps are defined. The wound is closed to allow healing and neovascularization of the skin margin. If necrosis occurs, another operation can be done to benefit the skin. It is certainly safer to do this procedure and delay the total knee replacement so that skin healing can be assured. For tight skin having little subcutaneous tissue, a tissue expander may help permit closure of the incision after implantation of a total knee replacement. Frequently, the limb is lengthened slightly during knee replacement and significant tension on the skin flaps may result in hypovascularity and necrosis. A tissue expander can be implanted as an out-patient procedure and it creates enough redundant skin to facilitate closure of the wound.

Slight wound drainage often requires no modification of the postoperative regimen. When profuse wound drainage occurs, the knee should be immobilized until it stops. Antibiotics should be given for superficial drainage for protection, although their administration may mask a latent deep infection. Wound drainage occurs in about 25% of the cases and may be further classified culture-negative or culture-positive. There appears to be no relationship between culture-positive wound drainage and subsequent deep infection. During the early postoperative period, there are a few patients who have persistent drainage, a tense knee effusion, and persisting pain. For this situation, open debridement, evacuation of the hematoma, copious lavage, and reclosure should be considered.

The organism most frequently obtained in an infected knee replacement is Staphylococcus aureus. Schoifet and Morrey (4) found that 58% of 31 infected total knee replacements cultured Staphylococcus aureus. Wilson et al. (5) observed S. aureus in 42 of 67 infected replacements. Staphylococcal organisms were responsible for infection in the majority of patients who had concurrent skin ulceration. Gram-negative organisms, such as Escherichia coli and Pseudomonas aeruginosa, have been found less frequently. A mixed bacterial infection is usually associated with actively draining sinuses through which bacteria may enter the knee joint. Patients who have been chronically treated with antibiotic suppression may develop resistant bacterial strains. Thus, it is important to have close surveillance of the clinical situation during the postoperative period.

Diagnosis of Deep Infection

Deep periprosthetic infection may be either early (within 3 months of surgery) or late (more than 3 months after surgery). An early infection is usually not difficult to recognize. The clinical course is abnormal, with prolonged pain, swelling, inflammation, and fever. The leukocyte count, C-Reactive protein level, and erythrocyte sedimentation rate remain elevated. Late hematogenous infection is much more common than early infection, and the diagnosis is usually straightforward unless antibiotics have previously been given. The patient usually presents with acute pain and swelling in the knee. Late infection usually develops from hematogenous spread of microorganisms from a distant site, such as an ulcer on the foot, infected in-grown toenail, urinary tract infection or diverticulitis with septicemia.

Severe knee pain should alert the surgeon to consider infection. In a study of 52 patients with total knee replacement infection, pain was present in 96% of the patients, 77% had swelling of the knee, 27% were febrile, and 27% had active drainage (16). The average erythrocyte sedimentation rate was 63 mm/h (range, 4 to 125 mm/h). The average leukocyte count was 8,300/mm 9 range, 5,800 to 14,000/mm. Aspirated knee fluid was positive in all cases except one; in that case, no organism was cultured until aspiration was done at the time of the revision arthroplasty for what was thought to be aseptic loosening.

The diagnosis of an infection after total knee arthroplasty must depend on the examination of knee fluid aspirates under strict aseptic conditions. Knee radiographs may be unclear and show no clear signs of premature loosening, which may be expected, in an infected joint. Large radiolucencies usually indicate advanced stages of infection. Technetium and gallium bone scans also may not conclusively show presence of infection. Cultures of wound drainage, if present, often do not truly reflect the organisms found deep in the knee, since there is the likelihood of contamination of the fluid by other skin flora. Knee aspiration is the standard of care for conclusively determining whether there is deep joint infection. The aspi-

rated fluid is sent for direct smear, Gram stain, and routine cultures with antibiotic sensitivities for aerobic and anaerobic bacteria, acid-fast bacilli, and fungi (17, 18). If fluid is not easily obtained, a fluoroscopically assisted aspiration should be considered.

If enough fluid is aspirated from the knee, a complete blood count and a differential white blood count may also give valuable information. If the leukocyte count is more than 25,000/mm and there are greater than 75% polymorphonuclear cells, infection should be suspected.

Fluid should also be sent for glucose and protein levels. Normal synovial fluid contains protein levels about a third of serum levels. Glucose values in the synovial fluid are usually similar to those in plasma. In infection synovial glucose values are decreased and the protein levels are increased.

Frequently, patients referred from other institutions are already receiving antibiotics, which may suppress the infection enough to render knee aspiration falsely negative. It is important to obtain the organism on culture so that the infectious disease consultant can more precisely treat the infection with proper antibiotic agents. If the patient is receiving antibiotics, they should be immediately discontinued, and serial aspirations of the knee should be done at weekly intervals until a positive culture is obtained. It may take up to 1 month before a positive culture is obtained. Once an organism is obtained, the surgeon will be more confident in yielding a positive culture from the wound during surgery that accurately reflects the organisms involved.

Procrastination and the prolonged use of oral antibiotics should be condemned, particularly when infection is suspected but not confirmed by bacteriologic evidence. The end result is likely to be an indolent subclinical infection and a painful prosthesis. Additionally, it may make subsequent culture of the organism very difficult even after the components have been removed, so that appropriate antibiotic therapy is impossible and ultimate salvage of the arthroplasty by reimplantation becomes much less likely.

Intraoperative frozen section can also prove meaningful. In a study of 175 specimens, a positive predictive value of infection increased from 70 to 89% when the criteria went from 5 to a level of 10 white blood cells per high powered field. The negative predictive value of 98% was achieved when both indices were absent. Intraoperative frozen sections certainly suggest infection when 10 WBC's per high powered field are observed (19, 20).

Polymerase chain reaction is another method that has been recently utilized in obtaining evidence of infection. There are messenger DNA strands that can identify particular species of bacteria and precisely identify the organism that is present in the joint. However, the technique is expensive and slow with a turn around time in the operating room of about 2 hours. There has also been an observation of false positive results. The technology is still progressing and in the future this technique may be able to give the clinician a precise knowledge about the presence of the infection and the offending organism.

Treatment Options

The treatment options for an infected total knee replacement (21) include 1), antibiotic suppression alone (22, 23, 24); 2) aggressive wound debridement, drainage, and antibiotic suppression therapy (25, 26); 3) resection arthroplasty (27, 28); 4) arthrodesis (29, 30); 5) two-stage or one-stage reimplantation (31, 32); and 6) amputation (33, 34).

Because the knee joint is relatively superficial, treatment of the wound is preeminently important. Success of any treatment option will be severely compromised by inadequate wound care or inappropriate choice of incisions.

The original midline incision should be utilized whenever possible. It may be extended proximally and distally to improve surgical exposure of the knee joint. New incisions should be avoided at all costs. Well-healed medial or lateral incisions from operations that predated the total knee replacement should not be reopened, even if wound drainage develops in those areas. These wounds and draining sinuses should be debrided, but the appropriate incision should be utilized to best remove all infected debris from the knee joint. Frequently, drainage stops and the wound heals nicely after implant removal and thorough debridement. Large areas of skin necrosis should be treated by rotation of a gastrocnemius muscle pedicle graft or free vascularized muscle transfers. Although infrequent, the complete exposure of a total knee replacement after severe wound dehiscence and necrosis should be aggressively treated by flap coverage and irrigation. There is 75% chance of successful salvage of the re-

placement by this treatment without having to remove the implants for subsequent infection (35).

Antibiotic Suppression Alone

The rheumatology literature has shown that treatment of knee sepsis may be accomplished adequately by serial aspirations and antibiotic treatment. However, treatment was successful in knees in which a total joint replacement was not implanted. The implant and acrylic cement act as foreign bodies that limit the ability of the immune system to adequately combat the infection. However, infection is not confined to cemented total knee replacements. Wilson et al. found that infection developed in 2.8% of 35 uncemented total knee prostheses, 1.5% of 138 hybrid total knee replacements (with uncemented femoral component), and 1.6% of 3,998 total knee replacements with totally cemented components. Thus, infection is possible regardless of the method of implant fixation.

The success of this treatment method is quite limited (2, 22, 23, 24). However, antibiotic suppression alone may be the only option for a patient who is a poor surgical candidate and does not have other total joint replacements that would be at risk of becoming infected by hematogenous spread of the original infection. Usually organisms with extreme sensitivity to antibiotics, such as Streptococcus species and Staphylococcus epidermidis, can be treated in this way. This treatment method, however, may create resistant bacterial strains, which may cause eventual painful loosening of the prosthesis. Thus, this method is reserved for the medically compromised patient who would not be able to undergo the rigors of surgical intervention.

Debridement with Antibiotic Suppression Therapy

Vigorous wound debridement and antibiotic therapy with retention of the components has demonstrated limited success (36). Success is greater if infection is diagnosed within 3 weeks of implantation of the original device. Schoifet and Morrey specifically studied this treatment method. The overall success rate was still only 23%. Borden and Gearen also found that this method was more successful than more radical treatment options when the infection was diagnosed within 2 weeks of total joint implantation.

Organisms such as Streptococcus viridans and Staphylococcus epidermidis may be successfully treated with this method. However, the patient will still have to take oral antibiotics for the rest of his or her life. Resistant bacterial strains may develop and cause breakthrough infections that are chemically difficult to treat.

Patients with replacements in other joints are not good candidates for debridement and suppression due to the risk of hematogenous seeding of a future resistant strain to the noninfected total joint replacements,

More radical options may become necessary if infection persists. In general, one attempt at this treatment option could be made. However, if the infection persists repeated attempts usually prove futile and the prosthesis should be removed. Repeated attempts at debridement may compromise skin viability and increase scar formation making it difficult to treat the infection when implant removal becomes necessary. Although this method of treatment has been mildly successful in some surgeon's hand, if repeated arthrotomies and debridements fail, a two-stage procedure is still necessary and will require a full 6 week course of antibiotic therapies between the removal and reimplantation stage. Also, the bacteriology may change and super-infections may occur.

The debridement may be done by arthroscopy or arthrotomy. However, regardless of the surgical method used, a thorough debridement is done. Frozen tissue section, Gram stains, cultures of the tissue should provide diagnostic information. The wound is closed over suction drains that remain in place for 36 to 48 hours. Under no circumstances should the wound be left open to close by secondary formation of granulation tissue. Ingress and egress irrigation systems should also not be used as this creates the risk of a superinfection

The wound is inspected after 2 weeks and is reaspirated under strict aseptic conditions. If the wound is benign and the cultures are negative, antibiotic therapy is continued for a further 4 weeks followed by prolonged oral antibiotic treatment. When this is not the case, reoperation with removal of the prosthetic components and all cement is performed. This decision should be made quickly before further compromise of the underlying tissues develops.

Resection Arthroplasty

Due to the limited success of antibiotic suppression, more radical surgical options are usually necessary to eradicate the deep infection. Resection arthroplasty involves the complete removal of all components of the knee replacement, acrylic cement, scar tissue, and synovium (27, 28).

This option as a definitive procedure is generally reserved for medically fragile patients who cannot tolerate another major operation (37). It may serve as an intermediate step for the patient who has reservations concerning arthrodesis. Falahee et al reported on 28 knees that underwent resection arthroplasty because of infection after total knee arthroplasty. The patients who had had the most severe disability before total knee arthroplasty were the most likely to be satisfied with the functional results of resection arthroplasty. Conversely, the patients who had had the least severe disability were more likely to find the results of resection arthroplasty unacceptable. Fifteen patients could walk independently without assistance. Thus, resection arthroplasty is very useful for the severely disabled person with a very sedentary lifestyle. The advantage of resection arthroplasty is that some motion is preserved to allow sitting and to facilitate transferring into and out of automobiles and aircraft. The disadvantage is the possibility of persistent pain and instability on walking.

Arthrodesis

Arthrodesis may be the only option for treating the infected total knee replacement when other forms of treatment are contraindicated (29, 30). Successful arthrodesis depends mainly on technique and the availability of adequate bone to accomplish fusion. The success of arthrodesis can be as low as 50% (infected hinged prostheses), and as high as 90% (infected surface replacements).

The indications for arthrodesis are 1) complete destruction of the extensor mechanism by infection, rendering the patient incapable of actively extending the knee; 2) a resistant bacterial infection that requires high toxic doses of antibiotics to reach adequate levels; 3) a knee with inadequate bone stock for placement of a new total knee prosthesis; 4) a knee with inadequate soft-tissue coverage and multiple incisions that may compromise future wound healing; 5) a young patient in whom the likelihood of subsequent infection or revision is great, and 6) patient choice.

Arthrodesis may be accomplished by different techniques. Adequate bacteriologic control of the wound should be obtained beforehand. We do not recommend performing arthrodesis at the time of the original debridement, as the risk of persistent infection is high in the setting of active wound sepsis when metallic implants are needed to accomplish fusion. Thus, arthrodesis is generally done in a staged manner (38). Some authors, however, advocate immediate arthrodesis.

External fixation and intramedullary rod fixation are two methods of arthrodesis that are best suited to this clinical situation. External fixation is particularly appropriate in patients who have an ipsilateral total hip replacement above the affected knee joint and in patients with an especially virulent microorganism.

Whenever possible, intramedullary arthrodesis is preferable, as the healing rates are higher than those for external fixation and the method is better tolerated by the patient. Although Puranen et al. believes that no secondary bone grafting is needed with this technique, adequate bone may be obtained from the anterior tibial flare or the patella to aid fusion. Adequate bone contact should be present between the femur and the tibia. With this method the patient can begin ambulating immediately. Puranen et al. reported the success of intramedullary arthrodesis in 33 patients. There were four broken nails. He advocated protected weight-bearing until evidence of fusion is seen radiographically.

The advantages of arthrodesis as treatment for an infected total knee replacement are that it is a definitive treatment for the infection with little chance of recurrence and that it promises reasonably good long-term function without the risk of future mechanical failure. The disadvantages of arthrodesis are 1) inability to bend the knee; 2) difficulty in transferring from a car or sitting in a small space, such as an airplane; and the 3) large increase in the energy required to walk with a stiff knee, which is particularly a problem for patients with cardiovascular or pulmonary problems. However, arthrodesis will provide the patient with a sturdy platform on which to walk, despite inability to move the knee.

Two-stage Reimplantation

The most successful functional results for the treatment of late infection of a total knee

replacement are obtained by the technique of two-stage reimplantation of a new total knee replacement, with success rates averaging 90% (3,16,17,18,31). This method represents the procedure of choice to definitively eradicate the infection and preserve knee function (39).

Adequate preoperative planning is necessary and the availability of special instruments is recommended. Removal of the prosthetic components and acrylic cement can be difficult, particularly if the septic process is of recent onset. In this case, the prosthetic components will most likely be well fixed, and removal of the tight interdigitation between bone and cement demands meticulous technique in order to prevent unnecessary loss of bone stock. The removal of hinged total knee replacements with intramedullary stems in the femur and tibia can also prove difficult. For these cases, special cement osteotomes and a high-speed cement drill are helpful.

Surgical Protocol

The protocol involves three stages. The patient must be in good general medical health to withstand the rigors of all the stages.

The first stage of the protocol involves complete debridement of all infected tissues, along with removal of the implants and all cement. All scarred, inflamed, and devitalized tissues should be thoroughly excised, leaving viable, healthy, well-vascularized tissues. Primary wound closure can usually be performed over closed suction tubes, which are removed after 24 to 48 hours. The knee is immobilized in a bulky dressing with plaster splints. A central venous catheter or peripheral infusion catheter (PIC line) is inserted to facilitate long-term intravenous therapy.

Surgical issues regarding this first stage involved careful exposure and complete debridement of all infected tissue. It is necessary to recreate and define the medial and lateral gutters and clear all cement debris from the knee. Sometimes, it is difficult to differentiate cement from sclerotic bone. A high-speed burr is necessary to carefully debride the bone.

The knee is generally kept immobile or allowed to move gently through limited flexion. Skeletal traction is not advised. Antibiotic-impregnated acrylic spacer blocks (with tobramycin or vancomycin) are placed in the knee joint to keep the soft-tissue sleeve under proper tension and provide an antibiotic-rich environment at the debridement site. In this way, the spacer block facilitates soft tissue exposure during the reimplantation stage (40).

The second stage involves a 6 week course of intravenous antibiotic therapy. The results of the intraoperative cultures and knee aspiration results determine proper choice of bacteriologic agents. Antibiotics that yield high bactericidal effects and low toxicity are chosen. An infectious disease consultant follows the minimum bactericidal concentrations at weekly intervals and assures a minimum 1:8 titer maintained for 6 weeks. The time is prolonged if this concentration is not maintained. Not infrequently, the patient may react adversely to an antibiotic during the course of administration. It is necessary to stop the antibiotic and begin a new one, still maintaining minimum bactericidal concentration titers of 1:8. It is sometimes necessary to make use of synergistic effects of the antibiotics to achieve even higher bactericidal concentrations. Methicillin-resistant Staphylococcus aureus and epidermidis have become more prevalent and are treated with Vancomycin (41).

After 6 weeks, if the wound is completely benign, a new total knee prosthesis may be inserted. If the wound is still not healing well, a brace is applied and the patient is discharged. The joint fluid can be serially aspirated to test the adequacy of the debridement. If growth of bacteria develops, the knee is debrided again and another course of antibiotic therapy is started.

The last stage of the protocol involves implantation of a new total knee replacement. Frequently, a modular prosthesis is used, which enables the surgeon to reconstruct any bone loss by adding metal wedges to the tibial component and distal and/or posterior augmentation to the femoral component. Frozen tissue sections and Gram stains are obtained at the time of surgery to assess tissue inflammation. The macroscopic appearance of the wound should be completely benign; all scarred and devitalized tissue is excised, leaving only viable, well-vascularized, tissue.

Exposure can sometimes be difficult after prolonged immobilization; there is a danger of avulsing the tibial tubercle while attempting to mobilize the patella and flex the knee. If this event seems likely, either a quadriceps snip or turn-down is used. One author recommends osteotomy of the tibial tubercle to gain sufficient exposure.

Preoperative planning is essential in order to have adequate prosthetic components available. A special custom-designed prosthesis is occasionally necessary. In most cases, proper alignment can be reestablished with adequate tissue tension and the use of press-fitted fluted intramedullary rods. The proximal end of the tibial component and the distal end of the femoral prosthesis are cemented. Some surgeons cement the prosthesis completely, but later revision, if necessary, will be difficult.

Excision of the patella has proved helpful in cases in which the skin closure was too tight. If the patella has insufficient bone stock to accept a prosthesis, it may be left unresurfaced. Normally, reconstruction can be achieved using standard designs that provide a substitution for the posterior cruciate ligament; in some cases, designs that preserve the posterior cruciate ligament are used.

The use of constrained components is often unavoidable. When this is the case, a constrained condylar knee prosthesis is selected; such a device has intramedullary stems on both components and restricts varus/valgus, anteroposterior, and rotary motions by means of a centrally positioned peg. Intramedullary stems are fitted in a modular fashion to the femoral or tibial prosthesis and are press-fitted into the intramedullary canal. While a stemmed component in the tibia, femur or both is required because of bone deficiency, constraint at the prosthetic surfaces is not automatically required unless there is uncontrollable ligamentous instability.

The use of antibiotic-impregnated cement has been recommended for reimplantation after infection (42, 43, 44). Although not statistically proven, most surgeons recommend its use to reduce as much as possible by any means the likelihood of reinfection. However, of 89 infected knee replacements that received prostheses, 25% of implants that were inserted without antibiotic-impregnated cement developed a recurrent infection, whereas only 4.7% developed recurrent infection when antibiotic-impregnated cement was utilized (45).

Clinical results after a first stage reimplantation is quite satisfactory

Postoperative Management

The postoperative management after reimplantation is the same as that used after a primary arthroplasty unless a quadriceps turndown was done to facilitate exposure. In this event the knee is immobilized in a splint and flexion is allowed after 3 weeks. If a quadriceps snip is performed, the closure is done in a routine manner and motion begins on the first postoperative day. Perioperative antibiotics are administered for 4 days until the final operative culture results are known to be negative after which they are discontinued. No further antibiotic treatment is necessary.

Results

A 97% success rate has been obtained at The Hospital for Special Surgery using this protocol. Thirty-seven of 38 knees had successful eradication of the original infection. Functional results reflected the difficulties that are usually encountered during revision arthroplasty. There were 11 excellent, 13 good, 6 fair and 7 poor results, based on the Hospital for Special Surgery Score. The reasons for the poor results were reinfection by a different organism and compromise of the extensor mechanism function with persistent pain. Overall function was well maintained in the group, with a range of motion averaging 95 degrees (range, 80 to 120 degrees). Twenty-three patients complained of some pain when walking, 15 patients had mild pain, 6 patients had moderate pain, and 2 patients had severe pain.

Although Insall et al. cautioned against using this protocol for reimplantation in the presence of Gram-negative infection, Windsor et al. has more recently showed that it is feasible to perform this protocol when certain sensitive Gram-negative infections are present. Escherichia coli and Pseudomonas aeruginosa infections have been successfully treated with this protocol, and the presence of newer nontoxic bactericidal agents has made it possible to eradicate these Gram-negative infections.

Others have tried to accomplish successful reimplantation by utilizing shorter periods of intravenous antibiotic therapy. However, Rand and Bryan found a 2-week course unacceptable. Borden and Gearen evaluated a small number of knees that were treated with a 4 week course of antibiotics. However, the overall results fell between those of Rand et al. and Windsor et al. Thus, a 6 week course overall yields the best results. Because of the economic burden that 6 weeks of antibiotic therapy places on the hospital and patient, some selected organisms (e.g., Streptococcal and Staphylococcus epidermidis) may possibly be just as successfully treated with a 4 week course of intravenous antibiotic therapy. However, there is so far little formal literature support for this

treatment plan, and treatment of the infected total knee replacement with a staged reimplantation procedure is, by far the most successful method and procedure of choice.

There has been some success with single stage reimplantation for infections caused by bacteria that are exquisitely sensitive to antibiotics. These comprise mostly gram + Streptococci species and Staphylococcus epidermidis. Goksan and Freeman reported 18 total knee replacement infections that were treated with this method. Sixteen were successfully treated and there was only one recurrence and one new infection (46). In this protocol, the knee is completely debrided of all necrotic tissue and cement. The implants are removed and the wound is copiously irrigated. Betadine soaked sponges are packed in the wound the incision is loosely closed. The tourniquet is released and antibiotics are allowed to flow through the limb for 30 minutes. The leg is re-draped and new sterile instruments are used to perform the implantation phase of the operation. Antibiotic-impregnated Palacos cement is utilized for fixation.

Other authors have also had limited success with one-stage reimplantation, but Scott et al. treated 10 of 17 infections with 3 recurrences. However, they applied the procedure to these 3 cases again and had success at eradication of the infection. They also treated 7 of 17 infected knee replacements by using the original prosthesis, sterilized again, as a spacer prior to reimplantation of a new knee replacement (47). This latter method still requires more literature support before the technique should be utilized in a widespread manner

Amputation

Amputation may be the final salvage procedure for severe infections that are associated with large-bone loss and compromised antibiotic treatment (33,34). This procedure was required most frequently in infected knee replacements with cemented, stemmed hinges, which for the most part have become obsolete. The remaining shell of bone was frequently inadequate for subsequent arthrodesis or reimplantation, making the limb essentially fail. Amputation may be the only option in patients with mixed infection for whom antibiotic treatment has proved inadequate or in whom there is such massive tissue destruction that knee function is unsalvageable. This frequently occurs with mixed infections in which multiple abscesses and sinus tracts are present and significant destruction of the surrounding soft-tissue sleeve and muscle occurs. If successful treatment cannot be accomplished in any other way, a successful above-knee amputation may provide the best function for patients who otherwise would have a functionless knee joint and distal extremity. The frequency with which the option used has substantially declined with the use of two-stage reimplantation protocols and modern antibiotics that are significantly safer over long-term use. Usually amputation is decided upon after failure of a two-stage protocol or inadequate debridements prior to removal of the implants where sinus tracts and abscess formation develops with severe localized soft-tissue destruction.

References

1) Deburge A, GUEPAR Group: Guepar hinge prosthesis: Complications and results with two years' follow-up. Clin Orthop 1976, 120:47-53.

2) Grogan TJ, Dorey F, Rollins J, et al: Deep sepsis following total knee arthroplasty: Ten-year experience at the University of California at Los Angeles Medical Center. J Bone Joint Surg; 68A:226-234, 1986.

3) Rand JA, Bryan RS: Reimplantation for salvage of an infected total knee arthroplasty. J Bone Joint Surg; 65-A: 1081-1086, 1983.

4) Schoifet SD, Morrey BF: Treatment of infection after total knee arthroplasty by debridement with retention of the components. J Bone Joint Surg; 72A:1383-1390, 1990.

5) Wilson MG, Kelley K, Thornhill TS: Infection as a complication of total knee-replacement arthroplasty: Risk factors and treatment in sixty-seven cases. J Bone Joint Surg; 72-A: 878-883, 1990.

6) Rand JA, Bryan RS, Morrey BF, et al: Management of infected total knee arthroplasty. Clin Orthop 1986, 205:75-85.

7) Garner RW, Mowat AG, Hazlemena BL: Wound healing after operations on patients with rheumatoid arthritis. J Bone Joint Surg; 55-B: 55:134-144, 1973.

8) Thomas BJ, Moreland JR, Amstutz HC: Infection after total joint arthroplasty from distal extremity sepsis. Clin Orthop 1983, 181:121-125.

9) Wilson MG, Kelley, K, Thornhill,RS. Infection as a complication of total knee replacement arthroplasty. Risk Factors and treatment in sixty seven cases. J. Bone Joint Surg. 72-A:878-883, 1990.

10) Lindqvist C, Slatis P: Dental bacteremia: A neglected cause of arthroplasty infections: three hip cases. Acta Orthop Scand 1985, 56:506-508.

11) Nelson JP, Fitzgerald RH Jr, Jaspers MT, et al: Prophylactic antimicrobial coverage in arthroplasty patients (editorial). J Bone Joint Surg; 72-A, 1, 1990.

12) Ainscow DAP, Denham RA: The risk of hematogenous infection in total joint replacements. J Bone Joint Surg; 66-B: 580-582, 1984.

13) England SP, Stern SH, Insall JN, et al: Total knee arthroplasty in diabetes mellitus. Clin Orthop 1990; 260:130-134.

14) Rae T: A study on the effects of particulate metals of orthopaedic interest on murine macrophages in vitro. J Bone Joint Surg; 57-B:444-450, 1975.

15) Schurman DJ, Johnson BL Jr, Amstutz HC: Knee joint infections with Staphylococcus aureus and Micrococcus species: Influence of antibiotics, metal debris, bacteremia, blood, and steroids in a rabbit model. J Bone Joint Surg; 57A: 40-49, 1975.

16) Windsor RE, Insall JN, Urs, WK, et al: Two-stage reimplantation for the salvage of total knee arthroplasty complicated by infection: Further follow-up and refinement of indications. J Bone Joint Surg; 72-A:272-278, 1990.

17) Borden LS, Gearen PF: Infected total knee arthroplasty: A protocol for management. J Arthroplasty 1987;2:27-36.

18) Insall JN, Thompson FM, Brause BD: Two-stage reimplantation for the salvage of infected total knee arthroplasty. J Bone Joint Surg; 655-A:1087-1098, 1983.

19) Lonner JH, Desai P, Di Cesare PE, Steiner G, Zuckerman JD. The reliability of analysis of intraoperative frozen sections for identifying active infection during revision hip or knee arthroplasty. J. Bone Joint Surg; 78-A:1553-1558, 1996.

20) Feldman DS, Lonner JH, Desai P, Zuckerman JD. The role of intraoperattive frozen sections in revision total joint arthrtoplasty. J. Bone Joint Surg; 77-A:1807-1813, 1995.

21) Rand, JA. Instructionasl Course Lectures. The American Academy of Orthopaedic Surgeons. Alternatives to reimplantation for salvage f the total knee arthroplasty complicated by infection. J. Bone Joint Surg; 75-A:282-289, 1993.

22) Johnson DP, Bannister GC: The outcome of infected arthroplasty of the knee. J Bone Joint Surg; 68-B:289-291, 1986.

23) Marsh PK, Cotler JM: Management of an anaerobic infection in a prosthetic knee with long-term antibiotics alone: A case report. Clin Orthop 1981;155:133-135.

24) Woods GW, Lionberger DR, Tullos HS: Failed total knee arthroplasty: Revision and arthrodesis for infection and non-infectious complications. Clin Orthop 1983;173:184-190.

25) Peled IJ, Frankl U, Wexler MR: Salvage of exposed knee prosthesis by gastrocnemius myocutaneous flap coverage. Orthopedics 1983; 6:1320-1322.

26) Sanders R, O'Neill T: The gastrocnemius myocutaneous flap used as a cover for the exposed knee prosthesis. JU Bone Joint Surg; 63-B:383-386, 1981.

27) Falahee MH, Matthews LS, Kaufer H: Resection arthroplasty as a salvage procedure for a knee with infection after a total arthroplasty. J Bone Joint Surg; 69-A:1013-1021, 1987.

28) Lettin AWF, Neil MJ, Citron ND, et al: Excision arthroplasty for infected constrained total knee replacements. J Bone Joint Surg; 72-B:220-224, 1990.

29) Hagemann WF, Woods GW, Tullos HS: Arthrodesis in failed total knee replacement. J Bone Joint Surg; 60-A:790-794, 1979.

30) Puranen J, Kortelainen P, Jalovaara P: Arthrodesis of the knee with intra-medullary nail fixation. J Bone Joint Surg; 72-A:433-442, 1990.

31) Rosenberg AG, Haas B, Barden R, et al: Salvage of infected total knee arthroplasty. Clin Orthop 1988; 226:29-33.

32) Whiteside LA. Treatment of Infected Total Knee Arthroplasty. Clin Orthop 1994; 299:169-172.

33) Pring DJ, Marks L, Angel JC: Mobility after amputation for failed knee replacement. J Bone Joint Surg; 70-B: 770-771, 1988.

34) Isiklar ZU, Landon GC, Tullos HS: Amputation after Failed total knee Arthroplasty. Clin Orthop 1994; 299:173-178.

35) Adam RF, Watson SB, Jarratt JW, Noble J, Watson JS. Outcome after Flap Cover for Exposed Total Knee Arthroplasties. A report of 25 cases. J. Bone Joint Surg; 76-B:750-753, 1994.

36) Burger RR, Basch T, Hopson CN: Implant Salvage in Infected total knee arthroplasty. Clin Orthop: 1991; 273: 105-112.

37) Lettin AWF, NEIL MJ, Citron ND. Excision Arthroplasty for Infected Constrained Total Knee Replacements. J. Bone Joint Surg; 72-B:220-224, 1990.

38) Ellingsen, DE and Rand JA. Intramedullary arthrodesis of the knee after failed total knee arthroplasty. J. Bone Joint Surg; 76-A:870-877, 1994.

39) Wilde AH, Ruth JT: Two Stage Reimplantation in infected total knee arthroplasty. Clin Orthop 1988; 236:23-35.

40) Trippel SB. Current Concepts Revirew. Antibiotic-impregnated cement in total joint arthroplasty. J. Bone Joint Surg; 68-A:1297-1302. 1986.

41) James PJ, Butcher IA, Gardner ER, Hamblin DL: Methicillin-Resistant StaphylococcusEpidermidis in Infection of Hip Arthoplasties. J. Bone Joint Surg. 76-B:725-727, 1994.

42) Carlsson AS, Josefsson G, Lindberg L: Revision with gentamycin-impregnated cement for deep infections in total hip arthroplasties. J Bone Joint Surg; 60-A:1059-1064, 1978.

43) Freeman MAR, Sudlow RA, Casewell MW et al: The management of infected total knee replacements. J Bone Joint Surg; 67-B:764-768, 1985.

44) Marks KE, Nelson CL, Lautenschlager EP: Antibiotic-impregnated acrylic bone cement. J Bone Joint Surg; 58-A:358-364, 1976.

45) Hanssen AD, Rand JA, Osmon DR: Treatment of the infected total knee arthroplasty with insertion of another prosthesis. The effect of antibiotic-impregnated cement. Clin Orthop 1994; 309:44-55.

46) Goksan, SB & Freeman, MAR. One Stage Reimplantation for Infected Total Knee Replacement. J. Bone Joint Surg; 74-B:78-82, 1992.

47) Scott IR, Stockly I, Getty CJM. Exchange Arthroplasty for Infected knee Replacements. A New Two-Stage Method. J. Bone Joint Surg; 75-B:28-31, 1993.

Chapter 18
Periprosthetic Fractures

Francesco Giron, Paolo Aglietti

IInd Orthopaedic Clinic of the University of Florence

Periprosthetic fractures of the knee are all those skeletal fractures that involve any one of the three joint ends of the prosthetized knee (femur, tibia, or patella) not more than 15 cm from the joint line.

Although they constitute a rare complication in orthopaedic surgery, precisely because of their closeness to a prosthetized joint, their treatment represents a serious problem. In cases such as these, in fact, the orthopaedic surgeon is not only forced to solve all of the problems inherent to correct reduction and osteosynthesis of a fracture, but when there is a modification, he must also recreate all of those conditions that allow for the perfect functioning and the good stability of the prosthesis. In recent years, furthermore, the incidence of fractures has increased at the same time as the rise in the number of prostheses.

Fractures of the Femur

Periprosthetic fractures of the femur are routinely distinguished in intraoperative and postoperative fractures.

Intraoperative Fractures

Etiopathogenesis

These constitute an unusual event, and one that occurs less frequently than postoperative ones, but nonetheless, some cases have been reported in the literature (1). Fractures of the diaphysis and supracondylar fractures are distinguished.

Fractures of the femoral diaphysis are often localized in the anterior cortical bone or they propagate in a disto-proximal direction from an intercondylar area. They may occur during insertion of the intramedullary guide because of the alignment of femoral cut and during the introduction of a femoral stem for stabilization (2, 3). Factors favoring the occurrence of fracture are represented by angular deformity of the diaphysis or by increased bone fragility consequent to severe osteoporosis. When angular deformity of the fracture is present, often consequent to an error in technique, it may easily be avoided by taking great care as regards the site where the hole is made to introduce the intramedullary guide, and widening the hole itself so as to allow for a certain leaway on the part of the guide inside the diaphysis during its insertion. In the same manner, a fracture caused by impaction of a slightly oversized stem, or one that is erroneously directed, may be prevented by paying close attention to the diameter of the intramedullary stem, correctly evaluating the angle of insertion, and, finally, in the case of osteoporotic bone, applying less impaction force.

These fractures often go unrecognized during surgery and they become an unpleasant surprise during postoperative rehabilitation when the patient begins to walk. Of great use in early diagnosis is radiologic monitoring at the end of surgery that allows for immediate treatment.

Condylar or supracondylar fractures are more frequent during revision surgery when severe loss of substance or weakening of the bone structure caused by osteolysis and osteoporosis is often present. In addition to these factors closely related to the quality of the bone, an important role is also played by errors in technique, such as notching of the anterior cortical bone, or medial positioning of the component, or the design itself of the component, such as in the case of posterior-stabilized prostheses, in which a larger bone resection to allow for lodging of the central box is required (2, 3).

Fracture most often involves the medial condyle, precisely because at this level stress produced by a position of the component that is too medial is concentrated, particularly in subjects who are not tall, or by a central cut that is slightly undersized in relation to the box of the component that is to be inserted.

Treatment

Treatment of diaphyseal fractures consists in the use of an intramedullary stem that exceeds the fracture rima and relieves the bone from stress.

A diacondylar screw is instead usually sufficient to adequately reduce a condylar fracture, also because the subsequent application of cement and of the component itself confer further stability. On the contrary, use of an intramedullary stem is preferable when the fracture is displaced, when it has multiple fragments, or when it is supracondylar. The stem is press-fitted, accurately keeping the cement from coming into contact with the fracture zone, which would, in fact, obstruct the formation of bone callus.

Postoperative rehabilitation in cases such as these is not much different from that of a normal knee prosthesis, as these fractures are rarely displaced or comminuted, they are not associated with trauma of the soft tissues, and synthesis is usually sufficiently stable to be able to tolerate mild loading during postoperative rehabilitation.

Results

Lombardi et al. (1) in comparing a consecutive series of 898 knee replacements with another series of 532 replacements of the same model, but implanted using different instrumentation for resection of the intercondylar box, observed an incidence of intraoperative fracture equal to 4.5% in the first series as compared to only 1 case that occurred in the second one. Non-displaced intercondylar fracture was revealed postoperatively in 35 cases; the fracture had been recognized at the time of surgery and it had alternatively required the use of screws or a stem for stabilization in 5 knees. In all of the cases, the fracture was consolidated with no variation in the standard rehabilitation protocol. Furthermore, long-term evaluation did not reveal any differences in clinical and functional results in patients with sequelae of fracture and in normal patients.

The authors concluded by emphasizing the fact that adequate instrumentation is indispensable for correct replacement and in order to avoid unpleasant complications. Nonetheless, also in the case of fracture, consolidation occurred without substantial changes in postoperative rehabilitation treatment, allowing us to obtain excellent results all the same.

Postoperative Fractures

Incidence and etiopathogenesis

Distal fractures of the femur after knee prosthesis have been reported in the literature with a frequency that varies from 0.3% to 2.5% in all implants (4-8).

Traumatic forms and those caused by stress are distinguished. Traumatic forms occur as a result of direct high-energy trauma or indirect trauma such as mobilization in narcosis. In the genesis of fractures caused by stress, instead, evident trauma is not always recognizable. In fact, there are numerous fractures that predispose the patient to fracture, and they often contribute to the occurrence of fracture.

Among systemic causes, a major role is played by osteoporosis, that to varying degrees is always present in patients that are submitted to prosthetic surgery, because of age, or because of a drug-induced effect, and also because chronic pathologies often coexist in these patients' pathologies. The importance of neurologic deficit, such as cerebellar ataxia (e.g., Sturge-Weber disease, tertiary syphilis, brain tumors, cerebral aneurysms, etc.) epilepsy, Parkinson's disease, the sequelae of poliomyelitis or severe myasthenia, have been revealed by Culp et al. (9). In fact, in reporting the long-term results of treatment in 61 supracondylar fractures of the femur after replacement surgery, the authors revealed the presence of a neurologic deficit in 3.6% of cases of fracture. Rheumatoid arthritis has also been described (5, 10-13) as a frequent systemic contributing factor because of its direct effect due to the chronic inflammatory process, or its indirect effect, consequent to the use of drugs such as steroids, that favor necrosis and bone resorption.

At a local level, all of those factors that lead to weakening of bone resistance may contribute, such as technical errors, notching of the anterior cortical bone (5, 9, 10, 12, 13) and malalignment of the components (2), or loss of bone stock due to repeated revision surgery (11), or to osteolysis caused by polyethylene wear (14). The influence of notching of the anterior cortical bone is nonetheless discussed, as those authors (5, 9, 10, 12, 13) who found a correlation between this radiographic sign and fracture are opposed by other authors (15) who deny any real importance, also because the femur during the postoperative period quickly undergoes remodeling.

Finally, the design of the prosthesis must avoid the production of surface stress at the prosthetic bone interface, or that implantation of the component require excessive bone resection.

Classification

Various classifications have been proposed with the purpose of standardizing treatment based on the severity of the fracture. Initially, the classification previously introduced by Neer (16) for supracondylar fractures of the femur was used, that defined three grades. Grade I included linear fractures, with little or no displacement, in which good stability could be obtained by simple manual reduction. Grade II fractures revealed displacement exceeding 1 cm and were divided into two categories, IIA and IIB, depending on whether the distal fragment was shifted medially or laterally. Grade III fractures grouped severe condylar T or Y fractures with marked comminution in the fracture site and major involvement of the soft tissues.

A different classification, again subdivided into grades, was recently proposed by Lewis and Rorabeck (2). Type I includes compound fractures in which the prosthesis proves to be whole and stable, type II displaced fractures, but always with stable prostheses, and type III fractures all those in which the prosthesis is loosened or shows evident signs of wear. To these three grades of fracture, according to Engh and Ammen (3), are associated a fourth in which to group all of the cases of failure of a previous attempt to stabilize the fracture.

Treatment

Two options of treatment may be used in this type of fracture: conservative and surgical.

The state of stabilization of the prosthesis must always be analyzed before deciding on any type of therapeutic approach. After fracture, it is often difficult to clearly evaluate the bone prosthesis interface using standard radiographic projections. The use of different projections and computed tomography, as well, may facilitate evaluation of the extent of fracture, and degree of comminution, as well as any loosening of the prosthesis. The quality of the bone is also a very important factor to consider.

Conservative treatment consists in immobilization in plaster or in a knee cast. It is indicated in types I or II fractures in which there is good stability, the prosthesis is not loosened, limb alignment, obtained after closed reduction, can be maintained, and the patient shows good muscle tone in the upper limbs and can walk with partial loading and the help of crutches in complete safety. Some authors suggest first the use of skeletal traction in order to maintain correct alignment, and then immobilization in plaster. Insall (17) suggests at least 4-6 weeks of traction, nonetheless, a longer period of time in bed may be necessary, keeping the knee immobile, factors that are not, however, tolerated by older patients. The final results are defined satisfactory only when final consolidation is accompanied by no pain and the degree of flexion is almost 90°. Up to 2 cm of shortening of the limb and axial deviation that measures less than 5° on the frontal plane and less than 10° on the sagittal one are acceptable.

The use of surgical treatment is instead necessary when stabilization of a more displaced type I fracture in patients that cannot tolerate plaster or the knee cast or in those incapable of standing on crutches, in type II fractures that present comminution or insufficient alignment of the segments, and in type III fractures where, although loosening of the prosthetic components is evident, revision surgery is postponed until consolidation is final.

There are numerous means of stabilization available for the internal fixation of a non-displaced or only slightly displaced type I fracture. Intramedullary nails, that do not interfere with the formation of hematoma in the fracture site, constitute the ideal solution. Rush nails (18), Zickel supracondylar nails (19, 20) and retrograde locked nails (7, 21, 22) may be used.

Alignment must be corrected in type II fractures, and the fracture must be stabilized to allow for mobility of the knee and walking without loading. The variables that must be taken into consideration when choosing a method of stabilization to be adopted must include the grade of displacement and the angulation of the bone fragments, alignment of the entire limb, the quality of the bone, the presence of previous bone deformities, and the type of prosthesis implanted. Finally, the extent of the skeletal injury in the condylar distal fragment is important when selecting a method of stabilization.

The means of stabilization available include plates and screws (23, 24, 25), external fixators (5), and retrograde intramedullary nails (7, 21,

22, 26). As for plates, various models are used successfully to treat these fractures. When a straight plate with screws is used, it is important to be sure that the distal fragment is sufficient in size to receive more than one screw and that the quality of the bone guarantees rigid stabilization. The closeness of the femoral component to the fracture must always be evaluated when choosing the plate to be used. A screw plate is probably the simplest device to use, but the screw is often large and it may be difficult to insert it when the size of the distal fragment is insufficient as in the case of very distal or comminuted fracture. A condylar buttress plate (Fig. 1) provides greater flexibility, but also less stiffness than stabilization. The use of a blade-plate is commonly considered the best solution since the blade can be inserted close to the femoral component. The fracture may be angulated with any one of these plates, but in the case of the blade-plate it is more difficult because the blade must migrate in the bone before causing a loss in alignment.

In cases where the stability obtained intraoperatively is doubtful, it is possible to increase the hold of the fixation, in the site of the distal fragment, by using bone graft or cement. Healy et al. (23) suggest opening a window on the lateral cortical bone of the lateral condyle. Thus, it is easier to impact the bone graft or inject the cement in the femoral metaphysis. Alternatively, it is possible to use a syringe to inject cement with low viscosity in the skeletal holes made to lodge the screws that are then inserted before the cement hardens. This method would confer solidity to the distal condylar fragment that at this point may be reduced and stabilized by fixing the plate proximally with the bicortical screws.

External fixators can be used successfully, but they are usually contraindicated in the treatment of these fractures. The purpose of their use is to achieve alignment and stability of the frac-

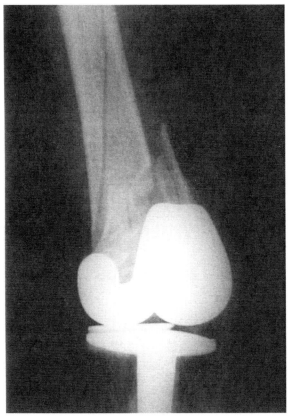

A

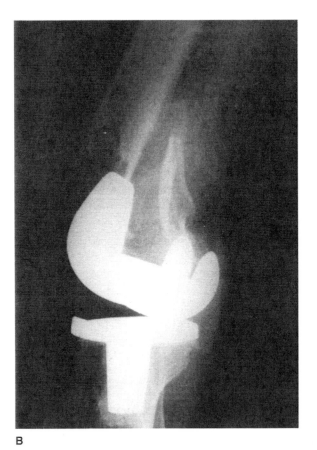

B

FIG. 1 (A,B,C,D) - Radiographic image in anteroposterior (A) and laterolateral (B) projections of displaced supracondylar fracture of the femur after knee replacement surgery. Postoperative radiographic image in anteroposterior (C) and laterolateral (D) projection of the same case treated by open reduction and osteosynthesis with plate and screws. The anatomical axis of the knee was restored and the fracture consolidated in about 4 months.

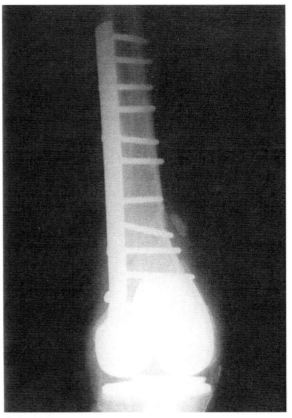

C

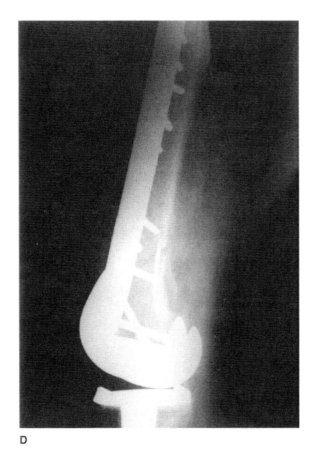

D

ture segments, so as to allow for the quick recovery of range of movement and walking with partial loading. But because the pins of the fixator pass through the muscle tissue of the quadriceps, they can obstruct recovery of mobility. The possible superficial infection of the sites where these wires are inserted consequently means a high risk of infection of the knee itself.

The supracondylar intramedullary nail represents an excellent solution in this type of fracture, as it does not interfere with soft tissues in the fracture site, and it is easily inserted by retrograde access through the intercondylar space left by the prosthesis. For this reason, it is very important to preoperatively identify what kind of prosthesis has been implanted, so as to be able to accurately define the intercondylar space available (Fig. 2). A minimum intercondylar distance of 12 mm is necessary; in general, it ranges from 15 to 20 mm. If the model of the prosthesis implanted cannot be identified in standard X-rays, the intercondylar space may be measured on a radiographic projection of the intercondylar notch. If this is not possible either, the fracture should be synthesized differently. Finally, two

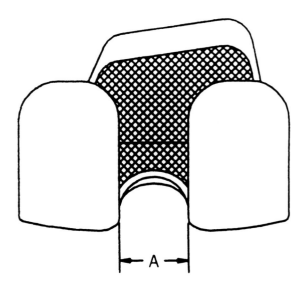

FIG. 2 - Method used to measure the intercondylar distance (A) of the femoral component of a knee prosthesis. To permit the insertion of a retrograde intramedullary pin, this distance must be at least 12 mm.

standard radiographic projections of the contralateral knee may be useful to correctly measure the diameter and the length of the rod to be inserted.

Using the approach used to implant the prosthesis, the fracture is reduced, and subsequently, with the knee flexed, the nail is inserted through a hole made in the roof of the intercondylar notch just before femoral insertion of the posterior cruciate ligament (Fig. 3). Once the nail is implanted, and correct alignment of the bone ends checked, with the use of an extramedullary guide the nail itself is blocked with at least two screws at the distal level and at the proximal one.

In type III fractures, where the prosthesis is loosened, treatment consists in doing revision and synthesis of the fracture in a single stage or in two separate stages (3, 7, 27, 28).

If revision is postponed, the means of synthesis used to treat fracture are not different from those described for type II fractures. Furthermore, this method offers two advantages. First, revision surgery on an anatomicallty consolidated fracture is technically easier. Second, it is possible to more frequently use a standard revision implant instead of a tumor prosthesis, a custom-made prosthesis, or an allograft that is large in size. The disadvantage of this choice in therapy, however, is constituted by the fact that the patient, in the interval between the two surgeries, is often confined to bed or at any case very limited in his or her activity, while waiting for fracture healing to take place.

In primary revision and synthesis, instead, intramedullary stems, custom-made prostheses, tumor prostheses or prostheses directly stabilized

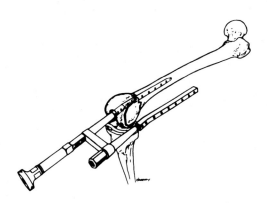

FIG. 3 - Once the fracture has been reduced, the intramedullary rod is inserted in the flexed knee through a hole made in the roof of the intercondylar notch before the insertion of the posterior cruciate ligament.

to the allograft may be used, if the distal femur is severely injured.

The use of femoral components with long intramedullary stems capable of bypassing the fracture constitutes the best way to treat most type III fractures; as already emphasized, it is very important that these patients, who are often elderly, and affected with associated systemic diseases, initiate rehabilitation treatment as soon as possible.

However, it is alway preferable to always have available an implant model or a sufficient quantity of bank bone to be able to fill or substitute femoral distal bone defect that is produced during the revision procedure. In fractures such as these, the bone quality is often poor, and removal of the femoral component means bone loss that is difficult to measure preoperatively. In fact, when severe bone loss is present, it becomes difficult to obtain good prosthetic stabilization. If condylar comminution is such as to make this attempt at synthesis useless, then the use of prostheses that substitute the condyles, such as in the case of prostheses for tumors, or an assembly is even more justified.

The tibial component, if stable, may be maintained as long as it presents the same design and it is correctly articulated with the femoral component, once the latter has been implanted. The same must be said for the patellar component. Usually, dome-shaped models do not need to be substituted, as they are compatible with most of the femoral components on the market.

Results

There are numerous authors in the literature who have studied the long-term results of the treatment of this kind of fracture (5, 6, 8-13, 18-33).

As far back as 1981, Hirsch et al. (10) reported 4 cases of supracondylar fracture of the femur after prosthesis. In all of the cases, fracture had been consequent to mild trauma. Three patients were affected with rheumatoid arthritis, while the fourth had been prosthetized following posttraumatic gonarthrosis. Fracture was compound and it was treated by immobilization in plaster in 1 case. Fracture was non-displaced unstable, but a conservative type approach was at any rate attempted in the remaining 3 cases. Malalignment defined acceptable persisted in 2 cases, while the third case was treated surgically. Consolidation was obtained within 6 months in all of the patients, achieving function that was comparable to that of the pre-fracture status. The authors concluded by affirming that in cases such as these it was possible to resort to open reduction with internal fixation, but that conservative type treatment always had to be attempted.

During the same year, Short et al. (29) reported 5 other cases. One patient was treated by primary surgery, while of the other 4, initially treated by immobilization in plaster or traction, only 2 showed signs of fracture consolidation 3 months after trauma. The authors affirmed that in this type of fracture, despite the complications related to the presence of the prosthesis, it was possible to obtain satisfactory results with open reduction and internal fixation.

In a series of 15 supracondylar fractures, Sisto and Insall (11) observed 3 types of treatment. Immobilization in plaster for 6-8 weeks and walking with partial loading allowed was used in 4 patients with compound fracture, or fracture that could be reduced under anaesthesia. Eight patients with fracture displacement were at first placed in traction and then immobilized in plaster. The remaining 3, who presented with severe fracture displacement, were treated by surgical reduction and internal fixation. At the end of the study, the authors suggested a treatment protocol initially based on closed reduction and traction of the limb. Surgery was to be reserved for those cases in which skeletal traction had proven to be ineffective in maintaining reduction.

Merkel et al. (5) in a retrospective study on 34 patients with 36 supracondylar fractures of the femur were the first to propose the Neer classification to describe this type of fracture. In this case, too, a distinction was made between 3 types of treatment: conservative, surgical with open reduction and internal stabilization, and surgical, with closed reduction and external stabilization. The first group included 26 grades I, IIA and IIB fractures; of these, 17 healed, while 9 required further surgery consisting in bone graft, internal stabilization, and revision of the prosthesis. In the second group, that included 5 cases of grade II fracture, there was a percentage of complications, such as infection, nonunion, and death, equal to 100%. In the third group, complete healing was obtained in all of the cases. The authors concluded that in grade I fractures the best possible treatment consists in immobilization in plaster for the first 4 weeks followed by the use of a knee cast. In grade II fractures, before proceeding to surgery, because of the high incidence of complications, it was recommended that an attempt be made to perform closed reduction associated with traction. Revision surgery was preferable in cases in which it was not possible to obtain stable fixation at surgery. Finally, surgical stabilization had to be attempted in all of the cases where consolidation had not taken place.

In evaluating the results obtained in 14 fractures of which 10 treated conservatively, Cain et al. (30) found a correlation between prosthetic alignment obtained after reduction and long-term results. In fact, if translation of the prosthetic axis was contained within 5 mm, long-term results in terms of function and stability were usually satifactory, while if translation exceeded 5 mm, results were invariably unsatisfactory.

In a series of 61 fractures, Culp et al. (9) used open reduction with internal fixation in 31 cases, while they used immobilization in plaster in the remaining 30 cases. In the group treated surgically 25 consolidated, while in the group treated conservatively satisfactory results were obtained in just a few more than half of the cases. For this reason, at the end of the study, the authors believed that open reduction with internal fixation could be considered the treatment of choice for all grades of fracture.

In reporting the results of the treatment in 24 supracondylar fractures after knee prosthesis, Figgie et al. (6) supported the conclusions previously drawn by Merkel et al. revealing the importance of the use of primary closed reduction with immobilization in plaster also for displaced fractures. Only in cases where the alignment achieved could not be maintained was surgery suggested.

Contrary to what is reported above, in 29 cases of supracondylar fracture after knee prosthesis Moran et al. (25) revealed that conservative treatment was effective only in compound fractures, while surgical treatment was mandatory in displaced fractures, allowing for a good success rate despite a high incidence of complications.

Zehntner and Ganz (24) and Healy et al. (23) in their series observed a low incidence of intra- and postoperative complications, and even suggested the use of internal fixation in all cases of supracondylar fracture. In fact, in their opinion satisfactory results could be obtained only with stable fixation.

There is no single opinion on the treatment of these fractures. Many authors agree that non-displaced supracondylar fractures may be treated with simple immobilization, while in cases in which there is severe comminution, or the prosthesis appears to be loose (Neer grade III and Lewis and Rorabeck grade III) surgery is required. Uncertainty persists as regards the best possible solution for treatment in cases where the prosthesis is stable, but fracture presents displacement that cannot easily be treated by simple closed reduction. In fact, conservative treatment often means healing with severe malalignment or sequelae in nonunion, while surgical treatment is burdened by a high incidence of complications such as deep infection, loss of stabilization, or death.

One solution was recently proposed with the introduction of the retrograde intramedullary nail. In fact, numerous studies (7, 21, 22, 26) report a high success rate with this means of stabilization whose function is similar to that of a prosthetic intramedullary stem without having to resort to revision of the femoral component. By bypassing the fracture zone, this nail would confer greater stability on the fracture itself; moreover, by crossing the locking both proximal and distal, it would restore correct alignment of the segments, and it would maintain the correct length of the limb, thus facilitating the bone consolidation process. In this case too, however, because of the high risk of infective complications, accurate sterility during surgery is mandatory.

Fracture of the Tibia

Intraoperative Fractures

Etiopathogenesis

Intraoperative fractures of the tibia are rarely observed, particularly at implantation. Vertical fractures of the metaphyseal portion may occur during an attempt to impact an oversized stem or a tibial component with small peripheral pegs or that is malaligned. Revision surgery and the possible use of osteotomy of the tibial tubercle to facilitate joint exposure further increase the risk of these fractures. Fractures of the diaphysis in general constitute the natural consequence of the conflict that takes place between the prosthetic intramedullary stem and the bone cortical at the time of impaction if the stem is introduced at an anomalous angle or in a position that is not centered in relation to the medullary canal. Generally, fractures such as these are not recognized at surgery, but only at postoperative radiographic monitoring.

Treatment

Fragments are usually anatomically reduced in metaphyseal fractures. A cancellous screw may be used for stabilization, although fixation of the tibial component with cement, in itself, is often sufficient to protect the fracture. Rehabilitation includes rapid recovery of the knee's range

of movement, with the use of a knee cast, while walking with partial loading must be maintained for at least 6-8 weeks. In the case of diaphyseal fracture, there may be angulation or displacement of the fragments if the fracture is not immediately recognized and loading is allowed with walking. Nonetheless, in fractures such as these, there is no severe involvement of the soft tissues typical of high-energy fractures and the periosteum is also often only slightly involved, so that fracture consolidation usually takes place without complications after closed reduction and the use of a plaster cast.

Postoperative Fractures

Etiopathogenesis

Postoperative fractures of the tibia are a rare event when there is no trauma. The literature reports data on the subject, and it mostly includes studies that concern the use of intramedullary stems in revision surgery (27). Cases of fracture after tubercle osteotomy have also been reported (2). The incidence of fractures of the tibial plateau, nonetheless, could be underestimated in association with the loosening of the tibial component.

Rand and Coventry (34) reported 15 cases of fracture caused by stress of the tibial plateau after implantation of old models of knee prostheses such as Geometric and Polycentric, whose components were inadequate in design. The fracture was consequent to fatigue failure of the tibia secondary to malalignment or erroneous orientation of the tibial component. In all of the cases, the correct treatment was revision of the implant.

Fractures caused by stress rarely occur if metal-back components that are correctly aligned are used. Nonetheless, fracture may occur when an attempt is made postoperatively to mobilize the knee in a patient that preoperatively was not capable of walking or that in any case presented with a limited range of movement. In patients such as these, the occurrence of strong pain in the knee during rehabilitation constitutes a warning signal that should not be overlooked, and radiographic follow-up excludes any doubts (3).

Treatment

Like in the femur, the choice of treatment in this type of fracture depends on two factors: the stability of interface and the quality of the bone. If the prosthesis is stable and the fracture is compound, and well-aligned, conservative treatment is recommended. In cases such as these, a plaster knee cast is used that may be substituted with an articulated knee cast when the fracture presents a sufficient degree of consolidation. Loading with walking will be allowed when consolidation is definite and at any rate not before 6 weeks have gone by.

Fractures of the diaphysis under the prosthesis that do not reveal signs of detachment may at times be treated conservatively. When there is instability or malalignment of the fracture segments, nonetheless, it is best to use surgical treatment with fixation by intramedullary access in a disto-proximal direction. This avoids the use of a plate, implying detachment of the soft tissues from the fracture zone, and considerably increasing the risk of infection of the implant.

Revision of the implant, finally, is indispensable when the tibial component is loosened or the quality of the bone is poor. In cases such as these, the use of an intramedullary stem whether or not associated with bone graft represents the treatment of choice.

Fracture of the Patella

Intraoperative Fractures

Intraoperative fractures of the patella may occur in a a patella with a significant amount of erosion, or whose component when inserted presents large anchor pegs so that the hole for bone lodging breaks the anterior cortical bone. Usually, these are vertical fractures that do not alter the integrity of the extensor apparatus so that treatment is not required either at surgery or postoperatively.

When inset type patellar components are used, peripheral fractures may occur. In this case, the treatment of choice consists in removing the fragment to avoid the possible cause of peripatellar pain postoperatively.

Postoperative Fractures

Incidence and etiopathogenesis

Postoperative fractures of the patella are reported to have a variable incidence, from 0% to 21% (35, 36). When the Insall-Burstein posterior-stabilized prosthesis is used, the incidence of fracture is decreased by an initial high 11% (37) to a more reasonable 2% (38), thanks to a more careful attention to patellar tracking and to modification (1982) of the anterior margin of the in-

tercondylar box of the femoral component. Stress fractures may also occur in the absence of a patellar prosthesis. In a comparative study, the incidence of these fractures was 0.05% as compared to 0.33% when the patella is resurfaced.

From an etiological point of view, these fractures were classified (40) as traumatic and atraumatic or stress forms. In fact, the forces that act on the femoropatellar joint are considerable. They vary with flexion and with the type of activity (41, 42), from a minimum of a fraction of body weight in walking at ground level (43) to three times the body weight in going up stairs and getting up from sitting, up to 20 times when jumping (44). This explains the occurrence of patellar fractures in the absence of real trauma. The probabilities then increase if one or more predisposing factors interact, such as: A) modified vascularity; B) modified patellar tracking; C) bone resistance; D) prosthetic design; E) prosthetic positioning; F) range of movement:

A) Vascularity

Vascularization of the patella depends on the supply of the following six arteries: the superior genicular, the lateral superior and the medial superior genicular, the lateral inferior and the medial inferior genicular, the anterior tibial recurrent artery. According to some authors (45, 46, 47) these form a peripatellar ring (Fig. 4) from with derive the branches that irrorate the anterior aspect of the patella, as well as the apical arteries (from the retrotendinous infrapatellar transverse branch). According to others (48) they form a rich anterior vascular plexus. Moreover, there is agreement in believing that the main vascular supply to the patella derives from the anterior perforating cortical arteries. The patellar ligament, the quadriceps tendon, the fat pad do not seem to contribute but minimally. Thus, the intraosseous plexus originates from the extraosseous anterior plexus through the foramina (49), and not from the periphery of the patella (except for the apical part). Hassenpflug also agrees with this theory and reveals that in relation to the patella, the main vascular supply derives from medial-proximal and lateral-distal (50).

Many authors agree on the need to try to reduce trauma and anterior patellar dissection, avoiding perforating the cortical bone and producing a large hole of central fixation for the patellar peg. The capsular incisions that are made to insert the prosthesis may compromise vascularization. This is true for the traditional anteromedial incision and it is aggravated if a lateral retinacular release and perhaps also excision of the fat pad are carried out. Experimental-

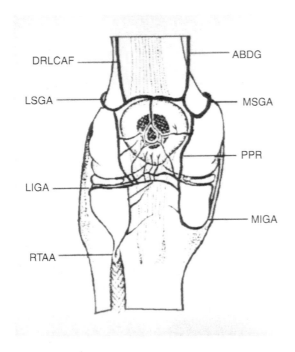

FIG. 4 - Vascular supply to the patella based on the theory of the peripatellar ring. The arteries that flow together to form the peripatellar ring (PPR) according to Kayler and Little (47) are the descendent ramus of the lateral circumflex artery of the femur (DRLCAF), the lateral superior genicular artery (LSGA), the lateral inferior genicular artery (LIGA), the recurrent tibial anterior artery (RTAA), the medial inferior genicular artery (MIGA), the medial superior genicular artery (MSGA), and the articular branch of the descendent genicular (ABDG).

ly in the dog (51) the anteromedial incision reduces the patellar flow measured by a Laser Doppler by 34%, a lateral release reduces it by 47%, and excision of the fat pad by another 58%. The cumulative effect is a reduction by 85%. Some authors confirm that excision of the pad provokes a reduction in flow (47, 52). Others, based on bone scan and clinical observation, respectively, have found the influence of the fat pad to be less (53, 54).

In order to preserve patellar vascularization, different types of surgical access have been determined, such as the anterolateral (55) one in the valgus knee, the midvastus (56), or the subvastus (57) and the tri-vector (58). The advantage to using these methods would also be the minor use of lateral release.

Many bone scan studies carried out early after knee replacement surgery reveal a reduced or absent vascularity of the patella, although with various incidences. Scuderi reports avascularity in 56% of knees with lateral release (59), McMahon in 54% (53), Wetzener in 9% (60),

Ritter in 0% (61), but in later bone scans. Recently, Ritter observed that lateral release is associated with a significantly higher incidence of fractures of the patella (4% vs 0,5%) and that saving the lateral superior genicular artery has no effect (62). Scott instead believes that bone necrosis of the patella may occur particularly after lateral release and that thus every effort must be made to preserve at least one of the genicular arteries (63, 64).

A further factor in necrosis could be the thermic effect caused by the saw and the cement used for fixation (39, 65), even if this should be limited to a few tenths of a micron (66, 67).

B) Patellar tracking

Patellar tracking in flexion-extension must be accurately verified during knee replacement surgery (68). If subluxation or lateral tilt (generally evident in 30-45° of flexion) are present, it is preferable to perform a lateral retinacular lysis rather than leave this element which is unfavorable in terms of patellar function and the genesis of the stress fracture. The way in which all of this is monitored is very important; we usually use the "no thumb technique," that is, without applying tension on the anterior rectus (with a Kocher) particularly in going from flexion to extension and maintaining the tibia in neutral rotation (69). An attempt will be made to monitor the presence or the absence of contact between the patella and the medial femoral condyle. In the valgus knee, the need to perform retinacular lateral lysis is more frequent (70, 71, 72). The execution of lateral lysis is compatible with the preservation of the lateral superior genicular artery with adequate attention to technique.

A very important factor is the thickness of the patella, that is, the bone-prosthesis combination. This thickness must not exceed the original one of the patella that is not prosthetized. This would result in an increase in lateral tilt due to increased tension in the lateral retinacula and an increase in the shear forces that act on the patella in a mediolateral direction as demonstrated by an in vitro study (73). Star has demonstrated in vitro that a progressive increase in thickness produces a significant increase in the femoropatellar compressive forces measured with a cell loaded from 70 to 95° in flexion (74). Even an increase by just 10% (2-3 mm) is important. Thus, it is necessary to evaluate with a caliper the initial thickness of the patella and then evaluate it once again after prosthetization. There are special instruments (patellar reamers) that allow for resection as far as the thickness desired. Oishi et al. (75) used cadavers to evaluate the compressive and shear forces that act on the patella. Above 45° in flexion, increasing thickness by +2 or +4 mm, there is a significant increase in total shear forces as compared to when the initial thickness is preserved.

C) Bone resistance

The qualities of the patellar bone are another factor to be taken into consideration. At times, osteoporosis associated with rheumatoid arthritis has been correctly believed to be a predisposing factor even if the incidence of fracture, according to some authors, is greater in arthritis (63).

Within this context, it must also be recalled that an excessive or asymmetrical resection of the patellar bone may be negative. It has been demonstrated that the anterior strain in the patella increases if the thickness of the residual bone after osteotomy is reduced (76). Fifteen millimeters seem to be the limit value (Fig. 5). Even an asymmetrical cut, sacrificing the lateral subchondral bone produces a reduction in bone stiffness (77) (Fig. 6).

The production of a central anchoring hole for fixation by a single peg of the prosthetic component appears to weaken the patellar bone and predispose it to fracture because of the production of a stress raiser, and because of a reduction in intraosseous vascularity (39, 78). If the large central hole can lead to fracture, one that is too small can lead to loosening, so that today the option of 3 small peripheral pegs is preferable, also because the vascular apparatus of the periphery appears to be very important in the patella.

D) Prosthetic design

Certainly one of the most important factors for the genesis of the fracture is the design of the prosthesis, meaning both the patellar and the femoral components.

As for the patellar component, the dome-shaped design, which is not anatomical, offers the advantage of being more tolerant as regards anomalies in centering that are always possible (a modest tilt is often noted in postoperative axial X-rays despite all of the efforts made to center the patella) (79). Thus, stress at the interface and on the patellar bone is reduced. This type of prosthesis is adapted to different shapes and sizes of knee, it eliminates any ambiguity of insertion (rotation, etc.), and it accepts tilting and twisting without modifying the contact area too much. The disadvantage is that contact occurs in a very reduced area, which is at times very small, at times only linear. This increases the stress on the polyethylene that in various activities can exceed the limits of tolerance (5-10 Mpa). The

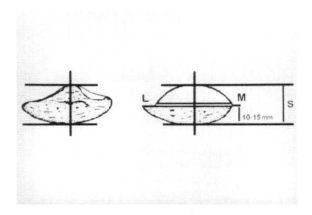

FIG. 5 - The thickness of the patella, that is, of the bone-prosthesis combination, must not exceed the original one of the non-prosthetized patella, while the remaining bone thickness of the patella must be at least 10-15 mm.

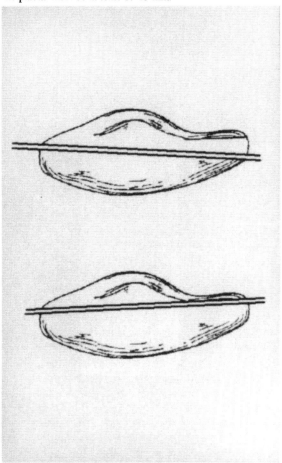

FIG. 6 - An asymmetrical cut, sacrificing the lateral subchondral bone, produces a reduction in bone stiffness.

anatomical implant instead allows for a contact area that is much greater and thus possibly greater duration, with minor wear of the plastic

(80). Today, modified dome-shaped prostheses are used (Mexican hat, sombrero type) that on one hand maintain several advantages of the dome, on the other, increase the contact area.

One particular type of design, the small inset prosthesis, has recently been exploited (81, 82, 83). In particular, it has been observed that the incidence of lateral release, patellar pain, stress fracture is less as compared to large onset prostheses after 5 years (83). Even congruent rotating-bearing prostheses appear to be very promising.

As for the design of the femoral component, it also seems important for a reduction in the incidence of stress fracture. It is essentially the anteroposterior diameter that is important. A prosthesis with a prominent "shoulder" increases stress on the patella. Many prostheses produce this effect. Often with the purpose of minimizing femoral bone resection and increasing the contact area in extension, designs with a less anatomical trochlea are used. The importance of the trochlea has been emphasized by many authors (85, 86), in order to avoid excessive prominence. Some prostheses, such as the Miller-Galante I, have a femoral component with a particularly prominent design. The incidence of complications, including fractures and subdislocations in this prosthesis as compared to the PFC, has been correlated to the design of the femoral component (87). The Miller-Galante II differs from the I primarily based on a more anatomical anterior trochlear groove. Even functionally, an increase in loading on the quadriceps while going up and down stairs with an increase in retropatellar forces has been documented, as patients with a trochlea that is not anatomical abnormally flex the knee during the late support phase in going up stairs. This design influences not just the kinematics, but also loading on the patella (88).

Recent prosthetic models pay very close attention to these parameters. In a comparison between three new prostheses (Genesis II, Nex Gen, PFC Sigma) inserted in a cadaver, evident improvement in the kinematics of the patella as compared to the past was seen, in the sense that, for example, lateral releases are not required for correct patellar tracking, but in all three designs there is an increased lateral tilt (although without differences in movement, shift or rotation) (89). The new Insall prosthesis with posterior-stability (Legacy, Zimmer) attempts to reduce anterior prominence by shifting posteriorly the mechanism of cam stability and reducing the walking arc (Insall J.N. personal communication, 1997).

Finally, even the question of the preservation of the posterior cruciate ligament and the use of a meniscal type prosthesis is of some importance. Fluoroscopic studies have shown the irregular kinematics of flat prostheses that preserve the posterior cruciate ligament (90). In fact, probably because of the absence of the anterior cruciate ligament there is abnormally posterior femorotibial contact in extension and the femur slides anteriorly towards the patella in flexion, thus increasing femoropatellar reaction forces (91, 92). As for meniscal prostheses, rotational freedom offered by the menisci or by the mobile platform may improve patellar tracking as the extensor apparatus may automatically find better centering in flexion-extension.

E) Prosthetic positioning

In general, there is a tendency to determine an alignment in the neutral zone in order to reduce the incidence of patellar problems and in particular of fractures of the patella. With the IB II posterior-stability prosthesis (93, 94) it has been seen that in the presence of major malalignments fractures are more severe. To establish the range of neutrality, numerous factors are evaluated, such as: 1) variation in the level of the joint line after surgery (up to 8 mm); 2) position in A-P of the tibial component (posterior to half the tibia); 3) height of the patella in relation to the joint line (between 10 and 30 mm) also emphasized by Fern et al. (95), 4) centralization of the tibial component in the M-L plane; 5) sagittal position of the femoral component (not too anterior); 6) valgus angle of the femoral component ($5° \pm 4°$); 7) tibial component at $90° \pm 2°$ in A-P and in L-L in relation to the tibial axis; 8) global mechanical axis in an X-ray 30 x 90 cm (malalignment must not exceed $4°$).

As for positioning of the patellar component, the positioning of M-L must also be evaluated. In fact, medialization seems to improve tracking and load distribution (73), thus reducing the incidence of lateral lysis (96). Yoshii et al. (97) have shown that improvement in tracking is obtained by medializing the patellar component and by deepening the trochlear sulcus.

As for the femoral component, it is important to evaluate both the valgus of the component that must not exceed $10°$ (98) and the mid-lateral and rotational positions. A more lateral position of the femoral component (+5 mm) is favorable to patellar tracking and it compensates for the prominence of the lateral labrum of the trochlea with the AMK prosthesis (99). Just as important is the rotational position. A mild external rotation in the posterior condyles improves patellar tracking and lateral stability of the knee (99, 100, 101). Positioning of the femoral component in a rotational direction is an important surgical problem. There are many options, beginning with reference to the posterior bicondylar axis that may however produce abnormal internal rotation if there is posterolateral erosion, as in valgus knee, external if there is posteromedial erosion. More favorable seems to be the method where reference is made to the resected tibial surface going parallel to it and keeping the collateral ligaments after adequate releases, or the determination of the Whiteside A-P trochlear axis (102). The method that we prefer is that in which the epicondylar axis is determined and we go parallel to it (103) (Fig. 7). This allows for automatic external rotation as compared to the posterior part of the condyles by about 3.5° in the varus knee and 4.4° in the valgus one (104). The incidence of lateral retinacular lysis with the IB PS prosthesis has been proven to be reduced from 55% to 13% with attention paid to the femoral rotation and to 2% with the use of epicondylar instruments (105).

Finally, with regard to the tibia, many authors agree that there is a need to correctly position the tibial component in order to obtain central patellar tracking. The rotational position is the most important. Internal rotation must be avoided (106). There are various methods to align the tibial component by rotation (107). The rotational position that is obtained may be very different. We prefer to use the tibial tuberosity and to align the component with the medial half of the same. According to some authors, it is also important to position the tibial component slightly more lateral in relation to the center of the tibial plateau (108).

F. Range of movement

Greater flexion, which is also desirable for the better function of the knee, nonetheless, exposes the patient to the risk of fracture (109).

Classification

Various types of classification have been reported in the literature to facilitate treatment of fractures of the patella in knee replacement.

Windsor et al. (40) distinguish between two types of fractures: traumatic and stress. Traumatic fractures are the consequence of severe trauma and are usually displaced. Surgery may be required to fix the fragments if they are very shifted and to suture the lesion at the retinacular level if there is insufficiency of the extensor apparatus. Stress fractures occur spontaneously when there is no evident trauma, they are often asymp-

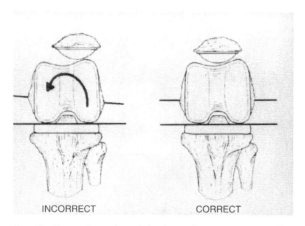

FIG. 7 - External rotation of the femoral component according to the epicondylar axis facilitates centralization of the patella, allowing for better tracking.

tomatic, and they are discovered by chance during follow-up. These fractures are subdivided into horizontal, vertical, comminuted and displaced. Horizontal fractures are usually consequent to improper tracking and they may be associated with dislocation of the patella. Vertical fractures nearly always involve the fixation hole, but they may heal spontaneously. Finally, comminuted or displaced fractures are often associated with two types mentioned above and in the absence of deficit of the quadriceps they may not cause important symptoms. They require surgical treatment if there is loosening of the component.

Goldberg et al. (110) have classified fractures of the patella after prosthesis of the knee based on type of treatment. Type I fractures (Fig. 8) do not involve the bone-cement surface or the extensor apparatus. This group includes marginal fractures (Fig. 10). Treatment is always conservative and results are good. Type II fractures (Fig. 8) instead involve the bone-cement and/or extensor apparatus surface. They are usually comminuted or displaced fractures and the use of surgery is indispensable even if the results are not always encouraging (Fig. 11). Type IIIA (Fig. 9) consists in fractures of the apex of the patella with associated rupture of the patellar tendon (avulsion) (Fig. 12). Surgical treatment often implies suturing of the patellar tendon to the proximal fragment and removal of the distal fragment. Type IIIB (Fig. 9) groups fractures-dislocations of the patella. The prognosis in most cases is disappointing even after suitable osteosynthesis (Fig. 13).

In a recent study by Tria et al. (111) the Goldberg classification was modified by distinguishing fractures of the patella non-displaced

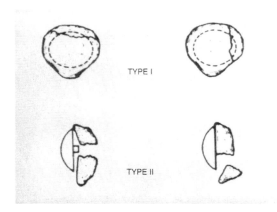

FIG. 8 - Types I and II fracture of the patella according to the Goldberg et al. classification (110).

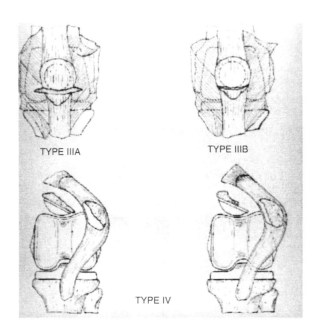

FIG. 9 - Types III and IV fracture of the patella according to the Goldberg et al. classification (110).

and displaced (>2 mm) with or without loosening of the polyethylene component and finally with or without associated lesion of the extensor apparatus.

Treatment

Treatment essentially depends on the type of fracture. When detachment, extensor deficit or severe displacement of the fragments are absent (±50% of cases), the treatment of choice is conservative, which usually consists in immobilization in plaster or in a knee cast, allowing for partial weight-bearing, and in the execution of isometric contraction exercises (particularly of the quadriceps). At this point, after about 6 weeks, the patient will begin a rehabilitation program to recover complete range of movement and strength of the quadriceps.

The use of surgery is advisable in all cases in which there is a lesion and insufficiency of the extensor apparatus, the fragments are displaced (> 2 mm), or if the patellar component is loosened. Although surgical fixation may seem impossible to avoid, open reduction and osteosynthesis have generally obtained poor results. The capacity for the bone to heal, in fact, may be compromised by avascularity and severe osteoporosis. In this case, the means of synthesis are hardly accepted, and solid fixation is not always obtained at surgery. In simpler cases, "8" wiring is preferable to the use of wiring in tension. In fractures of the apex of the patella this wiring may also include the tibial tuberosity so that the proximal insertion of the patellar tendon is not submitted to excessive tension during passive mobilization exercises that must be initiated immediately after

surgery. Movements in active flexion of the knee and reinforcement exercises of the quadriceps are allowed only when the fracture callus reveals a good state of consolidation.

In cases of severe associated lesion of the patellar tendon a useful technique consists in reinforcing the tendinous suture with transplant of the tendon of the semitendinosus passed through the transosseous holes on the patella and on the tibia. When the distal fragment cannot be fixed, it is preferable to remove it and suture the patellar tendon directly to the proximal fragment using the transosseous holes.

Excision of the detached fragment, in fact, is

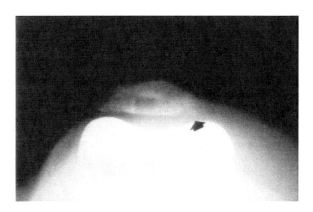

FIG. 10 - Radiographic example of the marginal fracture of patella after total knee replacement surgery.

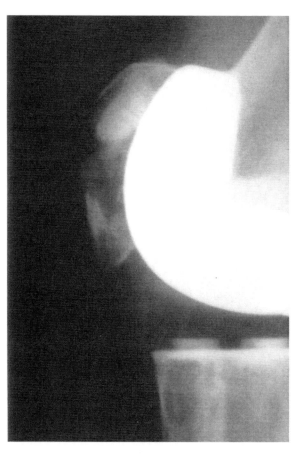

FIG. 11 - Radiographic example in laterolateral projection of a displaced fracture of patella after knee replacement surgery.

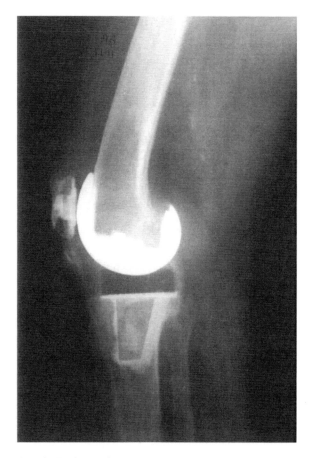

FIG. 12 - Radiographic example in laterolateral projection of detachment of the apex of the patella with avulsion of the patellar tendon.

useful not only at the apex of the patella, but also in all of those localizations in which it does not compromise the good function of the extensor apparatus. When there is loosening of the prosthetic component the same must be removed, arthroscopically and arthrotomically. When there is poor comminution of the bone, it is also possible to perform reimplantation of a new component. When, instead, because of the severity of the fracture, fixation is compromised and reimplantation of the prosthesis is not possible, reconstruction of the patella and partial patellectomy represent the best functional and biomechanical alternative to total patellectomy. In fact, total patellectomy must be exclusively reserved for those cases that cannot be adequately treated by surgery.

Results

The prognosis of fractures of the patella after knee replacement surgery is always uncertain; the type of fracture plays a role in the choice of the type of treatment and in the long-term results.

As early as 1980, Roffman et al. (112) showed this point reporting constrasting results in two cases of fracture of the patella after knee replacement surgery. The first patient, in fact, presented a compound fracture of the apex of the patella and 10° loss in active extension and obtained good results with the simple use of immobilization. In the second case, instead, the authors reported poor results, attempting to treat a fracture of the base of the patella associated with loss of the extensor apparatus equal to 60° with internal fixation and suture of the retinacula.

In going over a series of 6 patients, Clayton and Thirupati (78) confirmed the poor success rate of surgical treatment, reporting unsatisfactory results in all 5 cases that had been treated surgically.

Thompson et al. (113) conducted a long-term evaluation of 18 cases of fracture of the patella without shifting (4), with shifting (14), vertical

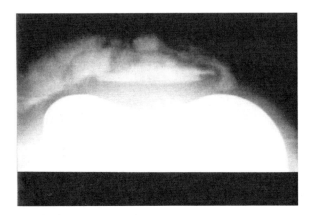

FIG. 13 - Radiographic example in axial projection of fracture-dislocation of the patella.

(10) or horizontal (4), extrapolated from an overall series of 1030 Total Condylar Knee replacements. Only 3 cases were consequent to effective trauma. Weight and height were above average. Treatment in each case depended on symptoms and degree of functional deficit more than on radiographic findings. In this series, too, the best results were observed after conservative treatment (10 cases excellent and 4 good) as compared to surgical treatment (3 cases good and 1 fair).

Scott et al. (63) presented a series of 1213 Duopatellar prostheses with 6 fractures. In 50% of cases (3 patients) it was not necessary to use surgery. In the remaining half of the knees, patellectomy (2 cases) and removal of the fragment (1 case) were performed, but satisfactory results were obtained in only 1 case.

Grace and Sim (39) observed 12 cases of fracture out of 8249 total knee arthroplasties. The choice of the type of treatment was based on grade of comminution and fragment displacement. Thus, fractures that presented with little or no comminution, shifting of fragments < 5 mm, and solid fixation of the patellar component were treated by immobilization for 6 weeks. Three of the 4 patients thus obtained satisfactory results. The remaining 8 fractures that presented extensive comminution, displacement of the fractures > 5 mm and/or loosening of the component were treated surgically in various ways including wiring and partial or total patellectomy. Satisfactory results were obtained in only 5 cases.

Hozack et al. (114) reported their data on 21 cases of fracture of the patella in patients with different types of prostheses models, and came to the conclusion that conservative treatment is indicated in non-displaced fractures and in displaced ones as long as there is no severe deficit of the extensor apparatus. Surgical treatment, instead, although necessary, provides poor results in all fractures with severe displacement and marked extensor deficit.

Goldberg et al. (114) reported 22 cases with excellent or good results and 14 fair or poor ones out of a total of 36 cases of fracture of the patella after knee replacement surgery. Using their own classification system, these authors found a correlation between type of fracture, type of treatment and long-term results. On radiographic examination, a correlation was also observed between the severity of the fracture and the criteria of alignment of the implant described by Figgie et al. (93). The type of fracture thus directly influenced treatment and results. Fractures that were not characterized by loosening of the component, lesion of the extensor apparatus, or severe errors in positioning of the prosthesis, were treated conservatively with success. Fractures that involved the complex bone-cement-prosthesis or apical fractures with complete lesion of the extensor apparatus, or, finally, fractures associated with dislocation of the patella were treated surgically. Satisfactory results were obtained in only 6 cases out of 20 knees. The authors also emphasized the importance of the possible occurrence of long-term complications. In fact, most (13 cases) of the 18 knees that on radiographic examination revealed errors defined to be major in positioning of the component had unsatisfactory results in the long-term; while all of the cases in which positioning of the component was within the neutral range or showed only minor errors reported satisfactory results. This fact was not however confirmed by other authors (111).

Windsor et al. (40) provided some indications as to the choice of the treatment of these fractures. When faced with comminuted or vertical fractures, regardless of the grade of displacement, in non-displaced fractures and in small proximal and distal avulsions, the authors suggest the use of immobilization in plaster for 6 weeks. They instead recommend the use of open reduction and internal fixation in transverse fractures characterized by displacement that exceeds 2 cm and that are associated with significant extensor deficit of the quadriceps. Removal of the component, partial patellectomy, and suturing of the extensor apparatus, finally, are indispensable in the treatment of comminuted fractures associated with deficit of the extensor apparatus and its loosening.

References

1) Lombardi A.V.Jr., Mallory T.H., Waterman R.A., Eberle R.W.: Intercondylar distal femoral fracture. An unreported complication of posterior-stabilized total knee arthroplasty. *J Arthroplasty* 10, 645-650, 1995.

2) Lewis P.L., Rorabeck C.H.: Periprosthetic fractures. In:*"Revision Total Knee Arthroplasty"*. Engh G.A., Rorabeck C.H.(eds.). Williams & Wilkins, Baltimore, 1997, pgg. 275-294.

3) Engh G.A., Ammen D.J.: Periprosthetic fractures adjacent to total knee implants. *J. Bone Joint Surg* 79-A, 1100-1113, 1997.

4) Rorabeck C.H., Angliss R.D., Lewis P.L.: Fractures ot the femur, tibia and patella after total knee arthroplasty: decision making and principles of management. *AAOS Istructional Course Lectures*, Volume 47, 449-458, 1998.

5) Merkel K.D., Johnson E.W.: Supracondylar fracture of the femur after total knee arthroplasty. *J Bone Joint Surg* 68-A, 29-43, 1986.

6) Figgie M.P., Goldberg V.M., Figgie H.E.III, Sobel M.: The results of treatment of supracondylar fracture above total knee arthroplasty. *J Arthroplasty* 5, 267-276, 1990.

7) McLaren A.C., Dupont J.A., Schroeber D.C.: Open reduction internal fixation of supracondylar fractures above total knee arthroplasties using the intramedullary supracondylar rod. *Clin Orthop* 302, 194-198, 1994.

8) Chen F., Mont M.A., Bachner R.S. : Management of ipsilateralsupracondylar femur fractures following total knee arthroplasty. *J Arthroplasty* 9:521-526, 1994.

9) Culp R.W., Schmidt R.G., Hanks G., Mak A., Estherhai J.L., Heppenstall R.B.: Supracondylar fracture of the femur following prosthetic knee arthroplasty. *Clin Orthop* 222, 212-222, 1987.

10) Hirsh D.M., Bhalla S., Roffman M. : Supracondylar fracture of the femur following total knee replacement. Report of four cases. *J Bone Joint Surg* 63-A, 162-163, 1981.

11) Sisto D.J., Lachiewicz P.F., Insall J.N. : Treatment of supracondylar fractures following prosthetic arthroplasty of the knee. *Clin Orthop* 196: 265-272, 1985.

12) Aaron R.K., Scott R. : Supracondylar fracture of the femur after total knee arthroplasty. *Clin Orthop* 219, 136-139, 1987.

13) Bogoch E., Hastings D., Gross A., Gshwend N.: Supracondylar fractures of the femur adjacent to resurfacing and McIntosh arthroplasties of the knee in patients with rheumatoid arthritis. *Clin Orthop* 229: 213-220, 1988.

14) Rand J.A.: Supracondylar fracture of the femur associated with polyethylene wear after total knee arthroplasty. A case report. *J Bone Joint Surg* 76-A, 1389-1393, 1994.

15) Ritter M.A., Faris P.M., Keating E.M.: Anterior femoral notching and ipsilateral femur fracture in total knee arthroplasty. *J Arthroplasty* 3:185-187, 1988.

16) Neer C.S., Grantham S.A., Shelton M.L.: Supracondylar fracture of the adult femur. A study of one hundred and ten cases. *J Bone Joint Surg.* 49-A: 591-613, 1967.

17) Insall J.N., Haas S.B.: Complications of total knee arthroplasty. In: *"Surgery of the knee"* Insall J.N. (ed.). Churchill Livingstone, New York, 1993, pp.891-934.

18) Ritter M.A., Keating E.M., Faris P.M., Mending J.B. : Rush rod fixation of supracondylar fractures above total knee arthroplasties. *J Arthroplasty* 10, 213-216, 1995.

19) Barker L.G., Ryan W.G., Paul A.S., Marsh D.R.: Zickel supracondylar nail to treat supracondylar fracture of the femur in patient with total knee replacement. *Internat J Orthop Trauma* 3: 183-85, 1993.

20) Rosenfield A.L., McQeen D.: Zickel supracondylar fixation device and Dall-Miles cables for supracondylar fractures of the femur following total knee arthroplasty. *Tech. Orthop* 6: 86-88, 1991.

21) Jabczenski F.F., Crawford M.: Retrograde intramedullary nailing of supracondylar femur fractures above total knee arthroplasty. *J Arthroplasty* 10, 95-101, 1995.

22) Murrel G.A.C., Nunley J.A.: Interlocked supracondylar intramedullary nails of supracondylar fractures after total knee arthroplasty. A new treatment method. *J Arthroplasty* 10, 37-42, 1995.

23) Healy W.L., Siliski J.M., Incavo S.J.: Operative treatment of distal femoral fractures proximal to total knee replacements. *J Bone Joint Surg* 75-A, 27-34, 1993.

24) Zehntner M.K., Ganz R.: Internal fixation of supracondylar fractures after condylar total knee arthroplasty. *Clin Orthop* 293, 219-224, 1993.

25) Moran M.C., Brick G.W., Sledge C.B., Dysart S.H., Chien E.P.: Supracondylar femoral fracture following total knee arthroplasty. *Clin Orthop* 324, 196-209, 1996.

26) Rolston L.R., Christ D.J., Halpern A., O'Connor P.L., Ryan T.g., Uggen W.M.: Treatment of supracondylar fractures of the femur proximal to a total knee arthroplasty. A report of four cases. *J Bone Joint Surg* 77-A, 924-931, 1995.

27) Cordeiro E.N., Cavalieri Costa R., Carrazzato J.G., dos Santos Silva J.: Periprosthetic fractures in patients with total knee arthroplasties. *Clin Orthop* 252, 182-189, 1990.

28) Kraay M.J., Goldberg V.M., Figgie M.K., Figgie H.E.III: Distal femoral replacement with allograft/prosthetic reconstruction for treatment of supracondylar fractures in patients with total knee arthroplasty. *J Arthroplasty* 7, 7-15, 1992.

29) Short W.H., Hootnick D.R., Murray D.G.:IpsilateralSupracondylar femur fractures following knee arthroplasty. *Clin Othop* 158, 111-116, 1981.

30) Cain P.R., Rubash H.E., Wissinger H.A., McClain E.J.: Periprosthetic femoral fractures following total knee arthroplasty. *Clin Orthop* 208, 205-214, 1986.

31) Nielsen B.F., Petersen V.S., Varmarken J.E.: Fracture of the femur after knee arthroplasty. *Acta Orthop Scand* 59, 155-157, 1988.

32) Di Gioia A.M., Rubash H.E.: Periprosthetic fractures of the femur after total knee arthroplasty. A literature review and treatment algorithm. *Clin Orthop* 271, 135-142, 1991.

33) Garvanos C., Rafiq M., Henry A.P.J.: Treatment of femoral fracture above a knee prosthesis. 18 cases followed 0.5-14 years. *Acta Orthop Scand* 65, 610-614, 1994.

34) Rand J.A., Coventry M.B.: Stress fractres after total knee arthroplasty. *J Bone Joint Surg* 62-A, 226-233, 1980.

35) Insall J., Scott N.W., Ranawat C.S.: The total condylar knee prosthesis. A report of two hundred and twenty cases. *J. Bone Joint Surg.*, 61-A, 173-180, 1979.

36) Cameron H.U., Fedorkow D.M.:The patella in total knee arthroplasty. *Clin. Orthop.* 165,:197-199, 1982.

37) Insall J.N., Lachiewicz P.F., Burstein A.H.: The posterior stabilized condylar prosthesis: a modification of the total condylar design. *J. Bone Joint Surg.* 64-A,1317-1323, 1982.

38) Larson C.M., Zhang A.X., Patrella A, Crosset L.S., Berger R.A., Rubash H.E.: Patellofemoral complications with the

IB-II P.S. total knee arthroplasty. Paper presentato al *64° Annual Meeting dell'AAOS*, 1997, San Francisco, California.

39) Grace J.N., Sim F.H.:Fracture of the patella after total knee arthroplasty. *Clin. Orthop.* 230,168-175, 1988.

40) Windsor R.E., Scuderi G.R., Insall J.N.:Patellar fractures in total knee arthroplasty. *J. Arthroplasty* 4 (suppl.), 63-67, 1989.

41) Aglietti P., Menchetti P.P.M.: Biomechanics of the patellofemoral Joint. In: *"The Patella"*. Scuderi G.R.(ed.). New York: Springer-Verlag, 1996, pp. 25-48.

42) Ahmed A.M.:Biomechanics of the patellofemoral articulation relevant to total knee replacement. In: *"Knee Surgery"*. Fu F.H., Harner C.D.,Vince K.G. (eds) Baltimora: Williams and Wilkins, 1994, pp. 1429-1450.

43) Reilly T.R., Martens M.:Experimental analysis of the quadriceps muscle reaction force and patellofemoral joint reaction force for various activities. *Acta Orthop. Scand.* 43,126-137, 1972.

44) Smith A.J.: Estimates of muscle and joint force at the knee and ankle during jumping activities. *J. Hum. Movement Stud.* 1, 126-137, 1975.

45) Scapinelli R.:Blood supply of the human patella. Its relation to ischaemic necrosis after fracture. *J. Bone Joint Surg.* 49-B,563-570, 1967.

46) Björkström S., Goldie I.F.:A study of arterial supply of the patella in the normal state,in chondromalacia patellae and in osteoathrosis. *Acta Orthop. Scan.* 51,63-70, 1980.

47) Kayler D.E., Lyttle D.:Surgical interruption of patellar blood supply by total knee arthroplasty. *Clin. Orthop.* 229,221-227, 1988.

48) Muller W.: *"The knee: form, function and ligament reconstruction"*. Muller W. (ed). New-York, Springer, 1983, fig. 198 pp.161.

49) Bonutti P.M., Mller B.G., Cremens M.J.: Patellar blood flow: evaluation of intraosseous blood supply. Paper presented at *64° Annual Meeting dell'AAOS*, 1997, San Francisco, California.

50) Hassenpflug J.: Presentation of intraosseous vascularization by sequential marcation. *Arch. Orthop. Trauma Surg.* 105, 73-78, 1986.

51) Tawakkol S., Haung T.L., Barmada R.: Quantification of the blood flow to the patella during surgical approach for total knee arthroplasty using a dog model. Poster presented at *64° Annual Meeting dell'AAOS*, 1997, San Francisco, California.

52) Ogata K., Shively R.A., Shoenecker P.L., Chang S.L. : Effects of standard surgical procedures on the patellar blood flow in monkeys. *Clin. Orthop.* 215, 254-259, 1987.

53) McMahon M.S., Scuderi G.R., Glashow J.L., Scharf S.C., Meltzer L.P., Scott W.N.:Scintigraphic determination of patellar viability after excision of infrapatellar fat pad and/or lateral retinacular release in total knee arthroplasty. *Clin. Orthop.* 260,10-16, 1990.

54) Abulencia A.E., Gibson D.H., Lynch K.J.: The effect of exercising the infrapatellar fat pad in total knee arthroplasty: a study of 161 patients. Poster exhibit presented at *64° Annual Meeting dell'AAOS*, 1997, San Francisco, California.

55) Keblish P.A.: The lateral approach to the valgus knee: surgical technique and analysis of 53 cases with over two-year follow-up evaluation. *Clin. Orthop.* 271, 52-62, 1991.

56) Engh G.A., Parks N.L., Ammeen D.J.: The influence of surgical approach on lateral retinacular releases in TKA.

Paper presented at *Scientific Meeting dell Knee Society*, 1996, Atlanta, Georgia.

57) Hofmann A.A., Plaster R.L., Murdock L.E.: Subvastus (southern) approach for primary total knee arthroplasty. *Clin. Orthop.* 269, 70- , 1991.

58) Donnachie N., Parkinson R.W., Hayward M., Bramlett K.: The tri-vector retaining arthrotomy versus the medial parapatellar arthrotomy for total knee replacement surgery. Paper presented at *Scientific Meeting della Knee Society*, 1996, San Francisco, California.

59) Scuderi G.R., Scharf S.C., Meltzer L.P., Scott W.N.:The relationship of lateral release to patellar viability in total knee arthroplasty. *J. Arthroplasty* 2, 209-214, 1987.

60) Wetzner S.M., Bezreh J.S, Scott R.D., Bierbaum B.E., Newberg A.H.:Bone scanning in the assesment of the patellar viability following knee replacement. *Clin. Orthop.* 199, 215-219, 1985.

61) Ritter M.A., Keating M.E., Faris P.M.:Clinical, roentgenographic, and scintigraphic results after interruption of the superior lateral genicular artery during total knee arthroplasty. *Clin. Orthop.* 248,145-151, 1989.

62) Ritter M.A., Herbst S.A., Keating E.M., Faris P.M., Mending J.B.: Patellofemoral complications following total knee arthroplasty. *J. Arthroplasty* 11, 368-372, 1996.

63) Scott R.D., Turoff N., Ewald F.C.:Stress fracture of the patella following duopatellar total knee arthroplasty. *Clin. Orthop.* 170,147-151, 1982.

64) Brick G.W., Scott R.D.:The patellofemoral component of total knee arthropalsty. *Clin. Orthop.* 231, 163-178, 1988.

65) Berman A.T., Reid J.S., Yanicko D.R., Sih G.C., Zimmerman H.R.:Thermally induced bone necrosis in rabbits: relation to implant failure in humans. *Clin. Orthop.* 186,284-292, 1984.

66) Jefferiss C.D., Lee C., Ling R.S.M.: Thermal aspects of self-curing polymethylmethacrylate. *J. Bone Joint Surg.* 57-B, 511-518, 1975.

67) Toksvig-Larsen S., Franzen H., Ryd L: Cement interface temperature in hip arthroplasty. *Acta Orthop. Scand.* 62, 102-105, 1991.

68) Insall J.N.: Surgical techniques and instrumentation in total knee arthroplasty.In: *"Surgery of The Knee"*. Insall J.N., Windsor R.E.,Scott W.N., et al. (eds) New York: Churchill Livingstone, 1993, pp. 739-804.

69) Kurzweil P.R.: Analysis of the no thumb rule to assess patellar tracking during total knee arthroplasty. Paper presented at *64° Annual Meeting dell'AAOS*, 1997, San Francisco, California.

70) Aglietti P., Buzzi R., Giron F., Zaccherotti G.: The Insall-Burstein posterior stabilized total knee replacement in the valgus knee. *Am. J. Knee Surg.* 9, 8-12, 1996.

71) Miyasaka K.C., Ranawat C.S., Mullaj A.: Total knee arthroplasty in the valgus knee: intermediate- term results and technique for ligament balancing. Paper presented at *Scientific Meeting della Knee Society*, 1996, San Francisco, California.

72) Goldfarb S.J., Bullek D.D., Scuderi G., Insall J.N.: The constrained condylar total knee arthroplasty for valgus deformity in the elderly patient. Paper presented at *64° Annual Meeting dell'AAOS*, 1997, San Francisco, California.

73) Miller M.C., Zhang A.X., Patrella A., Crosset L.S., Berger R.A., Rubash H.E.: A comprehensive in vitro study of the effects of component placement on total knee kinematics and patellofemoral load transfer. Scientific Exibit presented at *64° Annual Meeting dell'AAOS*, 1997, San Francisco, California.

74) Star M.J., Kaufman K.R., Irby S.E., Colwell C.W. Jr.: The effects of patellar thickness on patellofemoral forces after resurfacing. *Clin. Orthop.* 322, 279-284, 1996.

75) Oishi C.S., Kaufman K.R., Irby S.E., Colwell C.W.: Effects of patellar thickness on compression and shear forces in total knee arthroplasty. Clin. Orthop. 331, 283-290, 1996.

76) Reuben J.D., McDonald C.L., Woodard P.L., Hennington L.J.:Effect of patella thickness on patella strain following total knee arthroplasty. *J. Arthroplasty* 6, 251-258, 1991.

77) Josefchak R.G., Finlay J.B., Bourne R.B., Rorabeck C.H.:Cancellous bone support for patellar resurfacing. *Clin. Orthop.* 220, 192-199, 1987.

78) Clayton M.L., Thirupathy R.:Patellar complications after total condylar arthroplasty. *Clin. Ortrhop.* 170,152-155, 1982.

79) Aglietti P., Insall J.N., Walker P.S., Trent P.:A new patella prosthesis. Design and application. *Clin. Orthop.* 107, 175-187, 1975.

80) Hsu H.P., Walker P.S.:Wear and deformation of patellar components in total knee arthroplasty. Clin. Orthop. 246, 260-265, 1989.

81) Freeman M.A.R., Samuelson K.M., Elias S.G., Mariorenzi L.J., Gokcay E.I., Tuke M.: The patellofemoral Joint in total knee prostheses. Design considerations. *J. Arthroplasty* 4(suppl), 69-74, 1989.

82) Gomes L.S.M., Bechtold J.E., Gustilo R.B.: Patellar prosthesis positioning in total knee arthroplasty. A roetngenographic study. *Clin. Orthop.* 236, 72-81, 1989.

83) Sandquist P., Tao S.S., Nelissen R.G.H.H., Weidenheilm L.R.A., Mikhail M.N., Mikhail W.E.M.: Effect of patellar prosthetic design on tracking and incidence of lateral retinacular release, minimum follow-up five years. Poster presented at *64° Annual Meeting dell'AAOS*, 1997, San Francisco, California.

84) Buechel F.F, Rosa R.A., Pappas M.J.:A metal-backed, rotating-bearing patellar prosthesis to lower contact stresses. An 11-year clinical study. *Clin. Orthop.* 248, 34-49, 1989.

85) Petersilge W.J., Oishi C.S., Kaufman K.R., Irby S.E., Colwell C.W.Jr.: The effect of throclear design on patellofemoral shear and compressive forces in total knee arthroplasty. *Clin. Orthop.* 309,124-129, 1994.

86) Churcill D., Incavo S., Jewell R., Beynnonn B.: A comparison of patello-femoral contact loads in the normal knee and total knee arthroplasty. presented at *43° Annual Meeting della Orthopaedic Research Society*, 1997, San Francisco, California.

87) Theiss S.M., Kitziger K.J., Lotke P.S., Lotke P.A.: Component design affecting patellofemoral complications after total knee arthroplasty. *Clin. Orthop.* 326,183-187, 1996.

88) Andriacchi T.P., Yoder D., Conley A., Rosemberg A., Sum J., Galante J.O.: A relationship between patellofemoral mechanics and patient function following total knee replacement. Paper presented at *Interim Meeting della Knee Society*, 1996, Boston, Massachusset.

89) Chew J.T.H., Stewart N.J., Hanssen A.D., Zong-Ping Luo, Rand J.A., Kai-Nan An : Difference in patellar tracking and knee kinematics between three total knee arthroplasty designs. Paper presented at *Scientific Meeting della Knee Society*, 1996, San Francisco, California.

90) Sthiel J.B., Komistek R.D., Dennis D.A., Paxon R.D.: Fluoroscopic analysis of the kinematics after posterrior cruciate retaining knee arthroplasty. *J. Bone Joint Surg.* 77-B, 884-889, 1995.

91) Komistek K.R., Dennis D.A., Walker S.A., Northcut E.J.: In vivo determination of patellofemoral implant loading conditions. Paper presented at *64° Annual Meeting dell'AAOS*, 1997, San Francisco, California.

92) Komistek K.R., Dennis D.A., Walker S.A., Northcut E.J., Kettler P.: An in vivo determination of patellofemoral contact position. Paper presented at *64° Annual Meeting dell'AAOS*, 1997, San Francisco, California.

93) Figgie H.E., Goldberg V.M., Heiple K.G., Moller H.S., Gordon N.H.: The influence of tibial-patellofemoral location on function of the knee in patients with posterior stabilized condylar knee prosthesis. *J. Bone Joint Surg.* 68-A,1035-1040, 1986.

94) Figgie H.E., Goldberg V.M., Figgie M, Inglis A.E., Kelly M., Sobel M.: The effect of alignment of the implant on fractures of the patella after condylar total knee arthroplasty. *J. Bone Joint. Surg.* 71-A,1031-1039, 1989.

95) Fern E.D., Winson I.G., Getty C.J.M.: Anterior knee pain in rheumatoid patients after total knee replacement. Possible selection criteria for patellar resurfacing. *J.Bone Joint Surg.* 74-B, 745-748, 1992.

96) Lewonowski K., Dorr L.D., McPherson E.J., Huber G., Zhinian Wan: Medialization of the patella in total knee arthroplasty. *J. Arthroplasty* 12, 161-167, 1997.

97) Yoshii I., Witheside L.A., Anouchy Y.S.: The effect of patellar button placement and femoral component design on patellar tracking in total knee arthroplsty. *Clin. Orthop.* 275, 211-219, 1992.

98) Merkow R.L., Soudry M., Insall J.N.: Patellar dislocation following total knee replacement. *J. Bone Joint Surg. Am.* 67, 1321-1327, 1985.

99) Rhoads D.D., Noble P.C., Reuben J.D., Mahoney O.M., Tullos H.S.: The effect of femoral component position on patellar tracking after total knee arthroplasty. *Clin. Orthop.* 260, 43-51, 1990.

100) Rhoads D.D., Noble P.C., Reuben J.D., Tullos H.S.:The effect of femoral component position on the kinematics of total knee arthroplasty. *Clin. Orthop.* 285,122-129, 1993.

101) Anouchi Y.S., Witheside L.A., Kaiser A.D., Milliano M.T.: Effects of axial rotational alignment of the femoral component on knee stability and patellar tracking in total knee arthroplsty demonstrated on autopsy specimens. *Clin. Orthop.* 287,170-177, 1993.

102) Arima J., Whiteside L.A., McCarthy D.S., White E.S.: Femoral rotational alignment, based on anteroposterior axis, in total knee arthroplasty in valgus knee. *J. Bone Joint Surg.* 77-A, 1331-1334, 1995.

103) Berger R.A., Rubash H.E., Seel M.J., Thompson W.H., Crossett L.: Determining the rotational alignment of the femoral component in total knee arthroplasty using epicondylar axis. *Clin. Orthop.* 286, 40-47, 1993.

104) Poilvache P.L., Insall J.N., Scuderi G.R., Font-Rodriguez D.E.: Rotational landmarks and sizing of the distal femur in total knee arthroplasty. *Clin. Orthop.* 331, 35-46, 1996.

105) De Muth B.C., Scuderi G.R., Insall J.N.: The effect of the epicondylar axis on patellar tracking in total knee arthroplasty. Paper presented at *64° Annual Meeting della AAOS*, 1997, San Francisco, California.

106) Nagamine R., Witheside L.A., White S.E., McCarthy D.S.:Patellar tracking after total knee arthroplasty: the effect of tibial tray malrotation and articular surface configuration. *Clin. Orthop.* 304, 263-271, 1994.

107) Eckhoff D.G., Metzger R.G., Vandewalle M.V.: Malrotation associated with implant alignment technique in total knee arthroplasty. Paper presented at *Scientific Meeting della Knee Society*, 1995, Orlando, Florida.

108) Spitzer A.I., Vince K.G.:Patellar considerations in total knee arthroplasty.In: "The patella". Scuderi G.R. (ed). New York:Springer-Verlag,1995,pp. 309-331.

109) Insall J.N.: Complications of total knee arthroplasty.In *"Surgery of The Knee"*. Insall J.N., Windsor R.E.,Scott W.N., et al. (eds) New York: Churchill Livingstone, 1993, pp. 891-934.

110) Goldberg V.M., Figgie H.E., Inglis A.E., Figgie M., Sobel M.,Kelly M., Kraay M.J.:Patellar fracture type and pro-gnosis in condylar total knee arthroplasty. *Clin. Orthop.* 236,115-122, 1988.

111) Tria A.J., Harwood D.A., Alicea J.A., Cody R.P.: Patellar fractures in posterior stabilized knee arthroplasties. *Clin. Orthop.* 299,131-138, 1994.

112) Roffman M., Hirsh D.M., Mendes D.G.:Fracture of the re-surfaced patella in total knee replacement. *Clin. Orthop.* 148,112-116, 1980.

113) Thompson F.M., Hood R.W., Insall J.N.:Patellar fractures in total knee arthroplasty. *Orthop. Trans.* 5,516, 1981.

114) Hozack W.J., Goll S.R., Lotke P.A., Rothman R.H., Booth R.E.:The treatment of patellar fractures after total knee arthroplasty. *Clin. Orthop.* 236,123-127, 1988.

Chapter 19
Prophylaxis of Deep Vein Thrombosis After Total Knee Arthroplasty

Geoffrey H. Westrich - Steven B. Haas
The Hospital for Special Surgery - New York

Introduction

Patients who undergo elective total knee replacement are at a high risk for deep venous thrombosis, which can lead to potentially fatal pulmonary embolism. The incidence of deep vein thrombosis after total knee replacement has been reported to be between 50 and 88 % (1, 2, 3). While the majority of these thrombi occur in the calf veins and resolve without symptoms, up to 24% may propagate to the proximal veins (1). Approximately 3-10% of patient will develop proximal thrombi in the week following total knee replacement.

The occurrence of clinically significant pulmonary embolism is relatively uncommon and the symptoms are easily confused with other cardiac or pulmonary conditions found in the older population. The incidence of symptomatic pulmonary emboli detected by routine lung scans has been reported to be between 7 and 17% (1, 2). The reported incidence of symptomatic pulmonary emboli is generally reported to be 1-3% (100, 101), however, this is probably an underestimate since many pulmonary emboli do not occur until several weeks or even months following the surgery.

Clearly, prevention is the best solution for thromboembolic disease. This is especially true if one considers the risks involved in treatment of early proximal deep vein thrombosis and pulmonary embolism. Patterson et al (7) reported that heparin therapy used within the first five days following total joint replacement surgery was associated with a 51% complication rate. The morbidity and mortality associated with untreated symptomatic pulmonary emboli and proximal DVT is also high (8).

Deep venous thrombosis alone may or may not be symptomatic, but subsequent pulmonary embolism has the potential to be life threatening. Therefore, common knowledge about the prevention, diagnosis, and treatment of thromboembolic disease is essential to any physician who treats patients with disorders of the lower extremity. Furthermore, deep venous thrombosis should always be included in the differential diagnosis of pain and/or swelling in lower limb.

Thromboembolic Disease: Overview

While Virchow initially described venous thromboembolism in 1856 (10), the true morbidity and mortality in patients was not recognized until many years later. Approximately 90% of clinically important pulmonary embolism arise from proximal deep vein thrombosis of the lower extremities, and it is estimated that pulmonary embolism may be fatal in 50,000 to 100,000 individuals a year. This statistic results in 5% to 10% of all hospital deaths in the United States annually. Venous thromboembolism is the third most common vascular disease, following acute ischemic attacks and cerebrovascular accidents. Unfortunately, pulmonary embolism is difficult to diagnose and has the potential to be rapidly fatal. Among the patients who will eventually die of a pulmonary embolism, two-thirds will survive less than thirty minutes after the event, which is insufficient for most forms of treatment to be effective (28). Certainly, preventing deep venous thrombosis is preferable to treating the condition after the diagnosis is established. Fortunately, the presence of clinical risk factors can be used to identify patients at greatest risk (29). However, despite convincing evidence of the efficacy of a number of prophylactic agents, physicians have been slow to adapt these preventative regimens in patients at risk for thromboembolic disease.

Thromboembolic disease continues to pose a major threat for patients undergoing lower extremity surgery. A deep venous thrombosis occurs when one or more of the veins in the calf becomes obstructed to venous blood flow. In high risk patients, such as total joint replacement of the hip and knee, the incidence of deep vein thrombosis without postoperative prophylaxis diagnosed by venography has been reported as high as 88% (1, 2, 3). The majority of these thrombi occur in the deep veins of the calf; however, propagation of a calf thrombosis to a more proximal location in the popliteal or femoral veins is also known to occur. Using serial venous Doppler ultrasound, the rate of propagation after total knee replacement surgery has been documented at 23% (4). Therefore, one must be cognizant of the fact that a deep venous thrombosis in the calf has the potential to propagate, and one should follow these patients expectantly.

Pulmonary emboli result when a deep venous thrombosis in the lower extremity or pelvis embolizes through the right heart and into the pulmonary vasculature. As a result, a thromboembolism may lodge within the pulmonary artery, thus causing an obstruction of perfusion to the lung. While many pulmonary emboli are asymptomatic, such an event may be fatal. The size and location of the pulmonary embolism is related to the morbidity and mortality of the event with a large saddle-type embolism producing the greatest risk of mortality. After total joint replacement, the incidence of asymptomatic pulmonary emboli detected by routine lung scans has been reported to be between 10 to 20%, while the incidence of symptomatic pulmonary emboli is between 1 and 2% (5, 6). Many surgeons may ignore the possibility of thromboembolic disease, since the occurrence of clinically significant pulmonary embolism is relatively uncommon and the symptoms are easily confused with other medical conditions, such as cardiac or pulmonary problems.

Prevention of thromboembolic disease is essential to avoid the morbidity and mortality associated with this condition. A significant risk of hemorrhagic complications is associated with anticoagulation for thromboembolic disease in the immediate postoperative period. After total joint replacement surgery, Patterson et al. (7) reported that anticoagulation with heparin used within the first five postoperative days was associated with a complication rate over 50%. Unfortunately, the associated morbidity and mortality with untreated symptomatic thromboembolic disease is also significant (8).

Risk Factors for Thromboembolic Disease

Multiple risk factors have been identified that increase a patient's predisposition towards

Table 1: CLASSIFICATION OF LEVEL OF RISK

Thromboembolic event	Low risk (uncomplicated minor surgey in patients age > 40 with no other risk factors)	Moderate risk (Major surgery in patients age > 40 with no other risk factors)	High risk (Major surgery in patients age > 40 with additional risk factors)	Very high risk (Major surgery in patients age > 40 with history of thromboembolism, malignancy, major orthopedic surgery, cerebrovascular event or spinal cord injury)
Calf vein thrombosis	2%	10-20%	20-40%	40-80%
Proximal vein thrombosis	0.4%	2-4%	4-8%	10-20%
Clinical pulmonary embolism	0.2%	1-2%	2-4%	4-10%
Fatal pulmonary embolism	0.002%	0.1-0.4%	0.4-1.0%	1-5%

Adapted from Clagett et al.

the development of thromboembolism. While these factors will be discussed below individually, one should recognize that patients may have multiple risk factors that may further increase their propensity to develop a thromboembolic event. As such, patients should be classified as to their relative level of risk. (Table 1).

History of Thromboembolism

Patients with a history of thromboembolic disease are at a significant risk for repeat thromboembolism. In a hospitalized patient who has a history of thromboembolic disease, there is almost an eight-fold increase in acute thromboembolism compared with patients without such a history. As such, this is one of the more important risk factors for thromboembolic disease. Patients with a history of thromboembolic disease who undergo major surgery, immobilization, or a protracted hospitalization for serious medical illness must be considered very high risk. Thromboembolic disease prophylaxis is mandatory in this cohort of patients.

Elective Lower Extremity Surgery

Orthopedic surgery of the lower extremity is well appreciated as one of the most significant risk factors for development of thromboembolic disease. Without prophylaxis, over 50% of patients undergoing elective total joint replacement surgery may develop a deep venous thrombosis (34). Over 90% of proximal thrombi occur on the operated side in hip replacement. Twisting and kinking of the common femoral vein during the surgical procedure has been shown to occlude femoral venous return and also damage venous endothelium.

Patient Age

The incidence of thromboembolic disease increases exponentially between ages 20 and 80 (30). Although a patient age of 40 years has traditionally been used as an indication for an age-related increase in thromboembolic disease, the risk continues to increase after age 40, and nearly doubling with each successive decade. Thromboembolic disease is rare in children and usually occurs with high-risk situations, such as multiple trauma and lower extremity fractures.

Immobility

It is widely accepted that immobilization results in an increased risk for the development of thromboembolic disease. An autopsy study noted a 15% incidence of thrombosis in patients at bed rest for less than 1 week compared to 80% in patients at bed rest for greater than 1 week (39). Early mobilization of all patients following surgery or trauma is necessary to prevent thromboembolism. Immobilization secondary to traumatic spinal cord injury and paralysis of lower extremities has an associated risk of thromboembolic disease that approaches 40%.

Obesity

While obesity is usually cited as a risk factor for the development of thromboembolism, the actual risk is unclear. It is possible that obese patients with other risk factors may have an additive or synergistic risk for thromboembolism, however, this is speculation and has not been scientifically established. Furthermore, the term obesity is subjective and open to interpretation. One should use a percent over ideal body weight to truly study obesity.

Oral Contraceptives and Estrogen Therapy

While historically oral contraceptives were associated with an increased risk of thromboembolism, current preparations utilize less estrogen and are associated with a significantly lower risk of thromboembolic disease. Presently, the mortality from oral contraceptives is considered to be less than the risk of pregnancy itself. Although estrogen therapy may increase incidence of thromboembolism in patients with prostate cancer, estrogen replacement therapy in women appears not to be an additional risk factor (42, 43)

Hypercoagulable States

Lately, more attention has been directed to systemic hematological abnormalities that may predispose patients to thromboembolism. The presence of a lupus anticoagulant as well as deficiencies of protein-S, protein-C, and antithrombin III all reduce the fibrinolytic activity and put the patient at increased risk of thromboembolism.

Pathogenesis

The formation of deep vein thrombosis is multifactorial and best described by Virchow in 1846 (10). Virchow's Triad established the basis of our understanding of the pathogenesis of deep vein thrombosis and includes hypercoagulability, endothelial injury, and venous stasis (10). In the human vascular system, there is a delicate balance between thrombosis and fibrinolysis, and total knee replacement surgery affects all three aspects of Virchow's Triad. Hypercoagulability occurs due to activation of clotting factors with a decrease in anti-thrombin III levels and changes in platelet activity. Also, bone surgery produces the release of thromboplastins that further activate the clotting cascade. Surgery may also lead to endothelial injury of the vessels. Venous stasis occurs by two mechanisms: the use of a tourniquet or by postoperative immobilization thus inhibiting the normal venous return in the low extremity. Post operative swelling and limited ambulation further contribute to venous stasis and the establishment of a milieu that facilitates the formation of deep venous thrombosis.

Other co-morbidities further contribute to the formation of deep venous thrombosis or subsequent pulmonary embolism, and the surgeon should be aware of these risk factors preoperatively. Such risk factors include advanced age (over 40 years), female gender, obesity, immobilization, oral contraceptive use, superficial thrombophlebitis, a history of previous deep venous thrombosis or pulmonary embolism, cardiac disease. If one considers the fact that most patients undergoing knee replacement are elderly and many have co-morbid conditions, it is obvious that these patients are at extremely high risk for developing deep vein thrombosis.

Diagnosis of Thromboembolism

It must be understood that the majority of deep venous thromboses are asymptomatic, and therefore, not grossly apparent on physical examination. However, when the clinical suspicion of thrombosis in the lower extremity does exist, the accuracy of the physical examination for the diagnosis of deep venous thrombosis (i.e., Homan's sign, cords, edema etc.) is notoriously unreliable. Therefore, screening tests, such as a venogram or an ultrasound imaging study, are often utilized to establish if a deep venous thrombosis exists (86). In addition,

many current treatment protocols rely on the location and the extent of a DVT in the lower extremity as determined by the screening test.

Routine postoperative screening for deep vein thrombosis is performed in many institutions; however, the type of screening test varies considerably (72-86). In addition, the efficacy of such tests is dependent upon the technician that performs the study, as well as the radiologist that interprets the findings (72-86). This has become so variable that some authors have recommended that each institution should perform an internal validity study to assess the sensitivity, specificity, predictive values, and accuracy of the screening test that is utilized within that institution (38, 60). In addition, a "learning curve" has been noted with such techniques that warrant initial study and then subsequent study to document improvement in the reliability of the screening test (70). Some centers use routine deep vein thrombosis screening with duplex ultrasonography prior to discharge. The sensitivity of duplex ultrasound scanning varies widely, and has been shown to be extremely operator dependent (11). Since the sensitivity is lowest for calf thrombi, a follow-up duplex study may be beneficial for detecting distal thrombi that may propagate.

At the Hospital for Special Surgery, the efficacy of ultrasound compared to ascending venography for the detection of deep venous thrombosis after total knee arthroplasty was assessed after a two-year interval (104). Ascending venography was the considered the "gold standard" to which all ultrasound studies were compared. Overall, the sensitivity of ultrasound was 85%. Two years ago, our initial assessment of ultrasound for the detection of deep venous thrombosis in postoperative total knee arthroplasty patients revealed .a 75% sensitivity (99). Our initial assessment of color Doppler imaging for the detection of thrombosis in postoperative total joint replacement patients was less than satisfactory, but improved significantly after the technician gained experience. Due to the limitations of duplex ultrasound screening and its associated cost, we have almost eliminated routine screening after major orthopedic procedures and now routinely provide secondary post discharge prophylaxis for six weeks postoperatively.

Prophylactic Regimens

The ultimate goal of any prophylactic regimen is to prevent not only the formation of a deep venous thrombosis, but also the occurrence of symptomatic or fatal pulmonary emboli. However, the incidence of symptomatic and fatal pulmonary emboli is low, and as a result, a definitive evaluation of the various prophylaxis regimens would require many thousands of patients. Therefore, most studies have focused on the prevention of deep vein thrombosis. While there are limitations in this methodology, studies have shown that deep vein thrombosis places a patient at risk for pulmonary emboli (33, 34). Proximal thrombi represent the greatest risk; however, calf thrombi have also been shown to propagate to the proximal veins in approximately 23% of patients and have been correlated with the occurrence of both symptomatic and asymptomatic pulmonary emboli (31, 32). Numerous prophylactic regimens have been studied in orthopedic surgery and include pharmacological agents such as warfarin, low molecular weight heparins (LMWH) and aspirin as well as mechanical devices such as compression stockings and foot pumps.

Warfarin

Warfarin has become a popular form of prophylaxis following orthopedic surgery. Warfarin is an oral anticoagulant that inhibits the blood coagulation cascade by affecting the synthesis of active Vitamin K-dependent coagulation factors (factors II, 7, 9 and 10 as well as protein C). Since warfarin inhibits synthesis of active coagulation factors, it has no effect on existing circulating coagulation factors. Therapeutic anticoagulation is reached from 24-72 hours after the initial dose of warfarin. Most commonly 5 or 10 mg of Coumadin is started the night before or the night of surgery and then dosing is adjusted to maintain an INR (international normalized ratio) of 2.0 - 2.5.

Risks for using warfarin include bleeding and less frequently, warfarin induced skin necrosis. Bleeding complications have been reported in 0-4% of patients receiving warfarin prophylaxis (54, 55, 56). Another pitfall associated with the use of warfarin is the need to monitor the prothrombin time. The advantages of warfarin prophylaxis are that warfarin is administered orally and that it can be continued as treatment if deep venous thrombosis is detected.

Like most prophylactic regimens, the incidence of deep vein thrombosis using low dose warfarin varies considerably depending upon the patient population at risk. Although warfarin appears to be an effective agent in reducing the incidence of deep vein thrombosis after total hip replacement, its efficacy in knee replacement surgery is not clear. Warfarin may limit propagation and embolization of a thrombus after total knee arthroplasty, but it has not clearly been shown to decrease the occurrence of deep vein thrombosis.

Low Molecular Weight Heparin

Low molecular weight heparins are a relatively new form of prophylaxis that has been popularized in Europe and is currently being evaluated in the United States. Low molecular weight heparin was developed in the 1970s and has been shown to have very good anti-thrombotic activity, and when compared to standard heparin, the low molecular weight heparins have less bleeding per unit of equivalent anti-thrombotic effect. Low molecular weight heparins are the fractionated forms of heparin with a molecular weight ranging from 4000 - 6000 Daltons. There are several low molecular weight heparin compounds produced by various pharmaceutical companies, each differing in its fractionation technique and dosing schedule. However, all low molecular weight heparins contain a specific tetra-saccharide that binds anti-thrombin III. Because of their smaller size they can bind anti-thrombin III and this complex can inactivate coagulation factor Xa to a greater extent than factor IIa. Its small size also inhibits their combining with heparin co-factor II, a specific mediator that inactivates factor IIa. These compounds have a high bio-availability at low doses, unlike standard heparin, since they only bind to one circulating protein. low molecular weight heparins are administered in a fixed dose without daily monitoring of partial thromboplastin time.

Currently only Enoxaparin is approved by the FDA for deep vein thrombosis prophylaxis in patients undergoing orthopedic surgery or trauma. Dalteparin is approved by the FDA for general surgical use, but has not been approved for orthopaedic surgery at this time. The advantages of a low molecular weight heparin are that they are easily administered in the hospital with subcutaneous injection, and they do not require monitoring with partial thromboplastin times. Risks associated with using low molecular weight heparins include bleeding and heparin induced thrombocytopenia. Major bleeding complications have been reported in 0-2.8% of patients. Other disadvantages are that they are relatively expensive, they require self-injection or help with injection if administered following discharge, and that they have a known associated risk of bleeding.

Aspirin

Aspirin (acetylsalicylic acid) is a nonsteroidal anti-inflammatory agent that irreversibly inhibits the cyclo-oxygenase of platelets, thereby inhibiting the synthesis of thromboxane A2 (12). Thromboxane A2 causes platelet aggregation and vasoconstriction. Aspirin has been reported to be an effective antithrombotic agent in patients with ischemic heart disease and cerebrovascular disease. It gained popularity as a prophylactic modality in orthopaedic patients after early reports of success in total hip replacement (12). Follow-up reports and further evaluation revealed that aspirin is not an effective agent in preventing deep vein thrombosis in patients who had total joint replacement surgery or trauma.

Some authors have recommended the continued use of aspirin after hospital discharge as a secondary prophylactic agent (14). These authors note that aspirin is safe, associated with a low rate of pulmonary emboli and that most thrombi that occur with the use of aspirin are found in the calf veins. Risks of using aspirin include gastritis, gastric erosions and gastric ulcers. These side effects appear to be dose related. Most regimens employ aspirin by mouth, 325 mg to 650 mg twice daily.

We do not routinely use aspirin as a single prophylactic agent after major orthopedic surgery; however, we have noted that when aspirin is combined with routine venographic screening and treatment of detected thrombi, it is associated with a low rate of symptomatic and fatal pulmonary emboli.

Mechanical Devices

Mechanical devices and physical agents have been used for the prophylaxis of deep vein thrombosis after a variety of surgical procedures or trauma. Early mobilization, continuous passive motion machines, and graded compression stockings have all been advocated. A number of studies have demonstrated that mechanical devices designed to reduce venous stasis are effective in reducing the rate of deep venous thrombosis following total joint arthroplasty (31, 32, 45-51, 57, 60, 67-70, 72, 74, 76-

78, 84, 85, 89, 90, 93, 94, 97). Currently, marketed devices incorporate different parameters such as foot pumps, foot-calf pumps, calf pumps, and calf-thigh pumps, whereas some are single chamber yet others provide sequential chambers with a number of chambers. Although the optimal characteristics of these pumps to reduce deep venous thrombosis and pulmonary embolism are not yet known, it has been proposed that pneumatic compression devices are effective by two mechanisms: decreased stasis (accelerated venous emptying) and increased fibrinolysis (28, 32, 45-51, 60, 67-70, 72, 74, 76, 84, 85, 90, 94, 97). However, the relative contribution of these two mechanisms is unknown. Newer devices that produce impulse pumping, as opposed to a slow rise in venous return, have recently been introduced, and while some of these devices are thought to produce an increased peak venous velocity, it is unclear what is the optimal contribution of increased venous velocity or increased venous volume necessary to provide adequate deep venous thrombosis prophylaxis in the lower extremity (32, 45, 47-51, 67, 69, 70, 76, 90, 94, 97, 98). In addition, the fibrinolytic effect of such impulse pumping devices has not been elucidated.

Intermittent pneumatic devices include polyvinyl boots or leggings, stockings with inflatable bladders, multi compartment vinyl leggings and more recently foot pumps (15, 16). Generally pressures reach 35-55 mm of mercury and inflate in cycles of 60-90 seconds. The devices are intended to decrease stasis by augmenting venous flow in the lower extremities. In addition, studies have shown stimulation of the fibrinolytic system with the intermittent compression (17).

The boot or stockings can be applied to the non-operative leg preoperatively and postoperatively begun on the operative extremity. The pneumatic devices are continued until the patient is ambulating independently. The pneumatic devices can also be used in conjunction with continuous passive motion.

The incidence of deep vein thrombosis with the use of calf and thigh length devices has been reported to be between 7.5 and 33% after unilateral total knee arthroplasty (18, 19, 20, 21, 22, 23, 32). Haas et al. evaluated the efficacy of a multi chamber thigh length pneumatic compression stockings compared to aspirin in a randomized prospective study and found that the incidence of deep vein thrombosis was reduced to 22% with pneumatic stockings compared to

47% with aspirin (5). The greatest reduction was seen in large thrombi (greater than 6 cm) which were reduced from 31% with aspirin to 6% with the pneumatic stockings. Patients undergoing simultaneous bilateral total knee arthroplasty are at even higher risk for development of deep vein thrombosis. Despite the use of pneumatic compression stockings 48% of patients developed a deep vein thrombosis.

More recently there has been interest in the use of foot pump devices. These devices increase venous circulation by applying a rapid increase in pressure to the plantar plexus. Studies have shown that these devices can lead to a significant increase in venous flow in the lower extremity (51). Two studies have evaluated foot pumps in knee replacement. Westrich and Sculco evaluated the efficacy of the PlexiPulse (NuTech, San Antonio, Texas) device combined with aspirin compared to aspirin alone (24). The authors found a significant reduction in deep vein thrombosis with the use of a PlexiPulse; 27% of patients using the Plexipulse developed a deep vein thrombosis compared to 59% with aspirin alone. While no patient using Plexipulse developed a proximal thrombi, 14% of the patients using aspirin alone were found to have proximal thrombi. Westrich also evaluated compliance and found a relationship between deep vein thrombosis and the duration for which the device was used. Wilson et al. also evaluated the efficacy of foot compression after knee arthroplasty (16). They found a significant reduction in proximal thrombi; 19% in the control group compared to 0% with foot pumps.

Pneumatic devices have been shown in numerous studies to lower the incidence of both proximal and distal thromboses after total joint replacement. Additionally, these devices have been associated with an extremely low rate of complications. Generally, however, they are not recommended to be used on patients who have severe peripheral vascular disease. The devices are relatively inexpensive but compliance problems have been noted by some. The foot pump devices appear to be well tolerated and we are now using them routinely on our knee replacement patients at The Hospital for Special Surgery. The use of foot pumps or other mechanical compression devices after surgery or trauma of the foot and ankle may be difficult, since most of these patients are immobilized in a splint or cast. While "under cast" pads are available for mechanical compression, these devices have not been studied for their clinical efficacy.

Recommended Prophylaxis

It is well accepted that patients undergoing major orthopedic surgery are at very high risk for the development of thromboembolic disease, and they should receive an effective primary prophylactic agent to prevent this predicament. The type of prophylactic regimen, however, is dependent not only upon the patient's relative risks factors for the development of thromboembolism, but also the type and duration of surgical intervention. The ideal type of prophylaxis would inhibit all thrombus formation and allow healing of the surgical site without bleeding or other complications. Unfortunately, there is no such prophylaxis regimen currently available. As discussed in the previous section, the several prophylactic regimens that are commercially available and would satisfy the necessity for prophylaxis, do not inhibit all thrombus formation and also have some associated risks.

Despite primary prophylaxis, some patients will develop deep vein thrombi that are mostly limited to the calf veins. These patients therefore require secondary prophylaxis to prevent the propagation and embolization of these thrombi, as well as the prevention of late thrombi formation. We therefore feel that prophylaxis should be continued post operatively for a period of three to six weeks. We have used low dose warfarin for secondary prophylaxis following discharge although others have recommended the use of low molecular weight heparins or aspirin.

This author maintains that the surgeon is obliged to discuss the possibility of thromboembolism with any patient who plans to have knee replacement surgery and especially evaluate patients to determine who may be at increased risk. In patients with known risk factors such as previous thromboembolism, age greater than 40 years, history of malignancy, obesity etc., postoperative prophylaxis is strongly encouraged.

Meta Analysis

We recently conducted a meta analysis to evaluate the efficacy of various prophylactic regimens in total knee replacement (102). Meta analysis is a methodologic technique that employs a standardized and prospective method of data extraction and statistical analysis to integrate the results of numerous individual studies. The efficacy of four prophylactic regimens: pneumatic devices, warfarin, low molecular weight heparins (LMWH), and aspirin. A complete English literature search was conducted from January 1980 to June 1996. Studies which evaluated any of the four prophylactic regimens were used. Only studies that employed routine venographic screening for deep vein thrombosis or routine lung scans for pulmonary emboli were included. 130 studies were identified and 105 excluded, most commonly for lack of venographic screening. 25 studies which included 6,060 patients were included in the analysis. Pneumatic devices were associated with the lowest DVT rate 18%, followed by 30% with LMWHs, 44% for warfarin and 53% for aspirin. Asymptomatic pulmonary emboli occurred in 6% of patients who received pneumatic devices, warfarin 8% and aspirin 11%. No symptomatic pulmonary emboli were reported in the studies using pneumatic devices for prophylaxis compared to 0.3% for patients receiving LMWHs, 0.5% for warfarin and 1.2%.

Treatment of Established Thromboembolism

Treatment of deep vein thrombosis in the postoperative knee replacement patient is not without potential complication and the goals for treatment must be clearly defined. Preventing emobolization of the clot is the primary concern because of the possibility of fatal pulmonary embolism. Morbidity from post-phlebitic syndrome and pulmonary hypertension are also concerns. Numerous factors must be taken into consideration when deciding on the appropriate treatment including: the location of the thrombi, the patient's age, the underlying medical status, the history of previous thromboembolism, and time interval since surgery.

Treatment regimens for deep vein thrombosis include anticoagulants, vena caval interruption devices, or, in the case of calf thrombosis, serial clinical or ultrasound monitoring.

Anticoagulants

The most commonly used anticoagulants are heparin and warfarin; however, more recently LMWHs are being investigated for treatment of deep vein thrombosis. Medical patients without contraindication to anticoagulation are generally treated with initial administration of intravenous heparin along with the initiation of warfarin therapy. When the warfarin dosage is therapeutic with an INR (International Normalized Ratio) between 2.0 - 2.5 (Prothrombin time at 1.3 - 1.5 x normal) the heparin is discontinued. Warfarin is generally continued for a period of approximately six weeks to three months.

Unfortunately, intravenous heparin therapy in the postoperative period has been shown to be associated with a high incidence of complications. Such complications include: bleeding at the operative sight, gastrointestinal bleeding, thrombocytopenia, venous thrombosis, and arterial thrombosis. Patterson at al. found that when intravenous heparin therapy was administered within the first five days following joint replacement surgery, bleeding from the wound occurred in 50% of patients (32). The occurrence of wound bleeding dropped to 15% when heparin was started more than one week after surgery. Overall, heparin therapy had to be discontinued in 35% of patients because of local or systemic complications related to the heparin therapy.

The use of warfarin therapy appears to be associated with less complications than intravenous heparin. The risk of bleeding is however related to the intensity of the therapy. Hull et al. reported a decrease in bleeding complications from 22.4% to 4.3% when moderately intense regimen of warfarin (prothombin time between 16 to 18) was utilized (25).

Low molecular weight heparins administered subcutaneously have recently been advocated for use in the treatment of deep vein thrombosis. The LMWH compounds are generally administered with subcutaneous injection twice daily. Numerous studies indicate that the LMWH are at least as effective as intravenous heparin. Although not yet FDA approved for the treatment of deep vein thrombosis, LMWHs may prove to be a simpler and safer method of treatment.

Vena Caval Filter Devices

Numerous vena caval filters are available in the United States. These devices are generally placed by interventional radiologists or vascular surgeons. The filters are placed percutaneously in the inferior vena cava and stop the migration of emboli from the distal venous system to the lungs. These devices have been shown to be effective in reducing pulmonary embolism while maintaining adequate blood flow. Long term follow-up of the Greenfield Filter revealed a recurrent embolism rate of 4% and a patency rate of 98% (26). Indications for vena caval filter include: recurrent embolism despite anticoagulation, and deep vein thrombosis with a contraindication to or complication of anticoagulation therapy. Vena caval filters have also been advocated as prophylaxis in high risk patients undergoing total joint replacement surgery.

The filters have no effect on the dissolution of thrombi and, therefore, no effect on the risk of post-phlebitic syndrome. Complications are unusual but can occur. At insertion there is a risk of filter misplacement (2.6%) and a risk of bleeding at the insertion site. Although rare, migration of the vena caval filter can occur over time as well as bleeding secondary to perforation of the vena cava.

Thrombolytics

Thrombolytics, such as streptokinase and urokinase, dissolve thrombi and are used mainly for massive pulmonary emboli. Complete clot lysis occurs in 30 to 40% of patients medicated with these agents (27). Due to the extremely high risk of bleeding, there is almost no indication for thrombolytics in the postoperative knee replacement patient.

Surgical Intervention

Surgical intervention, i.e., venous thrombectomy or pulmonary embolectomy, is performed only in extreme cases. These cases include venous obstruction that leads to cerulea dolens and limits the viability of the leg, and cases in which patients with massive pulmonary embolization do not responded to other therapy.

Recommended Treatment

There is a general agreement that large proximal thrombi and symptomatic pulmonary emboli should be treated aggressively. (Fig. 1) In addition to medical treatment (i.e., intravenous fluids, oxygen, possible ventilation support, etc.) these patients require a vena caval filter or anticoagulation with heparin followed by long term warfarin therapy. The choice of whether to use a vena caval filter or anticoagulation must be individualized. If heparin is chosen in the early postoperative period, one must be cautious not to give large boluses of heparin that may transiently raise the partial thromboplastin time to greater than 100 seconds. We generally use vena caval filters for patients who develop proximal thrombi or symptomatic pulmonary emboli within the first five days after major orthopedic surgery. Warfarin should be continued for 3 to 6 months. Patients who are identified with large proximal thrombi or symptomatic pulmonary emboli after the first seven days are generally treated with intravenous heparin, followed by three to six months of low-dose warfarin therapy.

There continues to be controversy concerning the treatment of calf thrombi in the postoperative patient. At The Hospital for Special Surgery, we have previously demonstrated that patients who developed calf thrombi are at increased risk for pulmonary embolism. We recommend that patients who are identified postoperatively as having a calf thrombi should be treated with low-dose warfarin therapy for six

Table 2: SUGGESTED TREATMENT REGIMENS

	Treatment Regimen
Treatment of calf thrombi	Low-dose warfarin therapy for six weeks or Follow-up duplex ultrasound (to evaluate propagation)
Treatment of proximal thrombi	Anticoagulation with heparin/warfarin for three to six months or Vena Cava Filter
Treatment of symptomatic pulmonary emboli	Anticoagulation with heparin/warfarin for three to six months or Vena Cava Filter or Both

weeks following surgery. We do not feel that calf thrombi, detected in the early postoperative period, should be treated routinely with heparin because of the risk of complication with intravenous anticoagulation therapy. Lotke has recommended that patients identified as having calf vein thrombosis should be continued on aspirin therapy for six weeks postoperatively (6). Since the primary risk of isolated calf thrombi is through proximal propagation, Colwell has advocated serial duplex ultrasound scanning without the use of anticoagulants to detect for proximal migration (103). Anticoagulation therapy is only initiated if propagation of a calf thrombi to a more proximal thrombi occurs.

Conclusion

Thromboembolic disease in any patient population is potentially life threatening. As a result, the diagnosis of deep venous thrombosis should be considered in any patient who receives a total knee replacement. While the diagnosis of a proximal deep venous thrombosis mandates treatment, the management of a calf thrombosis is controversial. Deep venous thrombosis of the calf can be treated with anticoagulation or followed with serial ultrasound examinations to exclude propagation. Prophylaxis of deep venous thrombosis should be considered in this patient population and should be based upon relative risks of the specific patient.

References

1) McKenna R, Bachmann F, Kullshal SP, Galante JO. Thromboembolic disease in patients undergoing total knee replacement. J Bone Joint Surg 1976;58A(7):928-32.

2) Lotke PA, Ecker ML, Alavi A, Berkowitz H. Indications for the treatment of deep venous thrombosis following total knee replacement. J Bone Joint Surg 1984;66A(2):202-8.

3) Stulberg BN, Insall JN, Williams GW, Ghelman B. Deep vein thrombosis following total knee replacement. J Bone Joint Surg 1984;66A(2):194-201.

4) Grady-Benson, JC, Oishi CS, Hannson PB, Colwell CW Jr, Otis SM and Walker RJ. Postoperative surveillance for deep venous thrombosis with duplex ultrasound after total knee arthroplasty. J Bone Joint Surg. 1994;76-A,(11):1649-1657.

5) Haas SB, Insall JM, Scuderi GR, Windsor RE, Ghelman B. Pneumatic sequential compression boots compared with aspirin prophylaxis of deep vein thrombosis after total knee arthroplasty. J Bone Joint Surg 1990;72A(1):27-31.

6) Lotke PA, Wong RY, Ecker ML. Asymptomatic pulmonary embolism after total knee replacement. Orthop Trans 1986;10(3):490.

7) Patterson BM, Marchand R, Ranawat C. Complications of heparin therapy after total joint arthroplasty. J Bone Joint Surg 1989;71A(8):1130-4.

8) Barritt DW, Jordan SC, Brist MB. Anticoagulant drugs in the treatment of pulmonary embolism: A controlled trial. Lancet 1960;18:1309-12.

9) Kraritz E, Karino T. Pathophysiology of deep vein thrombosis. In: Leclerc JR. Venous thromboembolic disorders. Philadelphia:Lea and Febiger, 1991:54-64.

10) Virchow R. Neuer fall von todlicher emboli der kungerarteries. Arch Path Anat 1856;10:225.

11) Garino J, Lotke P, Kitziger K, Steinberg M. Deep Venous Thrombosis after Total Joint Arthroplasty: The Role of Compression Ultrasonography and the Importance of Experience of the Technician. J Bone Joint Surg 1996;78A:1359-65.

12) Hirsh J, Salzman EW, Harker L, et al. Aspirin and other platelet active drugs: Relationship among dose, effectiveness and side effects. Chest 1989;95(Suppl 2):12s-16s.

13) Mizel, MS, Temple, HT, Michelson, JD, Alavarez, et al. Clinically apparent thromboembolism following foot and ankle surgery. In: Foot and Ankle Annual Meeting, June 30, 1996.

14) Lotke PA. Aspirin prophylaxis for thromboembolic disease. In Instructional Course Lectures, The American Academy of Orthopedic Surgeons. Vol. 44, St. Louis, C. V. Mosby, 1995.

15) Tarnay TJ, Rohr PR, Davidson AG, Stevenson MM, Byars EF, Hopkins GR. Pneumatic calf compression, fibrinolysis, and the prevention of deep venous thrombosis. Surgery 1980;88:489-96.

16) Wilson NV, Das SK, Kakkar VV, Maurice HD Smibert JG, Thomas EM and Nixon JE, Thrombo-embolic prophylaxis in total knee replacement. Evaluation of the A-V impulse system. J Bone Joint Surg.1992; 74B

17) Knight MTN, Dawson R. Effect of intermittent compression of the arms on deep venous thrombosis in the legs. Lancet 1976;2:1265-7.

18) Lynch JA, Baker PL, Polly RE, et al. Mechanical measures in the propylaxis of post-operative thromboembolism in total knee arthroplasty. Clin Orthop 1990;260:24-9.

19) Hodge WA. Warfarin and sequential calf compression in the prevention of deep vein thrombi following total knee replacement. Presented at the Knee Society, Las Vegas, February, 1989.

20) Kaempffe FA, Lifeso RM, Meinding C. Intermittent pneumatic compression versus coumadin: Prevention of deep vein thrombosis in lower-extremity total joint arthroplasty. Clin Orthop 1991;269:89-79.

21) Graor RA, Davis AW, Borden LS, Young J. Comparative evaluation of deep vein thrombosis prophylaxis in total joint replacement patients. Presented at AAOS, Las Vegas, February, 1989.

22) Hood RW, Flawn LB, Insall JN. The use of pulsatile compression stockings in total knee replacement for prevention of venous thromboembolism: A prospective study. Presented at the ORS, New Orleans, January, 1982.

23) Hull R, Delmore TJ, Hirsh J, et al. Effectiveness of intermittent pulsatile elastic stockings for the prevention of

calf and thigh vein thrombosis in patients undergoing elective knee surgery. Thromb Resear 1979;16:37-45.

24) Westrich GH, Sculco TP. Prophylaxis against Deep Vein Thrombosis after Total Knee Arthroplasty. Pneumatic Plantar Compression and Aspirin Compared to Aspirin Alone. J Bone Joint Surg 1996;78A(6):826

25) Hull R, Hirsh J, Jay R, et al. Different intensities of oral anticoagulant therapy in the treatment of proximal-vein thrombosis. N Engl J Med 1982;307:1676-81

26) Greenfield LJ, Michna B. Twelve year clinical experience with the Greenfield vena caval filter. Surgery 1988;104:706-12.

27) Emerson RH, Cross R, Head WC. Prophylaxtic and early therapeutic use of the Greenfield filter in hip and knee joint arthroplasty. J Arthroplasty 1991;6:129-35

28) Donaldson GA, Williams C, Scannell JG, et al: A reappraisal of the application of the Trendelenburg operation to massive fatal embolism: Report of a successful pulmonary-artery thrombectomy using a cardiopulmonary bypass. N Engl J Med 1963: 268:171-174.

29) Anderson FA. Wheeler HB: Venous thromboembolism: Risk factors and prophylaxis. Clin Chest Med 1995; 235-251.

30) Anderson FA Jr, Wheeler HB, Goldberg RJ, et al: A population-based perspective of the hospital incidence and case-fatality rates of deep vein thrombosis and pulmonary embolism: The Worcester DVT Study. Arch Intern Med 1991; 151:933-938.

31) Rahr HB, Sorensen IV: Venous thromboembolism and cancer. Blood Coagul Fibrinolysis 1992:3:451-460.

32) Geerts W, Code KI, Jay RM, et al: A prospective study of venous thromboembolism after major trauma. N Engl J Med 1994;331:1601-1606.

33) Clagett GP, Reisch JS: Prevention of venous thrombosis in general surgical patients. Results of meta-analysis. Ann Surg 1988; 208-227.

34) Paiement GD, Bell D, Wessinger SJ, et al: New advances in the prevention, diagnosis, and cost effectiveness of venous thromboembolic disease in patients with total hip replacement. In: The Hip, Proceedings of the Fourteenth Open Scientific Meeting of the Hip Society. St. Louis, CV Mosby, 1987, pp. 94-119.

35) Sevitt S, Gallagher NG: Prevention of venous thrombosis and pulmonary embolism in injury patients: A trial of anticoagulant prophylaxis with phenindione in middle-aged and elderly patients with fractured necks of femurs. Lancet 1959;ii:981-989.

36) Clagett GP, Anderson FA Jr, Levine MN, et al: Prevention of venous thromboembolism. Chest 1992;102:391S-407S.

37) Green D, Lee Y. Ito VY, et al: Fixed- vs adjusted-dose heparin in the prophylaxis of thromboembolism in spinal cord injury. JAMA 1988; 260:1255-1258.

38) Warlow C, Terry G, Kenmure ACF, et al: A double-blind trial of low-dose subcutaneous heparin in the prevention of deep vein thrombosis after myocardial infarction. Lancet 1973;ii:934-937.

39) Gibbs NM: Venous thrombosis of the lower limbs with particular reference to bedrest. B J Surg 1957:45:209-236.

40) Nicolaides AN, Irving D: Clinical factors and the risk of deep venous thrombosis, in Nicolaides AN (ed): Thromboemboblism Etiology, Advances in Prevention and Management. Baltimore, University Park Press, 1975, pp 193-204.

41) Carter C, Gent M: The epidemiology of venous thrombosis, in Coleman RW, Hirsh J, Marder VJ, et al (eds): Hemostasis and Thrombosis: Basic Principles and Clinical Practice. Philadelphia, JB Lippincott, 1987, pp 805-819.

42) Lundgren R, Sundin T, Colleen S, et al: Cardiovascular complications of estrogen therapy for nondisseminated prostatic carcinoma. Scand J Ural Nephrol 1986;20:101-105.

43) Devor M, Barrett-Connor E, Renvall M, et al: Estrogen replacement therapy and the risk of venous thrombosis, Am J Med 1992;92:275-282.

44) Stewart, WP, Youngswick, FD: Deep vein thrombosis: Diagnosis, treatment, and prevention. J. Foot Surg. 1981: 20:232-238.

45) Agnelli G: Anticoagulation in the prevention and treatment of pulmonary embolism. Chest 1995; 107:39S-44S.

46) Jorgensen LN, Willie-Jorgensen P, Hauch O: Prophylaxis of postoperative thromboembolism with low molecular weight heparins. Br J Surg 1993;80:689-704.

47) Carter CA, Skoutakis VA, Spiro TE, et al: Enoxaparin: The low-molecular-weight heparin for prevention of postoperative thromboembolic complications. Ann Pharmacother 1993; 27:1223-1230.

48) Noble S, Peters DH, Goa KL: Enoxaparin: A reappraisal of its pharmacology and clinical applications in the prevention and treatment of thromboembolic disease. Drugs 1995;49:388-410

49) Frampton JE, Faulds D: Pamaparin: A review of its pharmacology, and clinical application in the prevention and treatment of thromboembolic and other vascular disorders. Drugs 1994;47:652-676

50) Collignon F, Frydman A, Caplain H, et al: Comparison of the pharmacokinetic profiles of three low molecular mass heparins- Dalteparin, enoxaparin and nadroparin- Administered subcutaneously in healthy volunteers (doses for prevention of thromboembolism). Thromb Haemost 1995;73:630-640.

51) Friedel HA, Balfour JA: Tinzaparin: A review of its pharmacology and clinical potential in the prevention and treatment of thromboembolic disorders. Drugs 1994.;48:638-660.

52) Menzin F, Colditz GA, Re-an MM, et al: Cost-effectiveness of enoxaparin vs low-dose warfarin in the prevention of deep-vein thrombosis after total hip replacement surgery. Arch Intern Med 1995;155:757-764.

53) Warkentin TE, Levine MN, Hirsh J, et al: Heparin-induced thrombocytopenia in patients treated with low-molecular-weight heparin or unfractionated heparin. N Engl J Med 1995;273:1032-1038.

54) Bern MM, Lokich JJ, Wallach SR, et al: Very low doses of warfarin can prevent thrombosis in central venous catheters. A randomized prospective trial. Ann Intern Med 1990; 112:423-428.

55) Wells PS, Lensin AWA, Hirsh J: Graduated compression stockings in the prevention of postoperative venous thromboembolism. Arch Intern Med 1994; 154:67-71.

56) Knight MTN, Dawson R: Effect of intermittent compression of the arms on deep venous thrombosis in the legs. Lancet 1976;ii: 1265-1267.

57) Nicolaides AN, Fernandes JF, Pollock AV: Intermittent sequential pneumatic compression of the legs in the prevention of venous stasis and postoperative deep venous thrombosis. Surgery 1980;87:69-76.

58) Fordyce MJF, Ling RSM: A venous foot pump reduces thrombosis after total hip replacement. J Bone Joint Surg 1992;74-B:45-49.

59) Ramos R, Salem BI, De Pawlikowski MP: The efficacy of pneumatic compression stockings in the prevention of pulmonary embolism after cardiac surgery. Chest 1996; 109:82-85.

60) Keith SL, McLaughlin DJ, Anderson FA, et al: Do graduated compression stocking and pneumatic boots have an

additive effect on the peak velocity of venous blood flow? Arch Surg 1992;127:727-730.

61) Fisher CG, Blachut PA, Salvian, et al: Effectiveness of pneumatic leg compression devices for the prevention of thromboembolic disease in orthopaedic trauma patients: A prospective, randomized study of compression alone versus no prophylaxis. J Orthop Trauma 1995; 1-7.

62) Jacobs DG, Piotrowski JJ, Hoppensteadt, et al: Hemodynamic and fibrinolytic consequences of intermittent pneumatic compression: Preliminary results. J Trauma 1996; 4:710-717.

63) Mohan CR, Hoballah JJ, Shari WJ, et al: Comparative efficacy and complications of vena caval filters. J Vasc Surg 1995;21:235-246.

64) Alexander JJ, Yuhas JP, Piotrowski JJ: Is the increasing use of prophylactic percutaneous IVC filters justified? Am J Surg 1994; 168:102-106.

65) Clagett GP, Anderson FA Jr, Heit J, et al: Prevention of venous thromboembolism. Chest 1995:108(Suppl):312S-334S.

66) Hirsh DR, Ingenito EP, Goldhaber SZ: Prevalence of deep venous thrombosis among patients in medical intensive care. JAMA 1995;274:335-337.

67) Keane MG, Ingenito FP, Goldhaber SZ: Utilization of venous thromboembolism prophylaxisin the medical intensive care unit. Chest 1994;106:13-14.

68) Cade JF: High risk of the critically ill for venous thromboembolism. Crit Care Med 1982;10:448-450.

69) Halkin H, Goldberg J, Modan M, et al: Reduction of mortality in general medical inpatients by low-dose heparin prophylaxis. Ann Intern Med 1982;96:561-565.

70) Gardlund B: Randomised, controlled trial of low-dose heparin for prevention of fatal pulmonary embolism in patients with infectious diseases. Lancet 1996;347:1357-1361.

71) Keaton C, Hirsh J: Starting prophylaxis for venous thromboembolism postoperatively. Arch Intern Med 1995; 155:366-372.

72) Ziomek S, Read RC, Tobler HG, et al: Thromboembolism in patients undergoing thoracotomy. Ann Thorac Surg 1993;56:223-227.

73) Nurmohamed NIT. Verhaeghe R, Haas S, et at: A comparative trial of a low molecular weight heparin (enoxaparin) versus standard heparin for the prophylaxis of postoperative deep vein thrombosis in general surgery, Am J Surg 1995; 169:567-571.

74) Kakkar VV, Cohen AT. Edmonson RA, et al: Low molecular weight versus standard heparin for prevention of venous thromboembolism after major abdominal surgery. Lancet 1993;341:259-265.

75) Caprini JA, Arcelus JI, Hoffman K, et al: Prevention of venous thromboembolism in North America: Results of a survey among general surgeons. J Vasc Surg 1994:20:751-758.

76) Janku GV, Paiement GD, Green HD: Prevention of venous thromboembolism in orthopaedics in the United States. Cln Orthop 1996;325:313-321.

77) Bergqvist D, Benoni G, Bjorgell O, et al: Low-molecular-weight heparin (enoxaparin) as prophylaxis against venous thromboembolism after total hip replacement. N Engl J Med 1996;335:696-700.

78) Warwick D, Williams MH, Bannister GC: Death and thromboembolic disease after total hip replacement. J Bone Joint Surg 1995;77-B:6-10.

79) Pellegrini DV, Laghans MJ, Totterman S. et al: Embolic complications of calf thrombosis following total hip arthroplasty. J Arthroplasty 1993;8:449-457.

80) Imperiale TF, Speroff T: A meta-analysis of methods to prevent venous thromboembolism following total hip replacement. JAMA 1994;271:1780-1785.

81) Leclerc JR, Geerts WH, Desjardins L, et al: Prevention of deep vein thrombosis after major knee surgery-A randomized, double-blind trial comparing a low molecular weight heparin fragment (enoxaparin) to placebo. Thromb Haeinost 1992;67:417-423.

82) Fauno P, Suomalainen AO, Rehnberg V, et al: Prophylaxis for the prevention of venous thromboembolism after total knee arthroplasty. J Bone Joint Surg 1994;12:1814-1818.

83) Frim DM, Barker FG, Poletti CE, et al: Postoperative low-dose heparin decreases thromboembolic complications in neurosurgical patients. Neurosurgery 1992;30:830-833.

84) Green D, Chen D, Chmiel JS et al: Prevention of thromboembolism in spinal cord injury: Role of low molecular weight heparin. Arch Phys Med Rehabil 1994:75:290-292.

85) Hamilton MD, Hull RD, Pineo GF: Prophylaxis of venous thromboembolism in brain tumor patients. J Neurooncol 1994:22:111-126.

86) Britt LD. Zolfaghari D, Kennedy E, et al: Incidence and prophylaxis of deep vein thrombosis in a high risk trauma population. Am J Surg 1996; 172:13-14.

87) Knudson MM, Lewis FR, Clinton A. et al: Prevention of venous thromboembolism in trauma patients. J Trauma 1994;37:480-487.

88) Upchurch GR, Demling, RH, Davies J. et al: Efficacy of subcutaneous heparin in prevention of venous thromboembolic events in trauma patients. Am Surgeon 1995;61:749-755.

89) Knudson MM, Collins JA, Goodman SB, et al: Thromboembolism following multiple trauma. J Trauma 1992:32:2-11.

90) Geerts WH, Jay RM, Code KI, et al: A comparison of low-dose heparin with low-molecular-weight heparin as prophylaxis against venous thromboembolism after major trauma. N Engl J Med 1996;335:701-707.

91) Eriksson BI, Ekman S, Kalebo P, et al: Prevention of deep-vein thrombosis after total hip replacement: Direct thrombin inhibition with recombinant hirudin, CGP 39393. Lancet 1996;347:635-639.

92) Cole CW, Shea B, Bormanis J: Ancrod as prophylaxis or treatment from thromboembolism in patients with multiple trauma. Can J Surg 1995;38:249-254.

93) Flinn NVR, Sandaraer GP, Silva MB, et al: Prospective surveillance for perioperative venous thrombosis. Arch Surg 1996; 131:472-480.

94) Grady-Benson JC, Oishi CS, Hanson PB, et al: Postoperative surveillance for deep venous thrombosis with duplex ultrasonography after total knee arthroplasty, J Bone Joint Surg 1994:76-A:1649-1657.

95) Wells PS, Lensina AW, Davidson BL, et al: Accuracy of ultrasound for the diagnosis of deep venous thrombosis in asymptomatic patients after orthopedic surgery.A meta-analysis. Ann Intent Med 1995; 122:47-53.

96) Pederson O.M, Aslaksen A, Vik-Mo H, et al: Compression ultrasonography in hospitalized patients with suspected deep venous thrombosis. Arch Intern Med 1991; 151:2217-2220.

97) Howell R, Fidler J, Letsky E, et al: The risks of antenatal subcutaneous heparin prophylaxis: A controlled Trial. Br J Obstet Gynaecol 1983;90:1124-1128.

98) Barbour LA, Pickard J: Controversies in thromboembolic disease during pregnancy: A critical review. Obstet Gynaecol 1995;86:621-633.

99) Westrich GH, Schneider R, Ghelman B, et al. The Incidence Of Deep Venous Thrombosis With Color Doppler

Imaging Compared To Ascending Venography In Total Joint Arthroplasty: A Prospective Study, Contemporary surgery, Vol. 51 (4), 1997:225-234.

100) Haas SB, Tribus CB, Insall JN, Becker MW, Windsor RE. The significance of calf thrombi after total knee arthroplasty. J Bone Joint Surg 1992;74B:799-802.

101) Lieberman JR, Huo M, Hanaway J, Salvati E, Sculco T, Sharrock NE. The prevalence of deep venous thrombosis after total hip arthroplasty with hypotensive epidural anesthesia. J. Bone Joint Surg.1994; 76-A: 341-348.

102) Haas S, Mosca P, Peterson, M, Westrich G. Meta Analysis of Thromboembolic Prophylaxis in Total Knee Arthroplasty. Presented at AAHKS Meeting, Dallas, TX, 1996.

103) Colwell C, Spiro T, Trowbridge A, Stephens, JW, Gardiner, GA, Ritter, MA. Efficacy and safety of enoxaparin versus unfractionated heparin for prevention of deep vein thrombosis after elective knee arthroplasty. Clin Orthop 1995; 321:19-27.

104) Westrich GH, Allen ML, Tarantino SJ, Derkowska I, Schneider R, Ghelman B, Ranawat C, Sculco TP: Ultrasound screening for deep venous thrombosis in total knee arthroplasty: Our two year reassessment of the learning curve, (Clin Orthop, Under Review).

Section 5

MISCELLANEA

Chapter 20
Blood Management in Knee Arthroplasty

B. Borghi
Rizzoli Orthopaedic Institute - Bologna

In major orthopaedic surgery, the patient must be managed so that his or her transfusional needs are covered entirely, or at any rate as much as possible, by autologous blood, not just to avoid the risks associated with the use of homologous blood products, but also in order to produce preoperative hemodilution for antithromboembolic purposes (1, 2).

Nonetheless, should homologous transfusion be indispensable, it will be necessary to follow several norms for the correct use of blood, in order to obtain optimal results with the least possible risk for the patient (3, 4).

Hemodilution may be considered a valid means of antithromboembolic prophylaxis (1, 2, 4, 5, 6). Because of the small number of studies conducted on the use of hemodilution as the only means of prevention (1), it is important to associate (for ethical reasons, as well) postoperative pharmacological prophylaxis. Given the complete uselessness of the preoperative administration of drugs in patients submitted to predeposit for hemodilution (7), pharmacological prophylaxis may only be initiated postoperatively. It must be kept in mind that hemodilution with a decrease in hematocrit and the concentration of plasma components may accentuate the effects of many drugs, particularly anticoagulants.

Drugs with antiaggregant and/or anticoagulant properties must be chosen so as to minimize any interference with hemocoagulative processes required for the repair and scar formation of the surgical wound: it is important to recall that in patients undergoing treatment with calcium heparin, postoperative bleeding occurring late may be considerable, and it may even lead to death (8).

In the wards connected to the Ist Service of Anaesthesia and Intensive Care at the Rizzoli Orthopaedic Institute, a transfusion protocol is carried out as routine, that is the result of 20 years experience (3, 4, 9, 10, 11), aimed at making major orthopaedic surgery as safe as possible. For major orthopaedic surgery (including knee arthroplasty), it is based on the following: predepositing for hemodilution; intraoperative salvage; postoperative salvage; external elastic compression bandage; deferred reinfusion of the unit of concentrated erythrocytes taken preoperatively during the first 3 days after surgery; use of homologous transfusions only in the presence of clinical intolerance to anemia and after excluding the presence of hypovolemia.

Predepositing

The number and frequency of blood units taken for predepositing in total knee arthroplasty is established by the anaesthetist with the transfusionist, according to the patient's clinical conditions (age, weight, basal Hb, any co-existing diseases). Routinely, two units of blood are predeposited, separated by centrifugation into concentrated erythrocytes and fresh frozen plasma.

Patients that are in generally good condition, characterized by no pathology of the cardiovascular apparatus, a value of Hb > 12.5 g dl^{-1}, body weight greater than 65 kg, and age under 65 years, can give blood at close intervals, every 2-3 days, until a value of about 10 g dl^{-1} of Hb has been obtained (11). Blood given for autotransfusion may also be increased or carried out in patients with hematological values at the limit, using human erythropoetin recombined to stimulate erythropoiesis, with the support of iron and hemoactive drugs.

In patients with basal values for Hb at around 10 g/dl and/or affected with rheumatoid arthritis, the administration of exogenous erythropoietin is required; to bring Hb to around 10 g/dl and maintain it at that value, doses of 50-70 U/kg of body weight are generally used (one 4.000 U vial) subcutaneously every 3 days for 1-2 weeks.

Patients affected by coronary ischemia and/or atherosclerotic pathology of the vessels afferent to the brain can give blood every 6-7 days.

To minimize preoperative hospitalization, predepositing is carried out on an out-patient basis, possibly at the Transfusion Center near the patient's home: the day of hospitalization the patient himself transports the units of autologous blood to the Transfusional Center of the Hospital in a container suitable for its preservation (4, 10). Final predepositing may be carried out at the time of hospitalization.

Limitations

Age: there are no theoretical limits in terms of age in carrying out predepositing.
Weight: there are no limits to body weight.
Situations that require specific evaluation, case by case:
- *previous myocardial infarction (echocardiogram is suggested with evaluation of the ejection fraction)*
- *cerebrovascular insufficiency (carotid Doppler echocardiograph to evaluate any stenosis)*
   - *chronic respiratory insufficiency*
   - *hepatic insufficiency*
   - *hemopathies and anemias of unknown origin*
   - *anticoagulant treatment underway*

Absolute **contraindications** to predeposit:
- *high fever*
- *bacteremia (documented or probable)*
- *hypovolemia that is not corrected*
- *cardiopathies:* • bradycardia or severe arrhythmias
   • unstable angina
   • angina caused by stress
   • low cardiogenic capacity
   • conditions that according to a clinical evaluation could become symptomatic with hypovolemia and acute hypoxia.
- *acute hepatic insufficiency*
- *generally poor conditions.*

Practically speaking, however, these clinical situations would also contraindicate knee arthroplasty.

Intraoperative Salvage

When intraoperative bleeding is expected to be such that homologous blood products will be needed, preparations are made for the blood to be collected from the surgical wound. The reservoir and sterile collection and clotting kit is always set up. When a decrease of $Hb> 2$ g dl $^{-1}$ or even lower occurs during surgery, if the risk of transfusion is very high (e.g., patients with anemia, coronary failure, low body weight) the kit for washing and reinfusing blood cells is assembled on appropriate apparatus (4). On machines manufactured in Italy used for intraoperative salvage (Dideco, Mirandola, MO) the passage of physiological solution for the washing of blood cells is alternated with the mixing of the contents of the bell, carried out by reducing the velocity of the centrifuge to less than 1000 rpm with the purpose of improving the quality of the washing with consequent minimization of the risk of hematuria caused by the transfusion of free hemoglobin.

Prevention of Bleeding and Postoperative Salvage

The prevention of postoperative bleeding begins during surgery with recovery of values for arterial pressure greater than basal ones (of about 10-20 mm Hg) 15 minutes before the onset of suturing (increase in infusions, administration of bolus of a vasoconstrictor, such as 1-2 mg of ethylephredine) to facilitate the surgeon in identifying the open vessels to be cauterized (3, 9, 10). Drainages, positioned along the entire wound to the two sides of the prosthesis, must be connected, by means of a connection with more than one path, to a system of recovery and possibly of monitoring of the postoperative blood loss, like the BT 797 Recovery Dideco. The blood cells salvaged using this system can be reinfused, following sedimentation and microfiltration, for 8 ± 2 hours. Sedimentation allows for the reinfusing of a concentrate of red blood cells, minimizing reinfusion of supranactant where products of hemolysis are contained, factors of the complement activated above all by the toxins C3 and C5a. BT 797 Recovery is constituted by a pressure transductor, that can be regulated from −100 to +50 mmHg, that starts up a peristaltic pump connected to drainages with a double line with differentiated calibers; the largest of these transports the blood from the drainages to the stock sack, while the smallest one has the task of making the anticoagulant flow (ACD) to the drainages at a ratio of 1:10. The display with memory shows the amount of hourly loss during the first 8 hours of functioning and the pressure applied to the drainages. The acustic alarm with which it is equipped is activated by blood loss exceeding 300 ml/hour, enabling immediate intervention when potentially dangerous early bleeding occurs. In a study carried out on consecutive patients submitted to hip and knee reimplantation, the acustic-visual alarm activated when bleeding exceeded 300 ml in less than 60' proved to be useful in singling out patients with bleeding underway and thus monitoring them more carefully (14). Thanks to this, the incidence of homologous transfusions and postoperative complications was nearly equal to that for the group of patients that did not reveal any episodes of bleeding.

External Elastic Compression Bandage

To prevent hematoma and postoperative bleeding an external elastic compression bandage is applied from the end of the limb to the iliac crest. The bandage also favors venous recovery, contributing to the prevention of DVT.

If bleeding exceeds 2-3 ml/min, the bandage pressure may be increased, and the negative pressure applied to the drainage tubes may gradually be decreased until it becomes positive.

Correct Use of Autologous and Homologous Blood Products

The reinfusion of the units of blood extracted before surgery is spread over the first 3 days after surgery to make up for the drop in Hb that normally occurs in this kind of surgery. The reinfusion of the units of autologous plasma takes place during the first 24-48 hours, or at the end of surgery, if intraoperative blood loss exceeds 30% of the circulating blood mass, avoiding, however, hypervolemia and hypertension that may increase postoperative bleeding.

The transfusion of fresh frozen homologous plasma is indicated when there is bleeding underway caused by deficit in the coagulation factors.

The value for Hb in the patient leads to different types of transfusion depending on whether autologous or only homologous blood is available: autologous transfusion is used each time Hb needs to be brought to about 11 g dl^{-1}; homologous transfusion is used only when anemia is not tolerated (4), at any rate carefully evaluating the benefits (immediate) as compared to the risks (immediate and long-term).

Anemia or Hypovolemia

The clinical examination of patients with Hb under 8-10 g dl^{-1} is particularly aimed at excluding the presence of clinical signs of bad tolerance to anemia such as: tachycardia, angina, dyspnea, cephalagia, vertigo, dizziness, or lipothymy to mobilization, postural hypotension, insomnia, state of confusion.

Lack of appetite and delays in digestion, even if they are concomitant with anemia, are helped by administering peristaltic drugs; as such they must not be considered an indication for transfusion.

The presence of one or more of the aforementioned clinical signs together with diastolic arterial pressure more than 15-20 mmHg below the basal level, should first suggest hypovolemia, so crystalloids or even plasmaexpanders are infused. If, after volemia has been restored to normal, shown by the normalization of diastolic pressure, clinical signs of intolerance to anemia persist, transfusion of red blood cells takes place one unit at a time until the signs disappear.

High frequency tachycardia with low Hb and without hypovolemia (PVC and diastolic pressure normal) would suggest left ventricle hypertrophy: the increase in cardiac range (range x frequency) required by the isovolemic decrease in Hb occurs above all due to the increase in systolic range with the increase in left ventricle diastolic volume; in patients with ventricular hypertrophy, the increase in diastolic volume is made more difficult by the reduced relaxability of the left ventricle wall and thus the increase in range occurs due to the increase in frequency (15).

The suspicion that the red blood cells salvages could have a shorter average life has been refused, first by Orr (16), who documented a higher osmotic resistance than homologous banked blood cells, by McShane (17) who observed a high concentration of 2,3 Diphosphoglycerate, a more physiological concentration of

Authors	Year	Type of surgery	Patient n.	Prede-posit	RIO	RPO	Autotrans-fusion alone
Thomson et al. (20)	1987	THA, TKA, SF	159	X			71%
MacFarlane et al. (21)	1988	THA, TKA	99	X			74%
Semkiw et al. (22)	1989	THA, TKA	74	X	X	X	83%
Groh et al. (23)	1990	TKA	25			X	92%
Gannon et al. (24)	1991	TKA, THA	239			X	87%
Slagis et al. (25)	1991	Monolat TKA	30			X	80%
		Bilat. TKA	22			X	46%
		THA	50			X	63%
Dieu et al. (26)	1992	TKA, THA	345		X	X	85%
Pluvinage et al. (27)	1992	TKA, THA	100		X		90%
Borghi et al (9)	1993	THA,TKA,HR	414	X	X	X	92%
Mercuriali et al (28)	1993	THA,TKA,HR	?	X	X		53%
Woolson et al. (29)	1993	TKA	65	X	X		92%
Rosencher et al (30)	1994	TKA	30			X	60%
Borghi et al (3)	1995	THA,TKA,HR	980	X	X	X	93.7%
Borghi et al (19)	1995	THA,TKA,HR	1576	X	X	X	90%
Oriani et al (31)	1995	THA, TKA	1578	X	X	X	89.6%
Caroli et al (10)	1996	THA, TKA, HR	1544	X	X	X	93,4%
Borghi et al (4)	1997	THA,TKA,HR	1785	X	X	X	92.7%
Borghi et al (32)	1998	THA,TKA,HR	2303	X	X	X	92%

THA= Total hip arthroplasty; HR= Hip revision; TKA= total knee arthroplasty;
Table I: Studies conducted on autotransfusion in orthopaedics

potassium and of the pH and a higher content of Hb, of blood prepared with the Dideco Auto-trans BT 795 system (Mirandola, Modena, Italy) as compared to that of the donor. Subsequently, Alleva (18) observed minor injury to the red blood cells salvaged intraoperatively with a Dideco STAT sytem and those salvaged postoperatively with a Dideco BT 797 Recovery system as compared to analogous ones predeposited in SAG-M and preserved in a refrigerator for 21 days at 4° C.

In the literature, some authors have proposed for use in orthopaedic surgery predepositing alone with only autologous blood variable from 71 to 74% (20, 21) of cases; others have proposed intraoperative salvage alone with the incidence of autologous blood in 90% (27) and postoperative salvage alone with results in terms of use of autologous blood ranging from 46 to 92% (23, 24, 25). The association of intraoperative salvage with predepositing or postoperative salvage allows us to achieve the result of exclusively using autologous blood from 53 to 92% (26, 28, 29).

The association between predepositing, intraoperative salvage, and postoperative salvage allows us to achieve better results with the use of autologous blood from 83 to 93.4% (3, 4, 9, 10, 19, 31, 32) (Table I). Based on an analysis of the literature and our experience, it may be observed that in non-selected patients, the techniques of blood saving, singly and associated, are not capable of reducing to zero the use of homologous transfusion (Table II); nonetheless, the integrated use of predeposits, intra- and postoperative salvage, applied according to the type of surgery and the needs of the patients, allows for a drastic reduction in the incidence of homologous transfusion.

The correct use of autologous and homologous hemoderivates is the result of 20 years of experience and an analysis of the literature is based on the following points:

1) predeposit for hemodilution possibly carried out on an out-patient basis near the patient's home, associated, if necessary, with medullary stimulation with exogenous erythropoietin;

2) in the absence of a tourniquet, sterile collection and possible salvage of blood lost intraoperatively with successive reinfusion of red blood cells in case of a decrease in Hb > 2 g/dl or between 1 and 2 g/dl for high-risk transfusion patients (coronaropathy, anemia, low weight) (3);

3) monitoring of postoperative bleeding both early and late and reinfusion of red blood cells lost during the first 8-10 hours following sedimentation or washing and microfiltering;

4) external elastic compression bandage or elastic stockings on both of the lower limbs;

5) antithromboembolic prophylaxis with low molecular weight heparin or indobufen at doses suited to body weight and to hemocoagulation;

6) dilation of reinfusion of autologous hemoderivates during the first 3 days after surgery,

7) transfusion of homologous red blood cells in the presence of anemia that is not well-tolerated, only after excluding the presence of hypovolemia by re-examining the evolution of the clinical conditions after each single unit transfused.

For the application of these points and the consequent minimization of complications related to knee arthroplasty, the active collaboration between anaesthetists, transfusionists, and surgeons in the perioperative management of the patient is required.

References

1) Vara - Thorbeck R, Rosssel Pradas J, Mekinassi KL, Et Al Prevention of thrombotic disease and post-transfusional complication using normovolemic hemodilution in arthroplasty surgery of the hip.Rev Chir Orthop1990:76(4):267-71

2) Bombardini T, Borghi B, Montebugnoli M, Picano E, Caroli GC. Normovolemic hemodilution reduces fatal pulmonary embolism: following major orthopaedic surgery. J. of Vascular Surg. New York, 1996:30(2):125-133

3) Borghi B, Bassi A, Grazia M, Gargioni G, Pignotti E. Anaesthesia and autologous transfusion. Int J Artif Organs 1995: 18(3):159-66.

4) B. Borghi, *E. Pignotti, M. Montebugnoli, ** A. Bassi, M. Corbascio, N. de Simone, K. Elmar, U. Righi, A.M. Laguardia, S. Bugamelli, F. Cataldi, R. Ranocchi, MA. Feoli, T. Bombardini, G. Gargioni, A.G. Franchini and GC. Caroli. Autotransfusion in major orthopaedic surgery: experience with 1785 patients.British Journal of Anaesthesia. 1997: 79(5): 662-4

5) Baron J.F . et al. Hémodiluition, autotrasfusion, hémostase. Arnette Paris 1989: 396

6) Messmer K. Haemodilution. Possibilities and safety aspects. A. Anaest. Scand. 1988; 32 (Suppl 89): 49-53.

7) Palareti G., Borghi B., Coccheri S. et al. Postoperative versus preoperative initiation of deep vein thrombosis prophylaxis with a replacement. Clinical and Applied Thrombosis/Hemostasis, 1996: 2(1):18-24

8) Borghi B, Bassi A, Grazia G, Feoli MA, Pignotti E.Evaluation of complication in major orthopaedics surgery: indobufen versus eparin calcium and low molecular weight heparin. Min. Anest., 1996: 62:95-100.

9) Borghi B, Bassi A, de Simone N, Laguardia AM, Formaro G. Autotrasfusion: 15 years experience at Rizzoli Orthopaedic Institute. Int J Artif Organs 1993: 16 S-5:241-6

10) Caroli GC., Borghi B., Bassi A. et all. Clinical aspects and results of blood saving at the Rizzoli Orthopaedic Institute. Min. Anestesiol. 1996: 62 (4, S1): 105-16.

11) Caroli GC, Borghi B, Pappalardo G, Oriani G, Valbonesi M, Ferrari M, Zanoni A, Miletto A, Mercuriali F, Conconi F, Mehrkens HH, Journois D. Consensus Conference. Risparmiare Sangue: quali i dubbi e i problemi? Min. Anestesiol., 1994: 60; 5: 285-93.

12) Borghi B, Bassi A, Montebugnoli M., Cataldi F., Bugamelli S. Low doses of recombinant human erythropoietin (EPO) to aid autotransfusion in orthopaedic surgery. Min. Anestesiol. 1994: 60 (9, S2): 26.

13) Bassi A., Borghi B., Brillante C., Mattioli R. Plasma predeposit: the role of productive plasmapheresis. Int. J. Artif. Organs. 1993: 16 (5): 253-6.

14) Borghi B, De Simone N, Facchini F, Fanelli G, Pignotti E: The control of postoperative bleeding and blood salvage. Min Anestesiol. 1996: 62, 4(S-1): 97-102.

15) Bombardini T, Borghi B, Caroli GC et al.: Short term cardiac adaptation to normovolemic Hemodilution in normal and hypertensive patients. An echocardiography study. European Heart J. 1994: 15: 637-40.

16) Orr MD, Blenko JW: Autotrasfusion of concentrated washed red cells from the surgical fields: a biochemical and physiological comparison of homologous cell transfusion. Proceeding of Blood Conservation Institute,1978:116-28

17) McShane AJ, Power C, Jackson JF, Murphy DF, Mac Donald A, Moriarty DC, Otridge-BW. Autotransfusion: quality of blood prepared with a red cell processing device. Br J Anaesth. 1987 Aug; 59(8): 1035-9.

18) Alleva R, Ferretti G, Borghi B, Pignotti E, Bassi A, Curatola G. Physico-chemical properties of membranes of recovered erythrocytes in blood autologous transfusion: a study using fluorescence technique.Transfus. Sci 1995: 16(3): 291-7.

19) Borghi B, Oriani G, Bassi A, Pignotti E,Corbascio M, Montebugnoli M, et al. Blood saving program: a multicenter Italian experience Int J Artif Organs. 1995: 18(3):150-8

20) Thomson JD., Callaghan JJ., Savory CG. et al.: Prior deposition of autologous blood in elective orthopaedic surgery. J. Bone Joint Surg. [Am] 69:320, 1987.

21) MacFarlane BJ., Marx L., Anquist K. et al.: Analysis of a protocol for an autologous blood transfusion program for total joint replacement surgery. Can. J. Surg. 1988:31:126.

22) Semkiw LB., Schurman DJ., Goodman SB., Woolson ST.: Postoperative blood salvage using the cell saver after total joint arthroplasty. J. Bone Joint Surg. [Am]. 1989:71:823.

23) Groh GI., Buchert PK., Allen WC.: A comparison of transfusion requirement after total knee arthroplasty using the Solcotrans autotransfusion system. J. Arthroplasty. 1990:3:281.

24) Gannon DM., Lombardi AV jr., Mallory TH. et al.: An evaluation of the efficacy of postoperative blood salvage after total joint arthroplasty. A prospective randomized trial. J. Arthroplasty 1991: 6:109.

25) Slagis SV., Benjamin JB., Volz RG., Giordano GF.: Postoperative blood salvage in total hip and knee arthroplasty. A randomised controlled trial. J. Bone Joint Surg. [Br] 1991:73:591.

26) Dieu P, Goulard M, Delelis D,Dumora D,Pascarel X. Blood saving inbone prosthetics surgery. A propos of 426 casesè. Cah-Anesthesiol. 1992; 40(6):403-5

27) Pluvinage C. Preant J.:Postoperative autotrasfusion in total hip and knee prostheses. Cah-Anesthesiol.1992; 40:241

28) Mercuriali F., Inghilleri G., Biffri E., Vinci A., Colotti MT Scalamogna R. Autotransfusion program: intefreted use of different techniques. Int J Artif Organs 1993; 16 S5: 233-40

29) Woolson ST., Pottorff G.: Use of preoperatively deposited autologous blood for total knee. Clinic. Orthop. 1993:137:141.

30) Rosencher N.,Vassilieff V., Tallet F., Toulon P., Leoni J., Tomeno B., Coinseller C.,: Comparison of Orth-Evac and Solcotrans Plus devices for the autotrasfusion of blood drained after total knee joint arthroplasty. Ann-Fr-Anesth-Reanim. 1994: 318-25.

31) Oriani G., Borghi B. et al. Il rischio trasfusionale nella chirurgia non cardiaca. Min. Anestesiol., 1995; 61 (9,S1): 395-402.

32) Borghi B, Pignotti E, Montebugnoli M, Bassi A, de Simone N, and Caroli GC.. Autotransfusion: role of perioperative blood salvage and predeposit. Anaesthesia 1998; 53 (S2): 28-30

Chapter 21
Rehabilitation Following Total Knee Arthroplasty

Sandy B. Ganz

The Hospital for Special Surgery - New York

Introduction

Reconstructive surgery has expanded tremendously with technologic advances in joint arthroplasty. Complex knee deformity with severe degenerative joint disease, associated bone deficits and soft tissue imbalances can now be successfully reconstructed with a myriad of modular knee implants that allows the surgeon to customize the prosthesis to the patient's specific problem. Technical advances and pressure of managed care have encouraged a more rapid advancement of patients and the associated need for more intense in patient rehabilitation. The orthopaedic surgeon, nursing, and rehabilitation staff must work together as a coordinated team with effective communication and common goals. It is paramount that the physical therapist be able to assess and modify the therapy program as indicated, utilizing basic knowledge of the surgical procedures.

Preoperative Evaluation

A preoperative physical therapy evaluation is crucial to the successful management of the total knee arthroplasty patient (4,6). It is extremely useful to perform a preoperative physical therapy evaluation on patients prior to their undergoing a total knee arthroplasty in order to identify and address potential problems postoperatively. Potential postoperative problems that are addressed preoperatively will enhance the rehabilitation process, and enable the health care professionals to plan for appropriate assistance at time of discharge (4,

5). While the long term outcomes are positive, the individual undergoing TKA surgery must cope with physical limitations in mobility, diminished ability to perform activities of daily living (ADL), and pain in the immediate postoperative period. Physical and Occupational therapy intervention are vital to assisting the individual to achieve his/her highest level of independence. Patient education whether individually or in groups has been shown to allay fears and enhance short and long-term outcome (11).

A preoperative physical therapy evaluation includes assessment of: gait, range of motion (ROM) and strength of all joints, neck and trunk, respiratory status, and, lastly, a functional assessment. The three most common types of gait analysis are 1) observational, 2) stride analyzer, 3) two/three dimensional.

Clinically an observational gait assessment is performed to determine the patient's functional status and degree of impairment. The therapist describes how the patient is ambulating; what assistive device is being used; type of gait deviation exhibited, i.e., coxalgic, antalgic; equal or unequal step lengths, type of gait pattern, i.e., heel—-> toe, and lastly, a description of how the patient ascends and descends stairs, i.e., reciprocally, non-reciprocally. Performance-based measures which address gait abnormalities and balance dysfunction which are easy to administer may be useful in objectively measuring a patient's functional ability pre- and postoperatively. One such measure is the Tinetti Gait and Balance assessment (17) which is a valid and reliable instrument that addresses both gait and balance ability in the geriatric population. It may be scored separately or together. It is easily administered and takes approximately 6-8 minutes to carry out (Table 1,2). Following the completion of a preoperative evaluation, the patient may be instructed in the proper use of the assistive device he/she will be using postoperatively. Two methods of gait analysis usually seen in academic research centers are the foot switch stride analyzer in which the patient's gait is analyzed using waist pack recorder, which analyzes cadence, velocity and single limb support time. Pre- and postoperative gait studies have been reported in TKA and have shown that both level walking and stairclimbing are influenced by the design of the prosthesis (Kelman). On ascending stairs, prostheses that retain both cruciates are closest to normal (Anderson). Andriacchi found that patients with less constrained TKA cruci-

ate-retaining designs have more normal gait during stair climbing than patients with more constrained cruciate-sacrificing designs (3,4). The second method is an automated three dimensional system that employs six video cameras strategically placed to capture all angles of the patient's gait. The cameras enable the therapist to view the patient while level walking or stair climbing and instantaneously capture the activity frame by frame to quantify specific elements of the gait cycle. Force plates are mounted in the floor and act as a sophisticated bathroom scale. As the patient steps on the force plate data is generated to the computer indicating the magnitude and direction of forces placed on the lower extremities during different phases of the gait cycle. The data collected during testing emerges on the computer as an animated stick figure that re-

Table 1 - Tinetti Gait

Tinetti Assessment Tool Gait			Date
1.Initiation of gait	Any hesitancy or multiple attempts	0	
	No hesitancy	1	—— —— —— —— ——
2.Step length and height	A. RIGHT swing foot		
	does not pass left stance foot with step	0	
	passes left stance foot	1	—— —— —— —— ——
	right foot does not clear floor		
	completely with step	0	
	right foot completely clears floor	1	—— —— —— —— ——
	B. LEFT swing foot		
	does not pass right stance foot with	0	
	step passes right stance foot	1	—— —— —— —— ——
	left foot does not clear floor		
	completely with step	0	
	left foot completely clears floor	1	—— —— —— —— ——
3. Step symmetry	Right & Left step length not equal	0	—— —— —— —— ——
	Right & Left step length are equal	1	
4. Step continuity	Stopping or discontinuity between steps	0	
	Steps appear continuous	1	
5. Path	Marked deviation		
	Mild/Moderate deviation or uses walking aid	1	
	Straight without walking aid	2	—— —— —— —— ——
6. Trunk	Marked sway or uses walking aid	0	
	No sway but flexion of knees or back or		
	spread arms out while walking	1	
	No sway, no flexion, no use of arms,		
	and no use of walking aid	2	—— —— —— —— ——
7. Walking Stance	Heels apart	0	
	Heels almost touching	1	—— —— —— —— ——
Total			/12 /12 /12 /12 /12

produces the patient's movement. (Fig. 1). These two methods of gait analysis are not only time consuming, but costly, and usually not reimbursable.

Range of motion measurement of all joints and gross manual muscle testing of the upper extremities and uninvolved lower extremity are performed to determine the functional ability of the patient and degree of overall impairment. Knowledge of the patient's functional status and impairment preoperatively allows the therapist to plan for the appropriate waking aids and other assistive devices that may be required postoperatively. Objective strength assessment may be performed biomechanically using isokinetic systems. Cybex°, Lido* and Kin-Com+ are the most common isokinetic systems used. A gross respiratory evaluation should include auscultation, and a measurement of the number of cubic centimeters a patient inspires and expires utilizing an incentive inspirometer, and blow bottle. Functional assessments are utilized to monitor progression during hospitalization and to track long-term outcomes. The SF 36, and the Hospital for Special Surgery Knee rating scale are instruments widely used in TKA patients. The SF 36 is a generic assessment of health, used widely in health care research. The visual analog scale, (VAS) is the easiest method to administer. Pain

Table 2 - Tinetti Balance

Tinetti Assessment Tool Balance			date ___ ___ ___ ___ ___
1. Sitting Balance	Leans, slides in chair	0	
	Steady, safe	1	___ ___ ___ ___ ___
2. Arises	Unable without help	0	
	Able, uses arms to help	1	
	Able without using arms	2	___ ___ ___ ___ ___
3. Attempts to Arise	Unable without help	0	
	Able requires > 1 attempt	1	
	Able to arise, 1 attempt	2	___ ___ ___ ___ ___
4. Immediate Standing Balance	First 5 seconds		
	Unsteady (swaggers, moves feet, trunk sway)	0	
	Steady but uses walker or other support	1	
	Steady without walker or other support	2	___ ___ ___ ___ ___
5. Standing Balance	Unsteady		
	Steady but wide stance (medial heels > 4 inches apart,		
	Uses cane or other support	1	
	Narrow stance without support	2	___ ___ ___ ___ ___
6. Nudged (feet as close together as possible, examiner pushes lightly on subjects sternum with palm of hand 3 times	Begins to Fall	0	
	Staggers, grabs, catches self	1	
	Steady	2	___ ___ ___ ___ ___
7. Eyes Closed	Unsteady	0	
	Steady	1	___ ___ ___ ___ ___
8. Turning 360 deg.	Discontinuous Steps	0	
	Continuous	1	___ ___ ___ ___ ___
	Unsteady (grabs, staggers)	0	
	Steady	1	___ ___ ___ ___ ___
9. Sitting down	Unsafe (misjudged distance falls into chair)	0	
	Uses arms or not a smooth motion	1	
	Safe, smooth motion	2	___ ___ ___ ___ ___
Balance score /16			**/16 /16 /16 /16 /16**

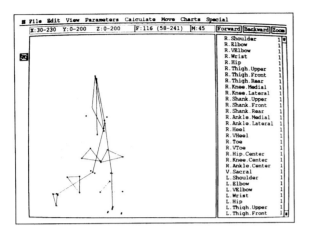

FIG. 1 - Gait computerized stick figure.

intensity is recorded for specific activities or a global rating can be obtained. Information regarding the social environment the patient will be returning to following surgery. For example, Does the patient live alone? Are there stairs in the home? Are the bathrooms accesible to a walking aid? Who does the cooking? It is necessary to determine the functional activities necessary to perform basic ADL: 1) lower extremity dressing, bathing, foot care, 2) transfer to and from bed, chair, toilet, tub, shower, and car, 3) current use of assitive device, and 4) limitations in activity tolerance or endurance with DL. Based on the assessment, the rehabilitation staff can begin to integrate the information obtained from the pre-op evaluation into an effective treatment plan. It should be recognized that the functional, environmental, and social components of the pre-op assessment can be a helpful predictor of discharge disposition.

In over three decades since the first total joint replacement was performed, methods and philosophies of rehabilitation have changed, but the primary goals of physical therapy have remained the same. To provide a stable joint with a functional range of motion, it is important to obtain from the patient what his goals are following TKA, to enable the health professional to determine if the patient-derived goals are realistic.

Total Knee Arthroplasty

Rehabilitation following total knee arthroplasty (TKA) has dramatically changed over the past three decades. Whether we are referring to a unicondylar or bicondylar TKA that is constrained, semi-constrained or unconstrained, cemented or uncemented, the primary goal is to provide a stable joint with a functional range of motion. Twenty years ago patients who underwent TKA remained in the hospital for three weeks and were immediately placed in cylinder casts, which remained on for a week to ten days before flexion was initiated. Today mechanical flexion is initiated within 24 hours postoperatively and average length of stay for an uncomplicated TKA is 5-7 days (4,5).

Continuous Passive Motion

Mechanical flexion most commonly referred to as continuous passive motion (CPM), is a method of passive flexion in the form of a machine that is applied to the knee joint. The CMP passively flexes and extends the knee at a designated speed and degree of knee flexion, that is set or programmed by the physical therapist, nurse, or physician. Widespread use of CPM following TKA began in the eighties (5). Much controversy exists regarding the efficacy of its use. Studies indicate that CPM may be beneficial in: counteracting the effect of joint immobilization, improving postoperative venous flow, maintenance of articular cartilage, a decreased hospital length of stay, increased range of motion at discharge (4, 7, 16). Coutts et al. performed a multi-institutional study in TKA patients, and found a more rapid gain in knee motion coupled with a decrease in length of stay in patients who received CPM compared with a control group that did not (4). Other studies have found diametrically opposed results: no difference in range of motion at discharge or hospital length of stay (7,15). Both short and long-term follow up studies reported no difference in patient ROM at 2 years postoperatively. CMP has been reported to decrease the incidence of deep vein thrombosis (18), but studies have reached contradictory results regarding the effects of CPM on swelling and postoperative blood loss (6, 14). Argument regarding use of CPM occurs throughout the country. Some physicians feel that CPM should be applied in the recovery room, others argue that CPM should be applied on the first postoperative day because the amalgamation of continuous passive-knee motion and freshly cut bone combine to procedure excessive blood loss within the first 24 hours postoperatively (9). Contraindications to use of CPM are: 1) sensory deficits **excluding** epidural anesthesia, 2) excessive wound drainage, 3) postoperative confusion, 4) significant knee flexion contracture, and 5) prothrombin time > 22 seconds and International Normalized Ratio (INR) >3 (Oertel). Patients whose active flexion is poor, who concomitantly have a knee flexion contracture should have limited time in the CPM with aggressive therapy to improve knee extension. A dynamic knee brace may also be indicated (5, 6).

CPM Guidlines

CPM application and use varies from institution to institution, and is usually dictated by the philosophy of the surgeon (1). If the CPM is applied in the recovery room, the primary compression dressing dictates the degree in which the CPM should be set (2). If the compression dressing is bulky, the CPM needs to be set at a lower range of motion i.e.: 0-45°. Bulky dressings tend to kink and create pressure areas on the posterior surface of the knee at higher degrees and pressure sores may result (3). If the compression dressing is thin, the degrees may be set to 90° or higher (5, 6).

The CPM is usually increased to the patient's tolerance. It is critical that the aides, orderlies, recovery room staff and nursing staff on the patient's floor have a thorough understanding of the mechanics of CPM and the proper placement of the limb in the machine. Through preoperative teaching the patient is made aware of the proper use of CPM and the need to combine functional activities, to gain the knee flexion needed for activities of daily living. Initiation of transfer activities, gait training, and active range of motion, are usually begun on the first postoperative day, and continued until the patient is discharged or achieves 90 degrees of active knee flexion. There is no consensus regarding discharging patients home with CPM.

Gait Training

There is no consensus regarding weight-bearing status following cemented/uncemented TKA, and patients are discharged from the hospital with a wide variety of weight-bearing status ranging from protected weight-bearing with crutches to full weight-bearing with a cane.

There have been no prospective randomized controlled trials which look at implant loosening as an outcome measure in patients with various weight-bearing statuses in the immediate postoperative period following TKA. Patients are advanced from a walker to a cane depending on their functional ability. They are instructed in ambulation on stairs, ramps and curbs prior to their discharge. If the patient exhibits an anthalgic gait pattern, then the cane should not be discarded.

Therapeutic Exercise

Following a TKA, there are three important factors that influence postoperative range of motion: 1) type of prosthesis, 2) preoperative deformity, 3) intraoperative bone resection (6). A thorough exercise program incorporates both open and closed chain exercises with emphasis on improving flexibility and strength. Exercises may consist of: active range of motion, active assisted range of motion, passive range of motion, isometrics (quadriceps and hamstring), straight leg raising, short arc quadriceps, patellar mobilization, and stationary bicycle or restorator. It is of paramount importance to have open communication between the surgeon and therapist as to what the expected postoperative ROM will be. The physical therapist must be cognizant that the expected degree of PROM one obtains postoperatively will be less than or equal to what the intraoperative PROM measurement was intraoperatively. Postoperative treatment should be aimed at increasing the patient's active knee flexion for the requirements for ADL (Table 3). The time frame for muscle strengthening is determined by the amount of time it takes for the capsule to heal. Cryotherapy in the form of a cryocuff, ice or cold pack is usually used concomitantly with exercise session to decrease swelling. Aggressive quadriceps-strengthening exercises should not be stressed during the immediaste postoperative period (1-2 weeks) for fear of damaging the capsular closure (9).

Historically-patients were discharged form the hospital with 90° of knee flexion, transferring in and out of bed independently, and ambulating with a cane unassisted on level surfaces and stairs. With managed care and Diag-

Table 3 - Range of Motion During Activities of Daily Living.

Activities of Daily Living (ADL)	Mean Knee Range of Motion
Walking (swing phase)	67°
Ascending stairs	83°
Descending stairs	90°
Rising from a chair	93°
Tying Shoe	106°
Lifting object from floor	117°

Keltenkamp DB e coll.: *An electrogoniometric study of knee motion in normal gait.* JBJS. 52A; 775-790; 1970.

nostic Related Group (DRG) pre-payment plans, patients are being discharged 4-6 days after surgery with much less than 90 degrees requiring home care services, outpatient physical therapy services or placement in short term rehabilitation centers. There is no consensus regarding the number of degrees of active knee flexion required for discharge. The gold standard had been 90 degrees, however, with shorter length of stays, and ROM at discharge less than a functional ROM, one may consider a CPM for home use. A standard multidisciplinary clinical pathway is essential for timely discharge (Table 4) Extension lags and inability to extend the knee to zero degrees are commonly seen following TKA. Functional electrical stimulation (FES) of the knee extensors can be used to increase quadriceps strength and decrease extensor lag. Haug and Wood looked at the efficacy of neuromuscular stimulation of the quad following TKA. They concluded that CPM combined with electrical stimulation in the treatment of TKA patients is a worthwhile

Table 4 - Total Knee Arthroplasty - Clinical Pathway.

HOSPITAL FOR SPECIAL SURGERY

DRG: 209 EST. L.O.S. 5 DAYS   STANDARD CLINICAL PATHWAY: TOTAL KNEE REPLACEMENT   SEPTEMBER 1996   DRAFT   (klu:\rl4\krep)

CARE DAY/PLACE	PRE-HOSPITAL P.S.S.	DAY OF SURGERY 4EN-->OR-->PACU-->INPT	P.O.D. #1	P.O.D. #2	P.O.D. #3	P.O.D. #4	P.O.D. #5
Consults/Assessments	Medical Clearance H&P Patient Data Base Consents Signed Physical Therapy Health Care Proxy Social Work Inpatient Alert PRN	Verify H&P Orthopedic Exam Review Data Base Anesthesia Pain Service Pastoral Care Dietician	Social Work Screen ---->	---------------->	Reassess need for home care/rehab/extended care placement/counseling	Finalize discharge plan/transportation with pt, family, team	DISCHARGE
Diagnostic	Urine: analysis/C&S, CxR, CBC, SMA 27, PT PTT, Type & Screen, SED Rate, EKG	Refer to Preoperative Flow Sheet	Lytes, H&H, PT daily if on Coumadin ---->	Lytes, H&H	Lytes, H&H	---------->	---------->
Medications	Check allergies Identify home meds, notify pharmacy if non-formulary, MAO's D/C NSAID 7 days prior	Antibiotic 1 hr prior to incision and continue x 24 hrs. Pain: IM or PCA	Antibiotic D/C Pain: IM or PCA ----> DVT Prophylaxis ----> - Coumadin - ASA Routine Meds, PRN's ---->	—Wean to p.o. ---->	---------->	Instructions for home meds ---->	Reinforce, clarify Meds ---->
Nutrition	N.P.O. 8 hrs prior to surgery	N.P.O. ----> clear based on bowel sounds	Clear liquids, progress to regular as tolerated	Regular diet---->	---------->	---------->	---------->
Treatment Plan	Autologous Blood Donation Pre-op THR Class: - Precautions - Exercises - Pain Management - Equipment/Treatments - Pre/Postoperative Planning - Operative Goals - LOS - Betadine Scrub - Enema Instructions	M.D. admitting orders: - Skin Prep - Shave - I.V. - Foley - TEDs - Oxygen - Drains Comfort Measures *Initiate* Standard Orders: - Post-op - Pain - Nursing Care Plan for TKR *Initiate* Nursing Protocols: - Management of pt in SDS/OR/PACU - Acute Pain: PCA or IM - Post-op Major Ortho - Elimination - High Risk Neurovascular - Blood PRN - Altered Mobility Physical Therapy: - TKR Protocol Ordered - CPM	Continue and individualize standard orders Continue and individualize Protocols ---------------> Ambulate x 1 -2 Initiate P.T. TKR Protocol Instruct: - Quad sets/Glut sets - Ankle pumps - Transfer: Dangle-->Stand - Begin ambulation Bedside Knee ROM CPM 4 - 6 hrs / day	D/C PCA D/C IV/I&O D/C Foley Ambulate x 2 Progressive ambulation per functional milestones-Walker	High Chair OOB for meals Bathroom Toileting Pain < 3/10 Ambulate x 3, observe gait Reinforce P.T. Progressive ambulation per functional milestones-Walker --> Cane	Assess wound healing S&S of infection Assistive devices Comfort Pain < 3/10 Ambulate x 3 - 4 Progressive ambulation per functional milestones-Cane, Stairs Instruct in Home Program	Discharge Teaching Wound healing No drainage Medically stable Afebrile Pain < 3/10 Achieve functional milestones: - in/out of bed Indep. - amb w/cane(s) - stair climbing - ≥80 degrees AROM flex - Indep. w/Home Program

adjunctive therapy when muscle re-education is needed (8). Patients whose pain cannot be controlled by medication, and who are unable to achieve optimal flexion, transcutaneous electrical nerve stimulation (TENS) may be used in conjunction with heat and cold modalities (5, 6). An in-patient therapeutic exercise usually consists of the following:

- Active range of motion (open and closed chain)
- Passive range of motion (open and closed chain)
- Straight leg raises/lateral leg lifts
- Quadriceps setting/gluteal setting/ankle circles
- Restorator/stationary bicycle

Strengthening exercises with ankle weights, therapy usually begins two weeks postoperatively with home care services or in an out-patient setting. Patients may be progressed to isokinetics as strength continues ot improve.

Home Care/Out-patient Services

Patients are usually discharged from the hospital between 5 and 7 days postoperatively. The goals of physical therapy following TKA, are to advance the patient to their maximal functional level. It is up to the physical therapist to design the appropriate exercise program to address these goals. Before progressing quickly to an aggressive strengthening program, one must guide the patient towards working on both a functional degree of knee flexion necessary to perform basic activities of daily living. Often medicare and insurance companies dictate how many visits a patient who has undergone a TKA is entitled to. It is crucial to keep this in mind when designing a comprehensive exercise program. Common questions asked of therapists are:

What are the guidelines for biking?
The patient MUST have enough knee flexion to complete a revolution on the bike. As soon as the patient has the range, biking is allowed and is usually started on a restorator, then advanced to a stationary bike, then a bicycle. Unlike a THA there are no precautions regarding cemented TKA. One must use common sense when prescribing an appropriate exercise program. If a patient has increased pain after his exercises regime, the program must be modified.

When should a knee immobilizer be used?
The purpose of a knee immobilizer is to maintain the knee in extension. If a patient is unable to maintain knee extension during ambulation due to muscle weakness a knee immobilizer is often used until the patient can actively control his quadriceps. If the patient does not have full extension in the supine position, a knee immobilizer is applied for sleeping in an attempt to facilitate knee extension and prevent further flexion contractures.

Is exercising in the water advisable and when is it allowed?
Most surgeons do not allow their patients to exercise in water until the sutures are removed. Hydrotherapy is not usually a part of the postoperative physical therapy program, however, most physical therapists will agree that exercising in the water is beneficial for getting increased motion to a painful joint.

Sports/Driving

The most common type of failure in TKA is mechanical loosening. By placing undue forces on the knee joint, the patient increases the chance of prosthetic loosening and endangers the overall success of the knee replacement (9). Patients are often instructed prior to and after surgery to avoid sports that would place excessive force on the prosthetic knee joint, i.e., running, jumping, singles tennis. Over 95% of orthopaedic surgeons who are members of The Knee Society allow their patients to play golf. Mallon and Callaghan studied the effects of golf on TKA and found that radiographic lucent lines occurred in 79.1% of cemented arthroplasties, 49% of uncemented arthroplasties and 53.9% of all TKA studies. Pain rates during and after play were significantly higher in golfers with left TKA's than for those with right TKAs. It is believed that this is a direct result of increased torque on the left knee in right handed golfers. It was recommended that patients use a golf cart while playing (13).

One of the most common questions patients ask following TKA is "when can I resume driving." Spalding studied the effect of driving reaction time on 40 patients and found that right TKA patients DRT did not return to normal for approximately 8 weeks post TKR. Left TKA patients, ability to brake was not impaired, suggesting that patients can return to driving as soon as they can depress the clutch pedal with sufficient force for their vehicle (17).

Measuring Functional Outcomes

A significant aspect in the rehabilitation of TKA patients is the ability to measure functional outcomes during hospitalization. Following both THA and TKA, the patients' level of activity rapidly increases. This rapid improvement in function must occur despite chronic shortage in hospital staff and fiscal constraints of managed care and diagnostic related grouping (DRG) reimbursement. It is necessary to carefully measure functional progression to assure that patients achieve specific functional milestones in a timely fashion. By consensual agreement of the in patient staff at The Hospital for Special Surgery (HSS), functional progression of TKA patients was documented on a TKA functional milestone form (Fig. 2). The HSS functional milestone forms are valid and reliable tools (11) used to determine the mean postoperative day of achievement of specific functional milestones that patients were required to achieve prior to discharge from the hospital. The specific functional milestones addressed were transfer in and out of bed, walker, cane, stair

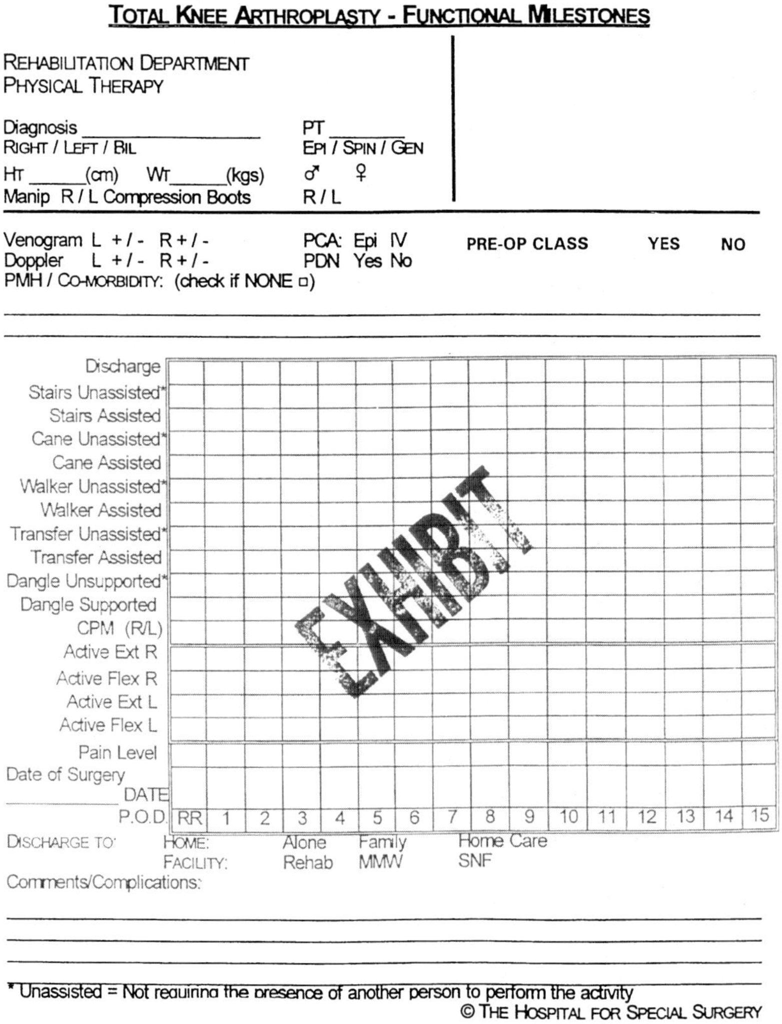
TOTAL KNEE ARTHROPLASTY - FUNCTIONAL MILESTONES

REHABILITATION DEPARTMENT
PHYSICAL THERAPY

Diagnosis ________ PT ______
RIGHT / LEFT / BIL EPI / SPIN / GEN
HT _____(cm) WT_____(kgs) ♂ ♀
Manip R / L Compression Boots R / L

Venogram L +/- R +/- PCA: Epi IV PRE-OP CLASS YES NO
Doppler L +/- R +/- PDN Yes No
PMH / CO-MORBIDITY: (check if NONE □)

	RR	1	2	3	4	5	6	7	8	9	10	11	12	13	14	15
Discharge																
Stairs Unassisted*																
Stairs Assisted																
Cane Unassisted*																
Cane Assisted																
Walker Unassisted*																
Walker Assisted																
Transfer Unassisted*																
Transfer Assisted																
Dangle Unsupported*																
Dangle Supported																
CPM (R/L)																
Active Ext R																
Active Flex R																
Active Ext L																
Active Flex L																
Pain Level																
Date of Surgery ______ DATE																
P.O.D.	RR	1	2	3	4	5	6	7	8	9	10	11	12	13	14	15

DISCHARGE TO: HOME: Alone Family Home Care
FACILITY: Rehab MMW SNF
Comments/Complications:

*Unassisted = Not requiring the presence of another person to perform the activity

FIG. 2 - HSS Total Knee Arthroplasty Functional Milestone Form

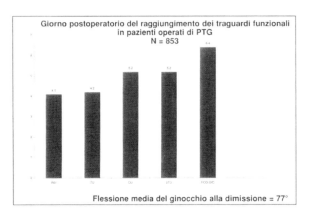

Flessione media del ginocchio alla dimissione = 77°

FIG. 3 - Functional Milestones of 853 Unilateral Total Knee Arthroplasty patients.

ambulation, active knee range of motion, and postoperative day of discharge. The milestones were characterized by two levels of achievement, assisted and unassisted. Assisted was defined as that requiring assistance from another person to perform the task, which included manual assistance, contact guarding, verbal cuing, supervision. The use of an ambulatory aid was not considered "assisted" as every patient was discharged with an ambulatory aid. The functional course of 853 patients who underwent uncomplicated unilateral TKA is illustrated in Figure 3.

References

1) Anderson G, Andriacchi TP, Galante JO: Correlations between changes in gait and in clinical Status after Knee Arthroplasty. Acta Orthop Scand 1981; 52:569.

2) Andriacchi TP, Galante JO, Fermier RW: The influence of total knee replacement design in walking and stairclimbing. J Bone Joint Surg 1982; 64:1235.

3) Coutts RD, Kaita J, Barr R, et al: The role of continuous passive motion in the preoperative rehabilitation of the knee. Orthop Trans 1982; 6:277-278.

4) Ganz SB, in: Insall: Surgery of the Knee, 2nd ed. Churchill-Livingston, New York, 1993.

5) Ganz SB, in: Sculco Surgical Treatment of Rheumatoid Arthritis, St. Louis: Mosby, 1992.

6) Goetz TH, Henry JH. Continuous passive motion after total knee arthroplasty. South Med J. 1986; 79: 1116-1120.

7) Gose JC: CPM in the postoperative treatment of patients with total knee replacement: A retrospective study. Phys Ther 1987; 67:39.

8) Haug J, Wood LT: Efficacy of neuromuscular stimulation of the quadriceps femoris during continuous passive motion following total knee replacement. Conn Med 498, 1985.

9) Insall: In: Insall JN, Windsor RE, Scott WN, Kelly MA, Aglietti P (Ed). Surgery of the Knee, 2nd Edition. New York: Churchill Livingstone, 1993.

10) Kroll MA, SB Ganz, Sl Backus, RA Benick, et al: A scale to Measuring Functional Outcomes After Total Joint Arthroplasty. Physical Therapy. Arthritis Care and Research: (July 1994).

11) Lichtenstein R, Semaan S. Development and Impact of a Hospital-based Perioperative Patient Education Program in a Joint Replacement Center. Orthopaedic Nursing Nov/Dec 1993;12(6):17-25.

12) Mallon WJ, Callaghan JJ: Total Knee arthroplasty in active golfers. Arthroplasty 1993; 8:299-306.

13) Ritter MA, Gandolf VS, Holston KS: Continuous passive motion versus physical therapy in total knee replacement. Clin Orthop. 1989; 244:239.

14) Romness DW, Rand JA. The role of continuous passive motion following total knee arthroplasty. Clin Orthop. 1988:226:34-37.

15) Salter RB, Clements ND, Ogilivie-Harris D, et al: The Healing of articular tissues through continuous passive motion. Essence of the first 10 years of experimental investigation. J Bone Joint Surg 1982; 64B:640.

16) Spalding TJW, Kiss J, Kyberd P, et al: Driver Reaction Times After Total Knee Arthroplasty. J Bone Joint Surg 1994;76B:754-756.

17) Tinetti ME, Speechley M. Prevention of falls among the elderly. N Engl J Med. 1989;320:1055-1059.

18) Vince KG, Kelly MA, Beck J, Insall JN. Continuous passive motion after total knee arthroplasty. J Arthroplasty. 1987; 2:281-284.

19) Ware J, Sherbourne C: The MOS 36 item short form health survey (SF-36). Med Care 1992;30:473-483.

Chapter 22
Revision Total Knee Arthroplasty

Thomas P. Sculco
The Hospital for Special Surgery - New York

Introduction

Revision knee replacement presents a complex surgical challenge to the orthopedic surgeon. Every phase of the revision procedure must be approached with careful planning to effect a sound functional result. Diagnosis of failure must be accurate, particularly to eliminate the presence of indolent infection. Mechanical causes of failure provide special problems of soft tissue balancing and bone loss and these must be thoroughly evaluated prior to proceeding with revision surgery. Comprehensive examination of the patient provides important preoperative information on the nature and utility of prior incisions, soft tissue deficits that may be problematic with wound closure, and ligamentous instability. Radiographs must be thoroughly evaluated to determine: (1) possible technical problems with implant removal, (2) prosthetic instability, (3) bone deficits that will need reconstruction after implant removal, and (4) patellofemoral failure and cause. Only after this type of comprehensive review can an operative plan be developed that will globally resolve all problem areas in the surgical treatment of the failed total knee replacement.

Ultimate clinical results of revision total knee replacement will be significantly influenced by the surgeon's ability to realize the preoperative plan at the time of the revision knee replacement. Therefore, the surgical treatment of the failed knee replacement can be divided into three phases: (1) exposure, (2) implant removal, (3) reconstruction, which includes soft-tissue balancing, management of bone deficits, proper implant selection and insertion. At the conclusion of the procedure the principles of primary knee reconstruction must be achieved: a well-aligned knee that is stable in an anteroposterior and mediolateral plane with proper and secure patellofemoral tracking.

I. Exposure

Exposure of the knee is pivotal to a successful knee revision. Prior incisions should be utilized whenever possible. Dissection should be directly through the subcutaneous tissue and excessive undermining of this layer to create large skin flaps should be avoided as devascularization of the skin flaps may occur and lead to wound slough and delayed wound healing. In a knee which has adequate preoperative range of motion exposure continues through the quadriceps tendon to the joint. Soft tissue elevation from the joint margins should always be performed subperiosteally and never in a transverse fashion. Injury to the collateral ligaments is prevented in this fashion. Periprosthetic exposure must be thoroughly performed to expose all surfaces of the implant. Particularly important is the ability to evert the patella and allow it to be subluxed laterally when the knee is flexed. A lateral retinacular patellar release can be performed from inside the joint to facilitate the eversion of the patella. This can be accomplished as part of the exposure process and is useful in obese patients and when motion is limited. The goal of the exposure is full visualization of the components, lateral subluxation of the patella, and the ability to anteriorly dislocate the tibia in front of the femur (Fig. 1). If any of these parameters is not possible, further dissection and soft tissue elevation is necessary.

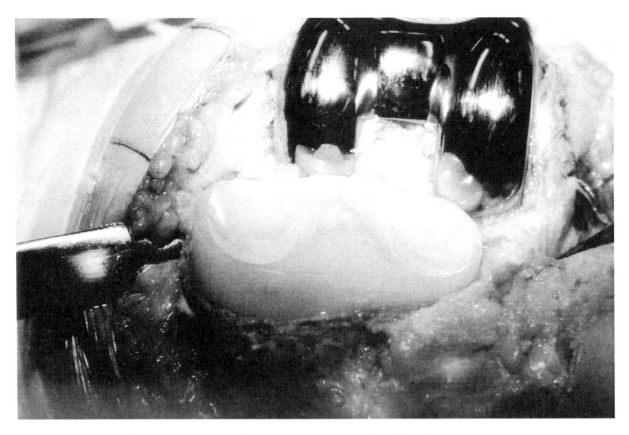

FIG. 1 - Proper exposure for revision total knee replacement surgery with complete subluxation of the tibia anterior on the femur.

A. The Stiff Knee

When the knee has a severely limited range of motion (less than 45 degrees) soft tissue periprosthetic dissection may not be adequate to expose the prosthesis. Also if the knee is very stiff the extensor mechanism is contracted and motion may not be possible once the revision implantation has been completed. The approach in these knees must be more radical in soft-tissue dissection than in the mobile knee. All intra-articular scar should be excised. The soft-tissue elevation should be extensive and skeletonize the distal femur and proximal tibia thoroughly.

The management of the stiff knee can be further accomplished by utilizing a proximal or distal lengthening. Distally the tibial tubercle can be elevated or the proximal tibia osteotomized to obtain exposure, or a proximal quadricepsplasty can be performed. The problem with tibial tubercle and proximal tibial osteotomy is that the contracture in the extensor mechanism is not addressed. The pathology in the stiff knee in extension is that the extensor mechanism is short-

ened and contracted and therefore I prefer to mobilize the extensor mechanism proximally. Depending on the degree of knee stiffness and extensor contracture proximal quadricepsplasty can be performed in the classic inverted V-Y manner or by a more limited quadriceps release by transversely cutting the quadriceps tendon laterally without full distal release. In the inverted V-Y quadricepsplasty (Fig. 2a, b, c) the release extends into the proximal quadriceps tendon and distally to both sides of the joint, medially and laterally. A tongue of quadriceps tendon can then be turned down distally and exposure is greatly enhanced. At the conclusion of the implantation, lengthening of the extensor mechanism is effected by allowing the tongue portion of the tendon to slide distally. The quadriceps is then repaired to itself proximally. Usually the quadriceps can be lengthened about 20-30 centimeters using this technique. The amount of lengthening is determined by flexing the knee to 40-45 degrees and suturing the quadriceps tendon at whatever level it reaches. This allows resultant mobilization of the very stiff knee to ap-

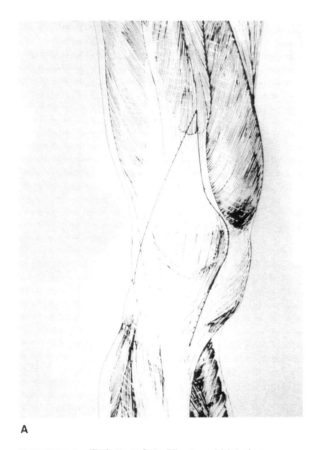

A

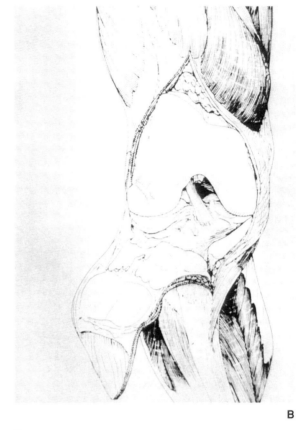

B

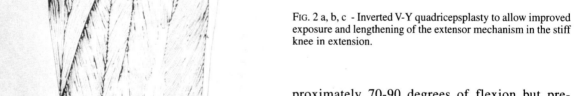

C

FIG. 2 a, b, c - Inverted V-Y quadricepsplasty to allow improved exposure and lengthening of the extensor mechanism in the stiff knee in extension.

proximately 70-90 degrees of flexion but prevents a persistent extensor lag. This extensive quadricepsplasty is required in the most severely contracted knees. In my personal experience with 14 knees with preoperative range of motion averaging 25 degrees (range 0-40 degrees) the average postoperative range of motion was 71 degrees (range 50-100 degrees). All patients had an extensor lag postoperatively, but it generally resolves at around 4-6 months. The average lag in this series was 15 degrees with a range of 0-45 degrees. There were two major complications in this series: a rupture of a patellar tendon during manipulation at three months postoperative and a deep periprosthetic infection.

In revision knees with preoperative ranges of 30-45 degrees, simply extending the proximal quadriceps incision laterally across the tendon may suffice to obtain exposure and allow mobilization of the tendon. The joint is then entered "like opening a book" with the entire extensor mechanism being everted laterally. After implantation, the quadriceps tendon can be lengthened slightly by repairing the tendon obliquely. This technique, in my experience, is not useful in the most contracted knees.

Tibial osteotomy as advocated by Whitesides (12) has several problems. Although exposure is facilitated by this approach, the contracted extensor mechanism is not lengthened and, therefore, motion remains limited. Additionally, fixation of the osteotomy is performed with circlage wires which may be suboptimal if the bone is osteopenic. Fracture may also occur through the site of the osteotomy.

In patients in whom the knee is stiff but fixed in flexion the exposure and management of the extensor mechanism is less complex. In these patients radical release of all periprosthetic soft tissues is necessary, but since the knee is in flexion the extensor mechanism is not severely contracted and a quadriceps lengthening is not necessary. The key surgical technique in these patients is a thorough posterior release of capsule from the posterior surface of the femur and tibia to allow the knee to be fully extended. Additional distal femoral bone may be resected if full extension cannot be achieved as this does not alter the soft tissue gap in flexion as an increased tibial resection does.

II. Implant Removal

The reconstructive aspects of revision knee replacement surgery become manifest once the implant has been removed. For this reason it is of the utmost importance that further damage to bone and soft tissues must not occur at the time of implant and cement removal. The prosthesis surfaces must be fully available if the implant is to be removed safely. Appropriate chisels should be used at the implant-cement interface to loosen the implant. Care must be taken not to lever on the underlying bone with chisels and elevators (Fig. 3). The bone is often osteopenic in these areas and will be crushed and deformed from the pressure of these instruments. A Gigli saw may be used beneath the femoral component beginning under the patellar flange, and by pulling toward the prosthesis and distally the cement-implant interface can be interrupted. A distracting slaphammer device (Fig. 4) may be used to dislodge the implant from the femoral and tibial surfaces by axial distraction with this device attached to the implant.

Once the femoral and tibial implants have been removed, cement chisels should be used to

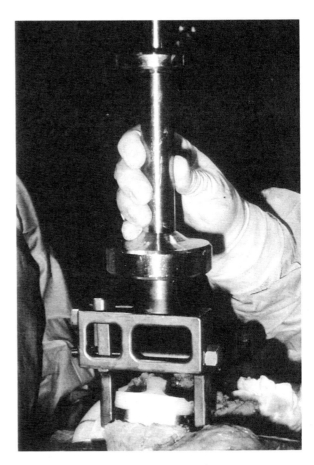

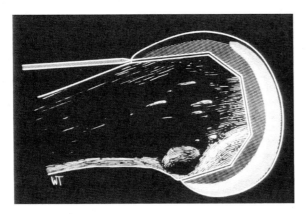

FIG. 3 - Chisel is used at the prosthesis-cement interface without levering on the bone.

FIG. 4 - Slaphammer used to remove the tibial and femoral component.

crack the remaining cement in a "mosaic" pattern. Levering techniques must be avoided or further bony damage will occur. High speed drills such as the Midas Rex are useful for cement removal at the base of the tibial peg hole/s if one is present but should be used sparingly otherwise. Care must be taken with these power drills as damage may occur if they are not cautiously used.

The patellar component is removed by using a power oscillating saw if the component is polyethylene, and transecting the base of the peg. High speed drills or curettes can be used to remove the polyethylene peg and remaining cement. If the patella is metal-backed osteotomes can be used to loosen the interface between the patellar component and the underlying bone and then curettes or drills used to remove cement.

In prostheses which are non-cemented similar techniques are utilized for femoral and tibial implant removal. Care must be taken to fully osteotomize the interface between the components and the underlying areas of bony ingrowth to reduce the amount of bone removed when the implants are extracted from the bone. If the tibial implant is fixed with a porous surface on the tibial fixation peg, the baseplate should be disengaged from the peg and a high speed cutting drill used around the peg to loosen it. If the implant cannot be disassembled, then axial distraction should be tried and if unsuccessful it may be necessary to cut the peg from the underlying baseplate.

III. Reconstruction

Once the implant and cement have been removed, a careful evaluation of the bone deficits and soft-tissue imbalance is made. These areas will be discussed separately in addition to the concepts of implant selection and augmentation. It is first necessary to prepare the underlying bony bed for implant insertion. The proximal osteotomy on the tibia should be made to correct any malalignment which has been created by the failure process. A minimal amount of bone should be removed to improve the tibial surface. Bone deficits if present should be treated as outlined below. Similarly the femoral surface should be prepared to improve the surface for prosthetic insertion. Minimal amounts of bone should be resected and areas of bone deficiency should be augmented with bone graft or prosthetic augmentation. Soft-tissue and remaining bony deficiency must now be resolved.

A. Soft Tissue

The approach is similar to the primary knee in that soft-tissue symmetry must be achieved and bone deficits must be corrected. Soft-tissue releases on the contracted side should be performed to effect soft-tissue symmetry. The releases are always performed by subperiosteally elevating the tight contracted soft-tissue structures on the tight side of the joint. When soft-tissue symmetry has been accomplished the implant then blocks open this symmetrical space and stability is achieved.

Soft-tissue asymmetry can persist despite attempts at balancing and then implants with constraining intercondylar augments must be used which provide additional medial-lateral and anteroposterior stability. Constrained condylar designs have increased polyethylene posts which articulate with an intercondylar deepened restraining box on the femoral component. These implants are useful if there is persistent medial or lateral instability or if the soft-tissue laxity is greater in flexion or extension as a result of the exposure and implant removal. Usually the flexion gap is greater than the extension gap and the increased stability of a constrained condylar design will provide a stable construct. If there continues to be flexion laxity despite the constrained design, the stemmed femoral component may be moved posterior in the femoral canal to allow the more posterior placement of the femoral condyles to close the flexion gap.

On occasion there is a complete absence of ligamentous support due to disruption as part of the prosthetic failure process. Constrained condylar designs, in my experience, are not adequate to stabilize the knee if there is no functional collateral ligament present. This is the only indication for the use of a hinge device which will provide complete fixed prosthetic stability. It is rarely necessary to use these hinged devices as almost always there is a component of the ligament remaining. However, the surgeon should be aware of the need for hinge in those cases where the knee is grossly unstable and be prepared to use it. Careful preoperative planning must insure it will be available.

B. Bony Deficits

Bony deficits present during revision surgery can be grafted or augments can be added to the implant itself. Bony deficits can be classified into five major categories based on the pattern of bone deficiency: (1) cystic areas of bone loss, (2) condylar or plateau deficits, (3) central or

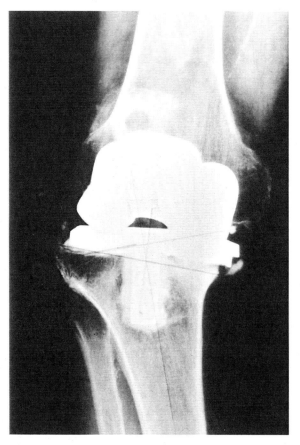

A

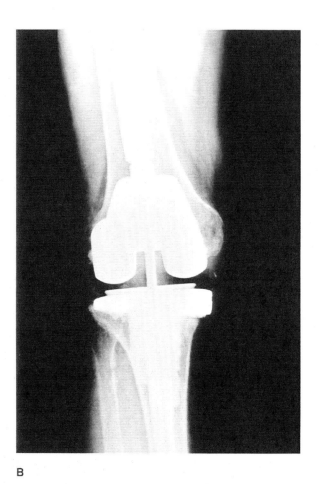

B

FIG. 5 a, b - Tibial plateau deformity treated by wedge augmentation of the tibial component.

cavitary deficits, (4) perforations or fractures of the distal femur or proximal tibia, (5) large segmental areas of bone loss. Each of these patterns is addressed differently but almost all bony deficiencies will fulfill criteria for inclusion into these categories.

Management of cystic bone loss which is usually produced at the time of implant removal, is easily addressed by filling these small areas with cancellous autogenous bone which is available at the time of the revision. Condylar and plateau deficits (Fig. 5a, b) usually occur as a result of collapse of underlying bone with resultant malalignment. Because of their wedge configuration on the tibial side where they are most common, wedge augmentation is the preferred treatment. Bone is resected into a planar surface and the appropriate wedge configuration used to fill the defect area (Fig. 6). On the femoral side a similar treatment is recommended. Distal augments added to the femoral component on the

collapsed side of the femur compensate for the bone loss and the deficiency is readily corrected.

Central cavitary lesions are most common on the tibial side of the joint and are present when stems or large tibial pegs are removed. These are best managed with allograft, both structural (femoral head) and morsellized bone to reinforce the area where the allograft coapts the underlying bone. A stemmed prosthesis should be used to bypass the graft area and transfer load to the intrameduallary area. For perforations and fractures of the distal femur and proximal tibia morsellized allograft can be used and a stemmed component to bypass the areas of bone compromise. Large segmental areas of bone loss will be discussed in a later chapter. These can be addressed with large segmental allografts or with prosthetic replacement of the resected area of bone (Fig. 7a, b). These are complex reconstructions and should only be performed by surgeons with great experience in revision knee replacement surgery.

C. Patellofemoral Joint

The patellofemoral joint is a significant cause of pain and dysfunction after primary total knee replacement and its management is even more complex in the revision knee replacement. Once the patellar implant has been removed there may be little bone available for implantation of another patellar prosthesis. In these circumstances the patella remnant can be debrided and shaped so that no sharp edges are persisting which may irritate the soft tissues about the patella. Once this patelloplasty has been performed the remaining patella is left in place.

If there is sufficient bone a patellar implant can be inserted again and cemented in place. Tracking must be carefully evaluated and often there is significant scarring in the lateral retinaculum which tends to pull the patella laterally. This lateral retinaculum and capsule should be released if there is a tendency for lateral subluxation of the patella. The lateral release is performed from inside the joint about one centimeter lateral to the patella. It should extend from the patellar tendon distally to the vastus lateralis muscle proximally. The superior lateral geniculate artery should be avoided during this release if possible. In knees with severe limitation of motion the skin and subcutaneous tissue may be adherent to the patella. In these cases the lateral release should be also performed from outside the joint by elevating the subcutaneous layer from the lateral retinaculum.

Rarely but in cases where patellar subluxation persists after an extensive lateral release it may be necessary to transfer the patellar tendon medially. This is uncommonly performed except in the most recalcitrant cases of patellar instability. Staples are used to hold the transferred tendon with a periosteal sleeve in its new position just medial to the tibial tuberlce. Postoperative rehabilitation proceeds more slowly when transfer of the tendon is needed. Full flexion is not allowed generally for four to six weeks from surgery.

IV. Prosthetic Selection

The Total Condylar III prosthesis was the first suitable revision non-hinged total knee replacement prosthesis and provided greater constraint and intramedullary fixation. Its design provided a deepened femoral intercondylar recess into which an elongated polyethylene peg articulated (Fig. 6). Because of the constraint

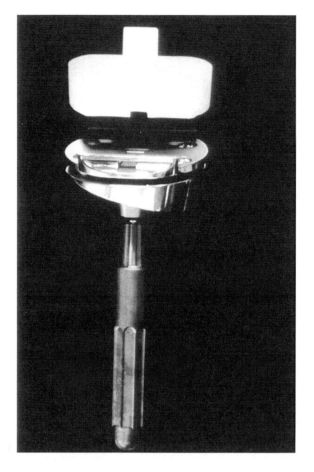

FIG. 6 - Wedge augmentation tibial component with fluted stem.

provided by this implant, mild to moderate degrees of anteroposterior instrability could be accommodated. Stems attached to the femoral and tibial component were cemented in place and provided transfer of load away from the femoral and tibial faces.

Although a useful implant in revision surgery where instability was marked, the Total Condylar III had its limitations. In situations where bone loss was significant and when asymmetrical soft-tissue instability was present, the Total Condylar III was suboptimal. To deal with the need for more flexibility for complex primary and revision knee replacement *modular* total knee systems were developed. These implants allow for the management of most of the surgical problems encountered with the more difficult knees. In the revision knee quality of bone is often inferior and deficient, particularly after implant removal both on the femoral and tibial implant surfaces. The tibial and femoral surfaces

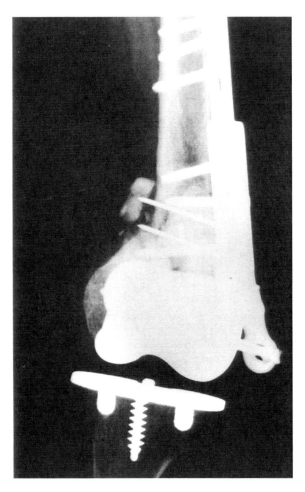
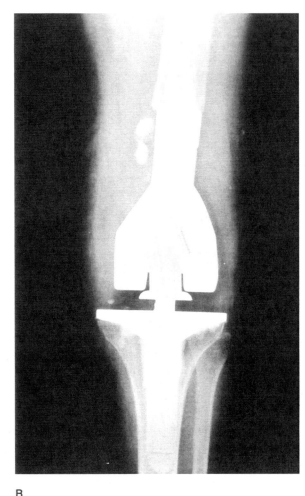

A   B

FIG. 7 a, b - Severe femoral bone loss managed with a segmental hinged knee prosthesis.

are therefore inadequate as the main load-bearing surfaces for the implant and fixation is poor into these surfaces because of their porotic and deficient character. Load must be transferred to the intramedullary area of tibia and femur in these circumstances. Stems, therefore, are necessary on the tibial and femoral component, which will transfer load into the medullary canals and modular stems added to the component allow variation in the length and thickness of the stem. Optimally, stems are fluted and press-fit and are not cemented to the medullary canals of femur and tibia. Stem length varies depending on degrees of transfer of load required based on the deficiency of bone at the tibial and femoral surfaces. With hinge revisions there may be considerable compromise of the upper tibia and distal femur and bone loss may extend

into the metaphyseal areas. In these clinical settings stems must be used that bypass these deficient areas, and gain purchase deeper into the more normal intramedullary bone.

Modular implants also allow for distal and/or posterior femoral augmentation as well as proximal tibial wedge augmentation. These may be used as necessary depending upon the bony deficit and its configuration (11). The tibial prosthesis, whether augmented with a wedge or just with a stem, will determine the alignment of the tibial component. Because this intramedullary stem will be placed into the tibial canal the implant should be squarely on the tibial surface to insure that a perpendicular cut has been made on the tibial surface and that the tibial component is properly positioned. If the tibial component does not sit on the tibial surface the tibial cut must be modified until the implant is closely coapted to the tibial bone. It essentially acts as a T-square and determines the alignment of the tibial component. Modification of this concept is necessary when there is tibial bowing present.

Several technical points must be kept in mind during implantation of these modular constrained implants. Stems should not be cemented and should be press-fit. Revision of cemented fluted intramedullary stems is extremely difficult and may lead to dramatic loss of bone during implant removal. Cement is therefore applied only at the femoral and tibial surfaces.

This means that reaming of the intramedullary canal should be performed until the reamer broaches cortical bone. A fluted stem can then be used that will gain purchase on the cortical bone. Revision of cemented intramedullary stems is onerous and may lead to dramatic loss of bone during implant removal. Cement is therefore applied only at the femoral and tibial surfaces.

Fabrication of the revision or complex primary implant at the time of implantation by modularity of the total knee augments greatly facilitates the operative procedure. Modifications in constraint deal with persistent ligamentous instability despite attempts at ligamentous balancing.

Augments solve the problem of bone deficits and asymmetrical flexion and extension laxity. Patella tracking and position are improved with these augments as joint position can be maintained. Stems of varying diameter and length transfer load away from deficient tibial and femoral surfaces. Customization has been transferred from the implant manufacturer to the surgeon depending on the needs at the time of the surgical intervention. This has led to more mechanically sound implant constructs in the revision knee replacement patient.

V. Results with Revision Knee Implants

Results of revision total knee replacement that are currently available represent a broad spectrum of techniques, implants and follow-up. Early studies of revision total knee replacement have demonstrated a success rate as low as 30%. (5). More recent studies have shown inferior results to primary knee replacement procedures but seem to be more encouraging. It is of importance to view these results in light of the evolving technical improvements in revision knee replacement surgery. Modular implants have been available relatively recently, and therefore re-

sults are still short-term. Many early revision procedures did not produce proper alignment and reconstruction of bone and soft-tissue deficits and the patella and its tracking were not carefully addressed.

Results with the Total Condylar III prosthesis were reported by Donaldson (1) and Sculco (9). Of 31 total knee arthroplasties, 17 were in severely damaged primary knees and 14 were for revision knee replacement. The overall group demonstrated a 77% good or excellent result but the revision group fared significantly poorer than the primary arthroplasties. Of the five overall failures all were in the revision patients, three for deep infection and two for aseptic loosening. Conversely, Goldberg (3) in a review of 65 revisions, 59 of which were followed for 5 years, found his best results in the Total Condylar III group. Overall only 46% of patients were good or excellent and 42% were poor or failed. There was a 4.5% deep infection rate in this series. Most of the failures were related to persistent instability postoperatively. The highest failure rate was in those patients revised to a total condylar prosthesis, 33% failed. In the Total Condylar III patients there was a 20% failure rate, the lowest of any implant used. Rosenberg (8) reported on 36 revision knee replacements with the Total Condylar III prosthesis followed after an average of 45 months. Twenty-five of the patients were rated good or excellent with six fair and four poor results.

Rand and Bryan (6) reported the Mayo Clinic experience with revision knee replacement with a non-constrained condylar implant as the revision implant. Only one-quarter of all their revisions fulfilled the criteria to use the condylar type design for the procedure. These revisions were among the least complex in that there was only mild bone loss, intact collateral ligaments and varus or valgus deformity of less than 30 degrees. Results reported on 50 revisions document 76% good to excellent results. Follow-up averaged 4.8 years in these patients. There were 17% significant radiolucencies. Complications included loosening of one or both components in three knees, hematoma in one knee, and a retained cement fragment that interfered with knee function in one patient. There were no infections or wound problems reported in this group of patients with the exception of the one wound hematoma. When comparing these patients to an earlier revision study (7) from the Mayo Clinic, results were better. Only 64% of the 427 revision total knee replacements in the earlier series were satisfactory after one revision, 59% after two revisions, and 50% after three revisions.

Elia and Lotke (2) reviewed a group of patients undergoing total knee revision with significant bone loss. This was defined as a deficit of at least one centimeter and at a minimum of 50% of the femoral or tibial plateau surface. In the overall series there were 40 revisions followed for 2 to 9 years. Good to excellent results were reported in 75% of patients. There was a 10% failure rate in these patients and these were mainly for loosening and instability. Additionally there was a 30% complication rate and wound complications were present in 4 patients. Two had severe wound sloughs and needed debridement and muscle flaps. The authors made the following recommendations for improved results: realignment must be restored, bone defects must be reconstructed, stems on the implant should be used for support, soft-tissue balancing must be accurately performed.

Stuart (10) reviewed the results of causes of failure in revision total knee replacements. In 45 patients 60 procedures were performed. The most common failure mechanism was extensor mechanism or patella problems in 19 knees (41%), loosening occurred in ten knees (22%), deep infection in nine knees (20%), wound problems in nine knees (20%), instability in eight knees (17%) and limited motion in four knees, (8%). Patients were followed after treatment for their failed revision for an average of 7.5 years. Twenty-four knees (52%) were recorded as failures because of persistent pain, limited motion, instability and infection.

Vince (12) has reported on results with newer modular components for revision total knee replacement. In a review of 44 revision total knee replacements the results with 13 with constrained condylar articulations are presented. Follow-up is from 2 to 6 years. Of these 13 patients, two have been revised for loosening, and one other patient has radiographic evidence of impending loosening. Interestingly all three patients were revised for deep prosthetic infection. There was no evidence of recurrent infection at the time of the second revision procedure.

Revision knee replacement is a complex surgical reconstruction that requires careful and thorough preoperative planning, atraumatic and accurate surgical treatment, and proper implant selection. Newer modular designs have facilitated knee revision, but the most important component in a successful revision procedure is the surgical reconstruction itself. Careless and poorly executed surgery will not be compensated by any prosthetic implant system. The failure for which revision surgery is performed still rests primarily with the surgeon's inability to align the knee properly, balance the ligamentous structures, and produce a patella that is stable and tracks properly. Failure of the implant itself has led to the need for revision but far less commonly than surgical imperfection. Revision surgery is far less forgiving and the underlying biological substrate greatly inferior than in the primary knee. Therefore planning and technique must be meticulous if a result is to be achieved which will provide painless function for an extended period.

References

1) Donaldson, WF III, Sculco TP, Insall JN, Ranawat CS. Total condylar III prosthesis: long term follow-up study. Clin. Orthop. 226:22-30, 1988.
2) Elia EA, Lotke P: Results of revision total knee arthroplasty associated with significant bone loss. Clin. Orthop. 271:114-122, 1991.
3) Goldberg, VM, Figgie MP, Figgie HE, Sobel M. The results of revision total knee arthroplasty. Clin. Orthop. 226:86-92, 1988.
4) Hanssen, AD, Rand JA. Comparision primary and revision total knee arthroplasty using kinematic stabilizer prosthesis. J. Bone Joint Surg. 70A: 491-499, 1988.
5) Hunter GA, Cameron HU, Welsh RP, Bailey WH. The natural history of the failed knee replacement. Orthop. Trans. 4:389, Abstract, 1980.
6) Rand JA, Bryan RS. Results of revision total knee arthroplasties using condylar prostheses. J. Bone Joint Surg. 70A:738-745, 1988.
7) Rand JA, Peterson LF, Bryan RS, Ilstrup, DM. Revision total knee arthroplasty. Instructional Course Lectures, 35:305-318, 1986.
8) Rosenberg AG, Verner JJ, Galante JO. Clinical results of total knee revision using the Total Condylar III proshesis. Clin. Orthop. 273:83-90, 1991.
9) Sculco, TP. Total Condylar III prosthesis in ligament instability. Orthop. Clin. North Am. 20:221-227, 1989.
10) Stuart, MJ, Larson JE, Morrey BF. Reoperation after condylar revision total knee arthroplasty. Clin. Orthop. 286:168-173, 1993.
11) Stulberg, D. Managing bone loss with augmentation. Orthopedics, 20(9): 845-7, 1997.
12) Vince, KG, Long, W. Revision knee arthroplasty. The limits of press fit medullary fixation. Clin. Orthop. 317:172-177, 1995.
12) Whitesides, LA, Ohl, MD, Tibial tubercle osteotomy for exposure of the difficult total knee arthroplasty, Clin. Orthop. 260:6-9, 1990.

Printed by Books on Demand, Germany